What midwives and mothers say about Bump

'I LOVE this book, just love it.'

'I totally love every detail, incorporating all those great scientific references! Super simple and effective descriptions, while the pics add an extra loving touch.'

'Fantastic! What an easy-to-understand explanation of all aspects of the process. Love it!'

'Informative and empowering. This is an epic work of love and deep understanding.'

'Awesome! Could these be the best cartoons I've ever seen?'

'I was gripped by it. Fab.'

'This work was done with soul.'

'Wow. This was just what I needed to read right now!'

'So entirely refreshing in the way women's bodies are described and portrayed.'

'This is just so wonderful – such a lovely way to describe how your body is designed to birth. I felt relaxed just reading it.'

'Wow! Love this!!! Love the drawings!! I really want to share this book with my daughters.'

'It's beautiful. I love it. I want all women and men and girls and boys to read this with lots of time to ask questions, reflect, and marvel!'

'I'll be recommending this to EVERYONE I know.'

'OMG!! Soooo beautiful and brought back the best memories of my children's births as well as a couple of tears! Thank you for this book.'

'Beautiful! It made me cry! (I may be a bit hormonal.)'

'As a midwife, can I say I love love love how you normalise birth, demystify the pro   o it! Nicely done!'

What midwives and mothers say about Bump

'I LOVE this! Such a powerful and beautiful portrayal of fertility and birth.
I teach active birth preparation and pregnancy yoga and will be recommending
this book to all my clients. Well done.'

'This will be a great book for my prenatal classes. While wanting to impart the
majesty of the birthing process, I am also not interested in shaming Mamas
who birth via Caesarean. This is brilliant! Bravo!'

'I want to give all my clients a copy!'

'Absolutely lovely – I wish this was written years ago. Reading this took me back
to why I trained as a midwife in the first place.'

'So accessible, fun, realistic and positive. *The Food of Love* is my favourite book
to leave with new mothers, and this will be a fantastic resource for pregnant
women and those trying to conceive.'

'It's a shame not everybody here in Brazil knows English but just the images
are already enough!! I'm sharing it on my Facebook page!'

'I loved it!! I hope you can get it translated to Spanish, so I can share it
with my friends. Greetings from Chile!'

'The illustrations are amazing. I'm a midwife in Taiwan.'

'A wonderful book! I will use this in my job as midwife in a Swedish hospital.'

'I was recently given a copy of *The Food of Love*, and if this book is anything like
as informative, comforting and funny then I will be snatching it up
in a heartbeat!'

'*Bump* is delicious and gorgeous and needed in this world. This purposeful and
fun book will gently educate, encourage and inspire people everywhere.'

'Huge applause for this beautiful, brilliant work.'

Life isn't a fairytale.
You won't necessarily meet
Prince Charming, he doesn't sweep
you off your feet, there are rarely any
white horses involved,
and never any dragons.

This book is about
the adventure of childbirth.

Life is more like a
pick-your-own-adventure story,
with divergent paths and choices
every step of the way.

If only! What if?

Maybe you'll have the two kids
you planned, or the five you didn't, or
you won't, and that'll be okay. Maybe
you'll get a water birth at home with
candles. Maybe you'll get a Caesarean
birth in hospital with screens and
hospital scrubs.

What you need is information,
about how your body works,
and what it's capable of.

Venture on!

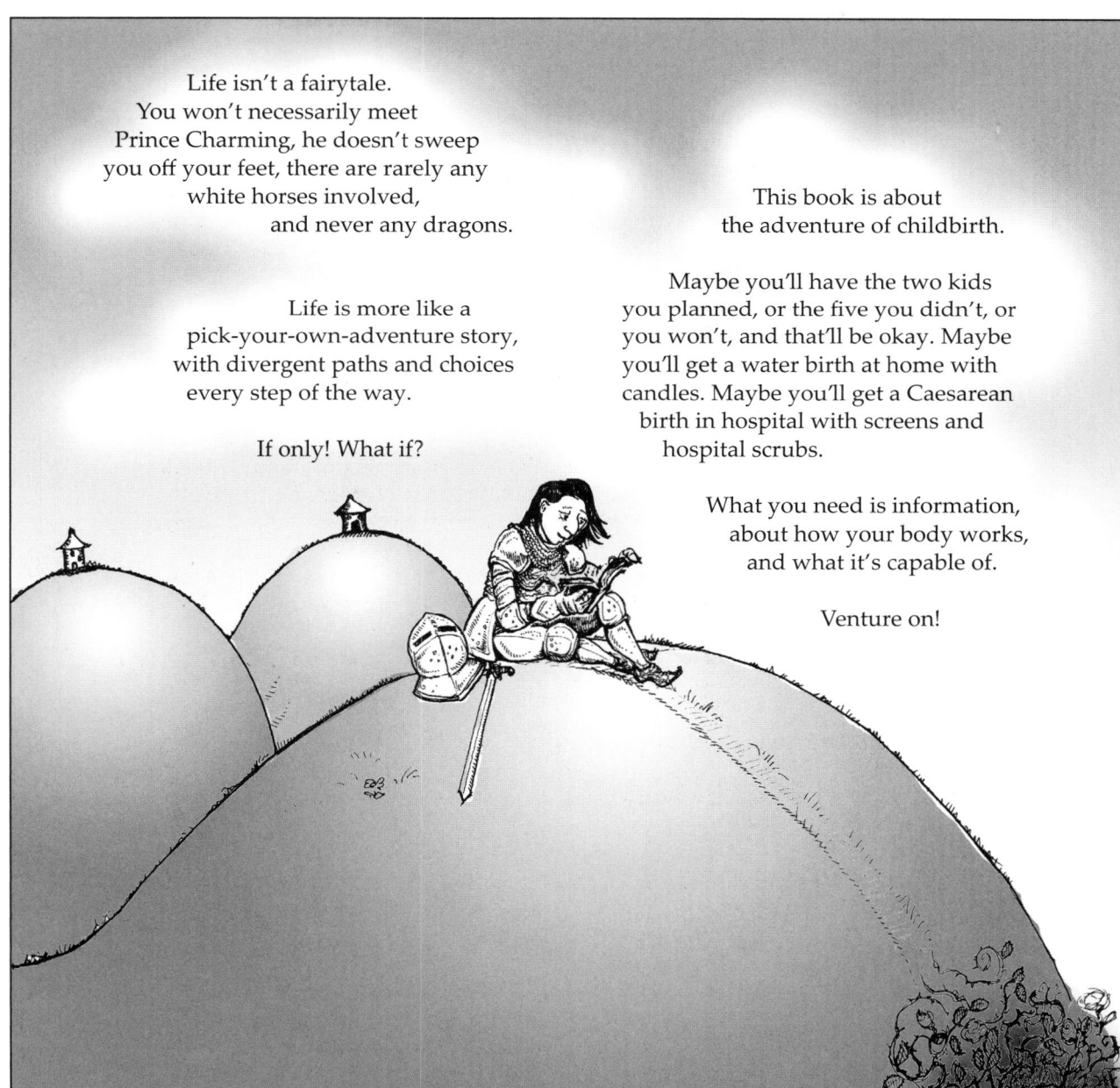

First published in 2014 by

Myriad Editions
59 Lansdowne Place
Brighton BN3 1FL, UK

www.myriadeditions.com

1 3 5 7 9 10 8 6 4 2

A CIP catalogue record for this book is available from
the British Library.

ISBN: 978-1-908434-35-7

Designed by Kate Evans

Printed in China on paper sourced from well-managed forests.
Honest. 'Cause someone checked. Yeah, right.

Bump

how to make, grow and birth a baby

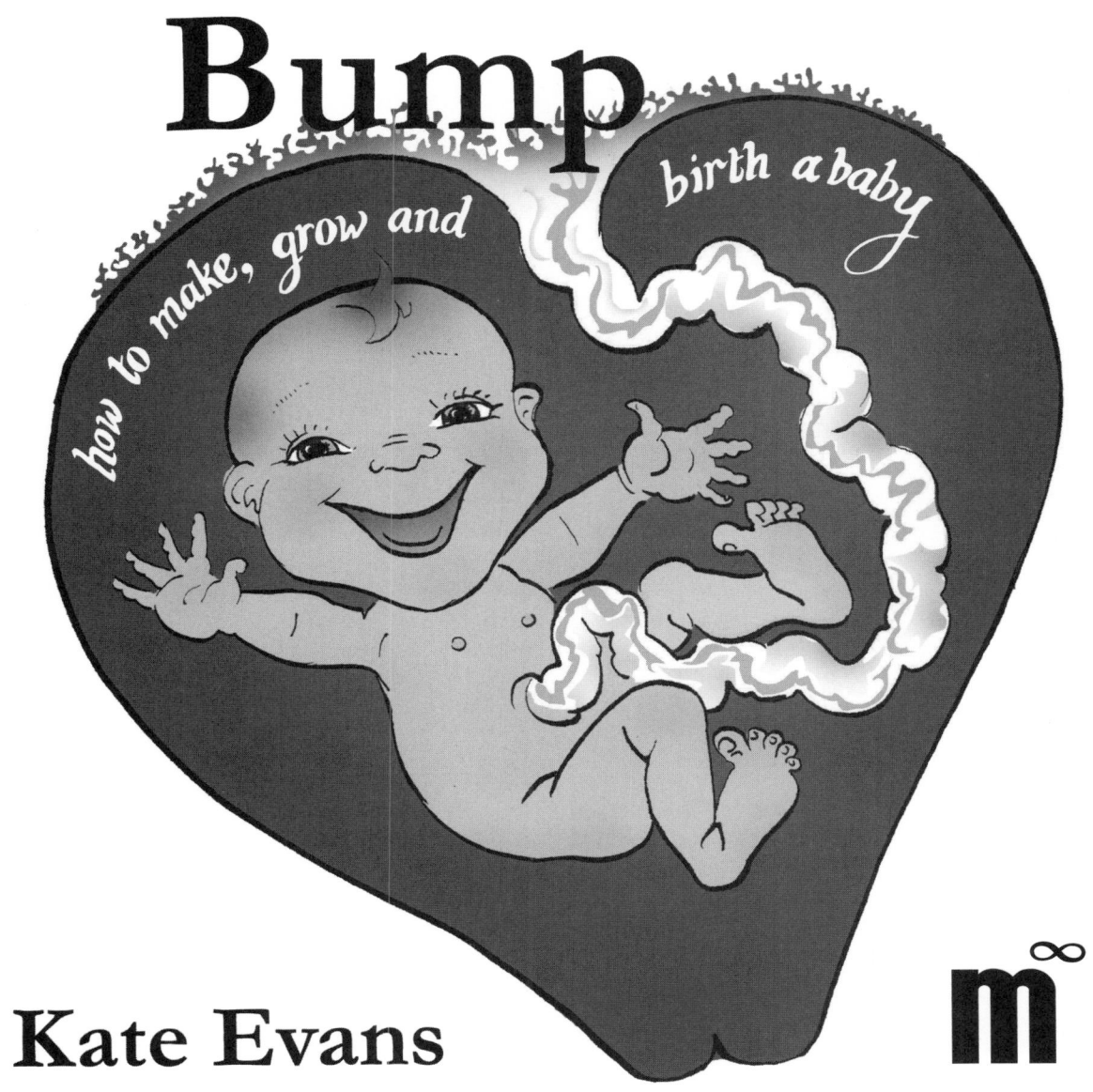

Kate Evans

m∞

Contents

Forward, forewarned...

This book is much more than a pregnancy manual. It's about womanhood. It covers every aspect of our biological destiny: choosing to have children, choosing not to have children, bearing children, losing children, blood, sweat and tears (you can read that last word with both pronunciations).

There's a lot in here that we don't talk about. As I wrote it, I had to fight against a sense that this knowledge is unimportant because it is unspoken, when, of course, the inverse is true.

But there is something I've left out. Men. So I'd like to apologise, guys. I have referred to your experiences only tangentially. In this book, when I write 'person', I mean 'woman' by default, not 'man', which is a complete reversal of the normal order of things. (Ha! Now you know how it feels!) More could be written about how fertility, pregnancy and birth feels from the male perspective. I'll lay down the gauntlet and hope that one of you picks it up.

And so I've ignored transgender men. There are men who have retained the biological ability to bear children from their previous sex. Good luck with your adventures, fellas. I hope you find some of this book relevant, but I found it hard to untangle sex, gender and female identity when I wrote it. In fact, I didn't want to, because so much of womanhood is uncharted territory.

I should also apologise to my children in advance: I'm going to make you turn off the computer now that I've finished writing this book.

There now follows a list of personal dedications that are irrelevant for a huge percentage of the readership. Thanks to Jabberwocky nursery for mothering my toddler while I've been busy authoring. Thank you, Mary Cronk, Denis Walsh, Joanna Ellington, Soo Downe, Rachel Reed, Emma Ashworth, Aurella Yussuf and Linda McQueen for your professional input. Thanks to Mipsy, Amy, Emma, Anna and Frankie Jo Magick, Anna Honesty, Mary, Ali, Joy Horner, Joy Hunt, Candida, Corinne, and Donach, I love you.

If you find nothing else to disagree with in this book, you may be dismayed by my use of the pronoun 'them' when referring to the singular unborn child. I thought it more elegant than the clunky 'she stroke he' and less impersonal than 'it'. We do need gender-neutral language, particularly when discussing the baby in the womb, whose personhood can be felt before their sex can be identified.

This book is dedicated to midwives everywhere.

PICK YOUR OWN ADVENTURE MOMENT!

Do you want to find out how babies are made?

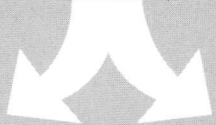

Yes, please.	No, thank you.
This sounds extremely interesting and potentially very useful.	I'm pregnant, and anatomy and physiology is one of the many things that might make me feel queasy. I'd rather skip straight to the funny cartoons.
Read on.	Turn to page 71.

Book the First

How to make a baby

1 The story of the egg and the fish

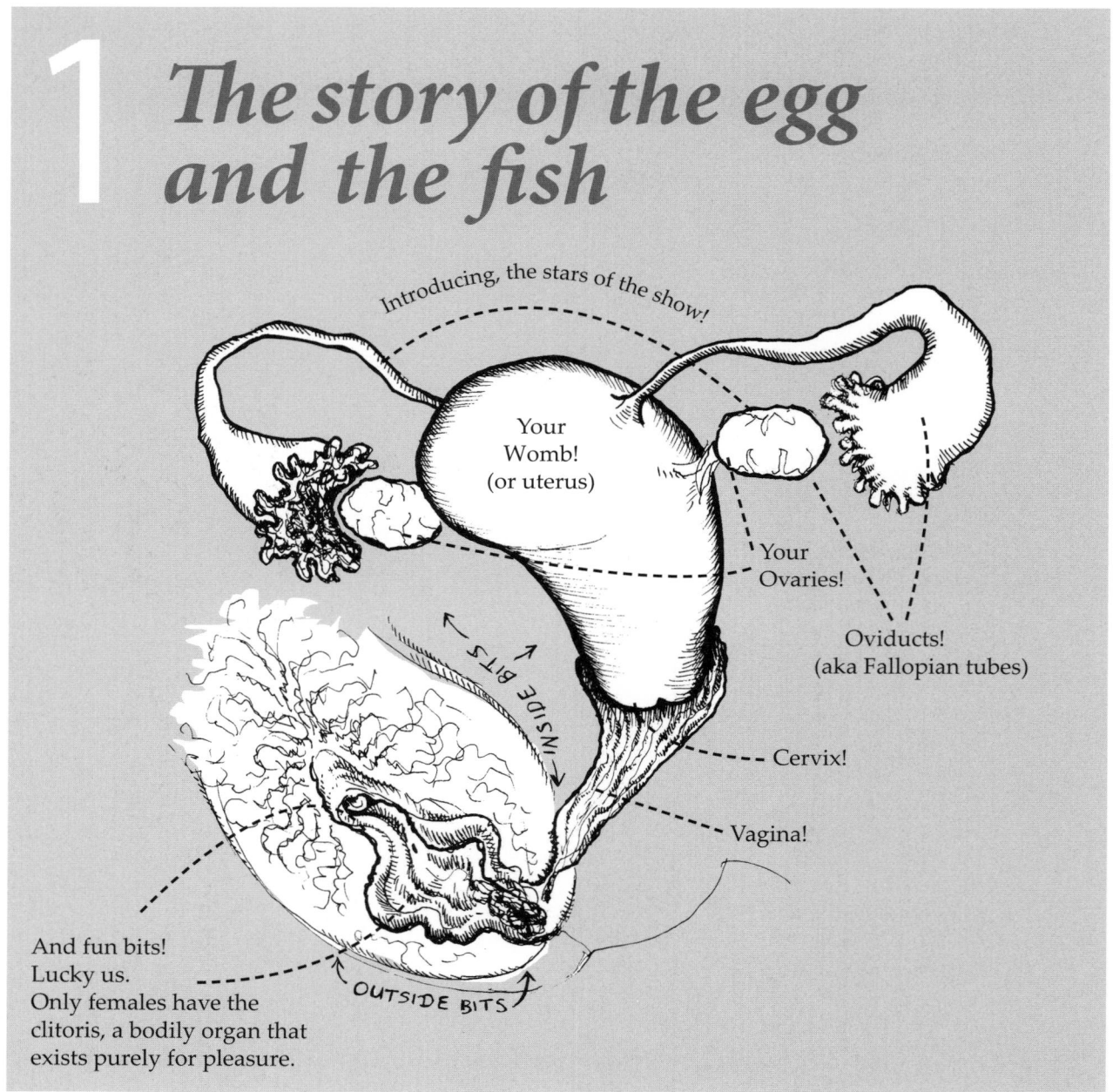

Introducing, the stars of the show!

Your Womb! (or uterus)

Your Ovaries!

Oviducts! (aka Fallopian tubes)

INSIDE BITS

Cervix!

Vagina!

And fun bits! Lucky us. Only females have the clitoris, a bodily organ that exists purely for pleasure.

OUTSIDE BITS

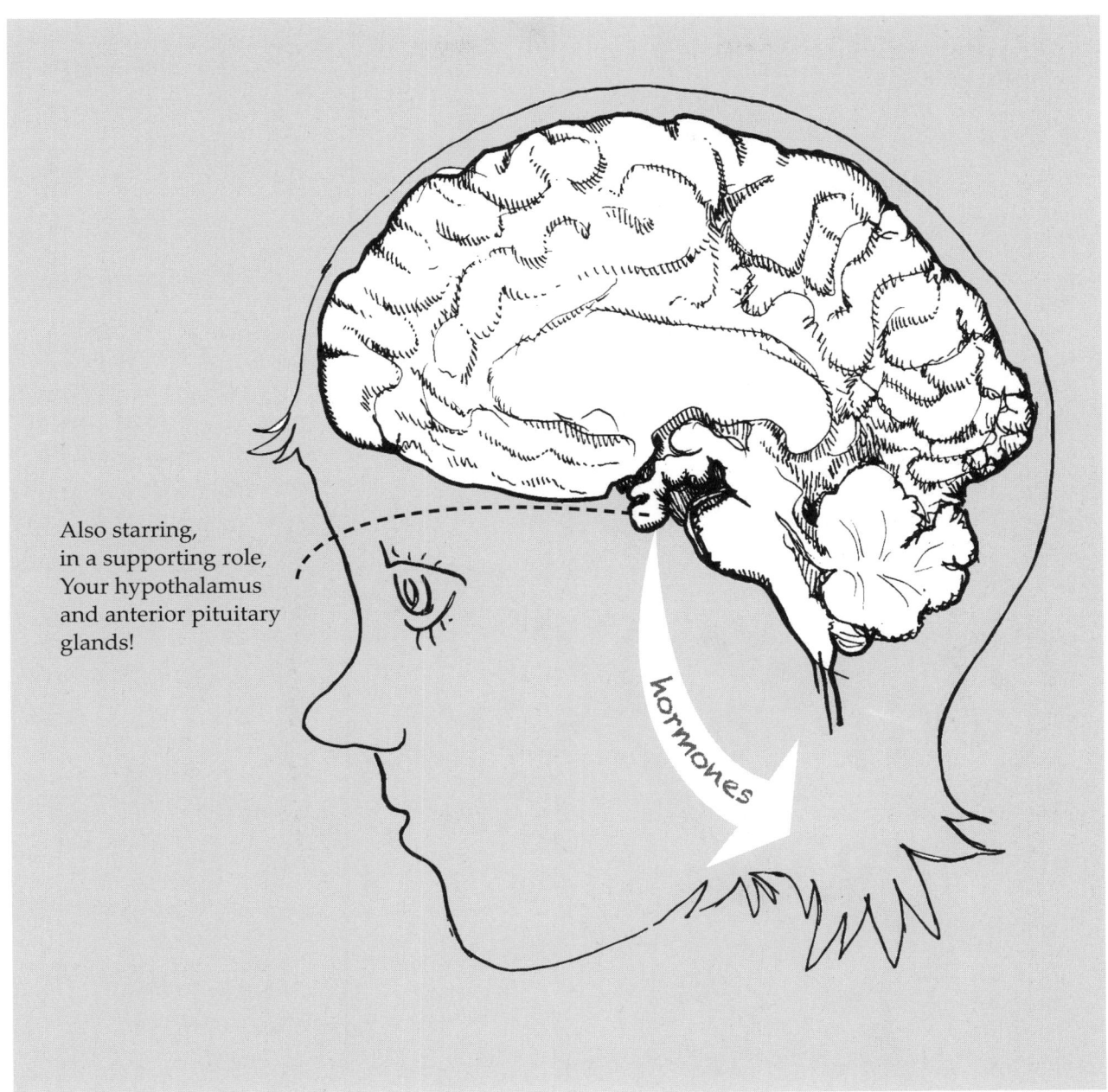

Also starring,
in a supporting role,
Your hypothalamus
and anterior pituitary
glands!

hormones

It's **Day 1*** of your menstrual cycle. You just got your period.

You know you're not pregnant, but your body is already plotting to change that.

Your ovaries have been gradually ripening up some eggs for months, and now a batch of about 12 of them is coming along nicely. Your pituitary gland starts to release increasing amounts of follicle-stimulating hormone (FSH), which stimulates the egg follicles to get busy, and then luteinising hormone (LH), which helps the eggs to mature.

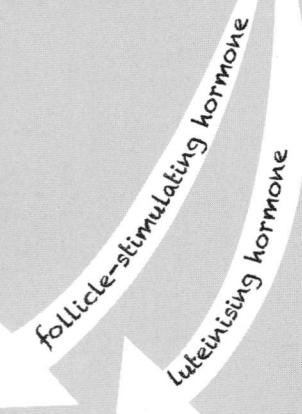

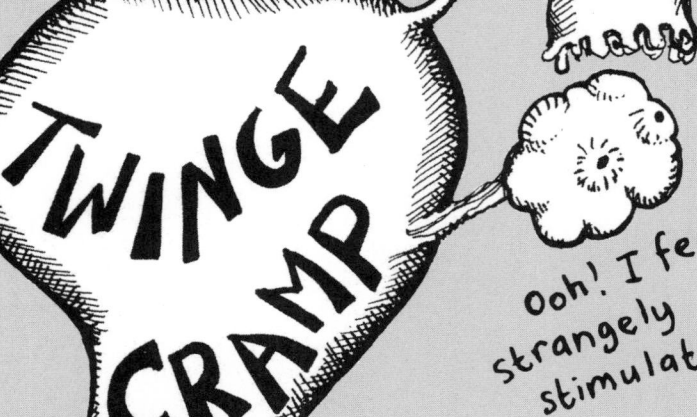

*(I'm using a 28-day 'perfect' menstrual cycle here, because it's the one that the doctors use. None of the timings is necessarily the same in real life.)

A week later, on **Day 7**, one of these egg follicles (sometimes two! very occasionally more!) has become fat enough to start to produce oestrogen. This is where things get juicy.

The oestrogen feeds back to the brain to tell it to stop producing FSH, so the other egg follicles wither and die away.

It starts a new, thick endometrial lining growing on the inside of your womb.

It gets the inner lining of your womb pulsating to help the sperm swim up it.

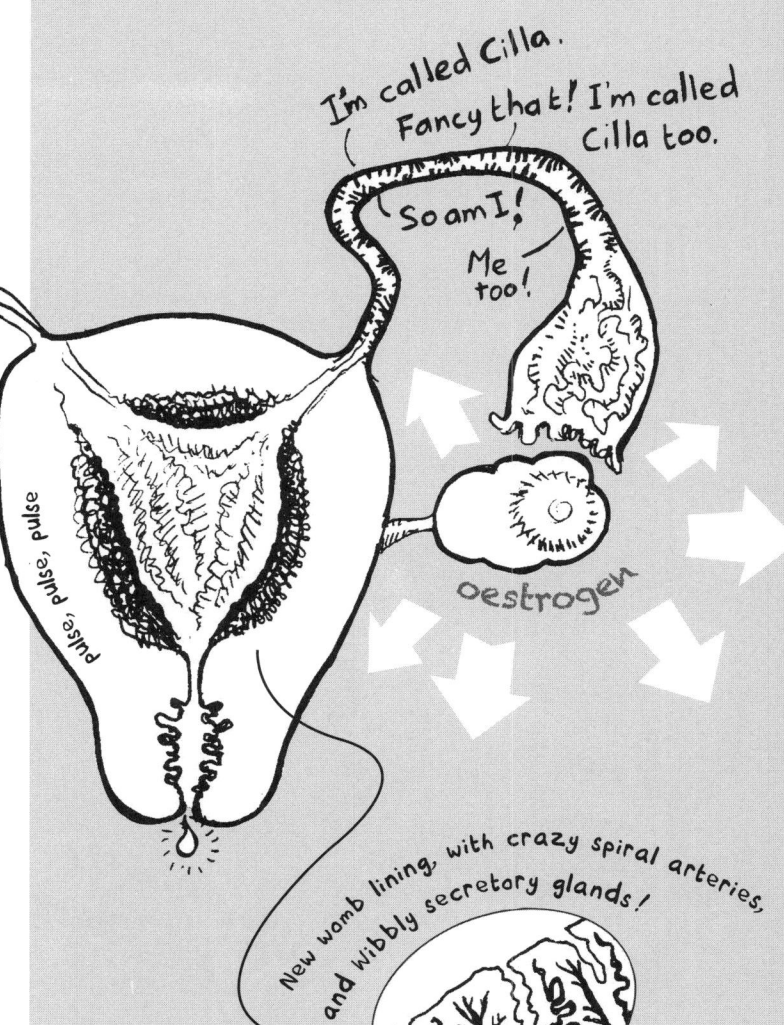

I'm called Cilla.

Fancy that! I'm called Cilla too.

So am I!

Me too!

pulse, pulse, pulse

oestrogen

New womb lining, with crazy spiral arteries, and wibbly secretory glands!

The little wavy hairs, or cilla, that line the insides of your oviducts grow longer, and cells within the tubes fill them with fluid (we will find out what that's for later).

And your cervix starts producing fertile juices.

Nobody talks about women's juices. We're largely ignorant of the amazing part they play in procreation. When they are mentioned, they are often referred to as 'mucus', which is inaccurate, and frankly insulting. A more neutral term is 'cervical fluid', but this is my book and I'm going to call it juice.

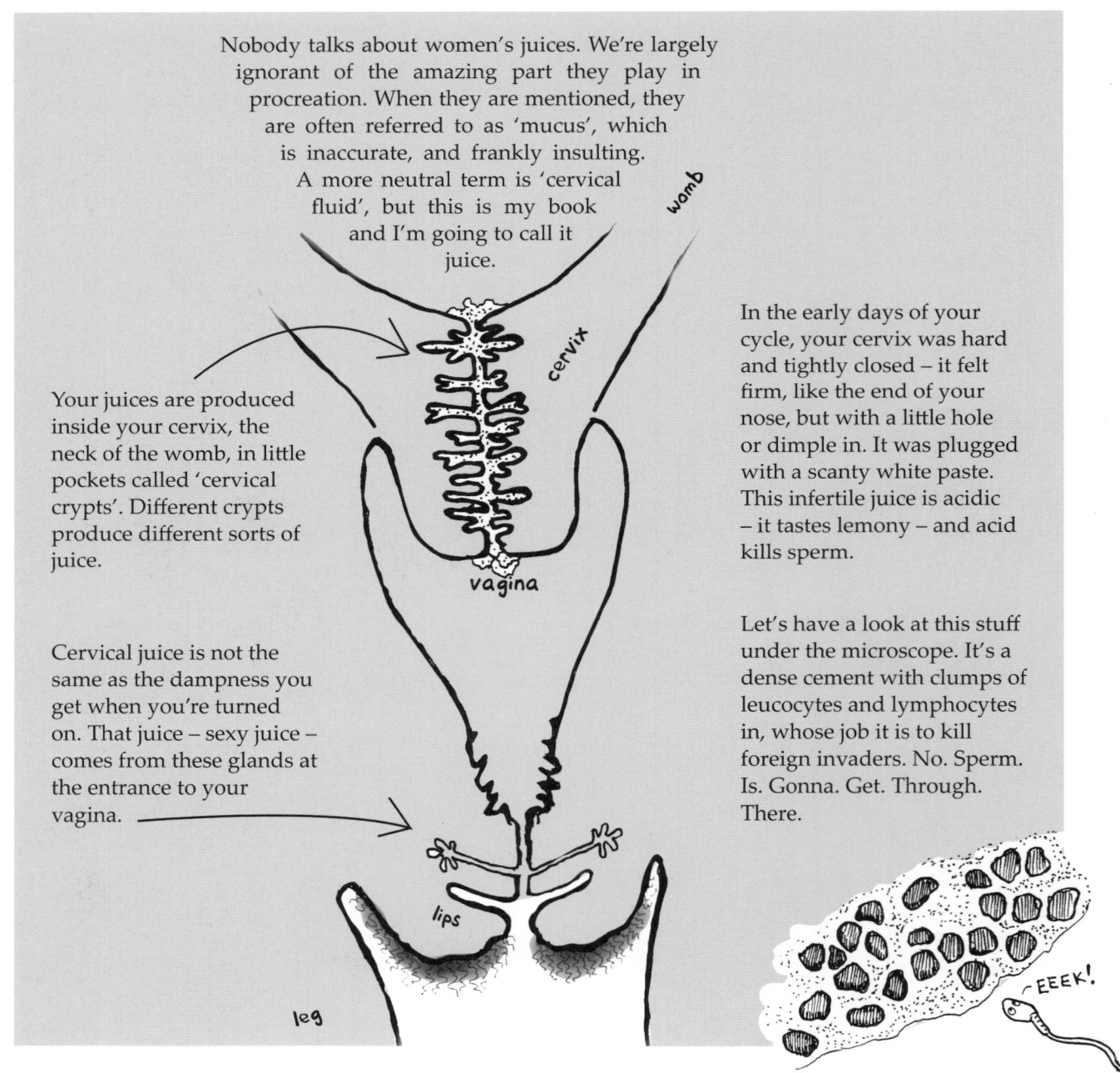

Your juices are produced inside your cervix, the neck of the womb, in little pockets called 'cervical crypts'. Different crypts produce different sorts of juice.

Cervical juice is not the same as the dampness you get when you're turned on. That juice – sexy juice – comes from these glands at the entrance to your vagina.

In the early days of your cycle, your cervix was hard and tightly closed – it felt firm, like the end of your nose, but with a little hole or dimple in. It was plugged with a scanty white paste. This infertile juice is acidic – it tastes lemony – and acid kills sperm.

Let's have a look at this stuff under the microscope. It's a dense cement with clumps of leucocytes and lymphocytes in, whose job it is to kill foreign invaders. No. Sperm. Is. Gonna. Get. Through. There.

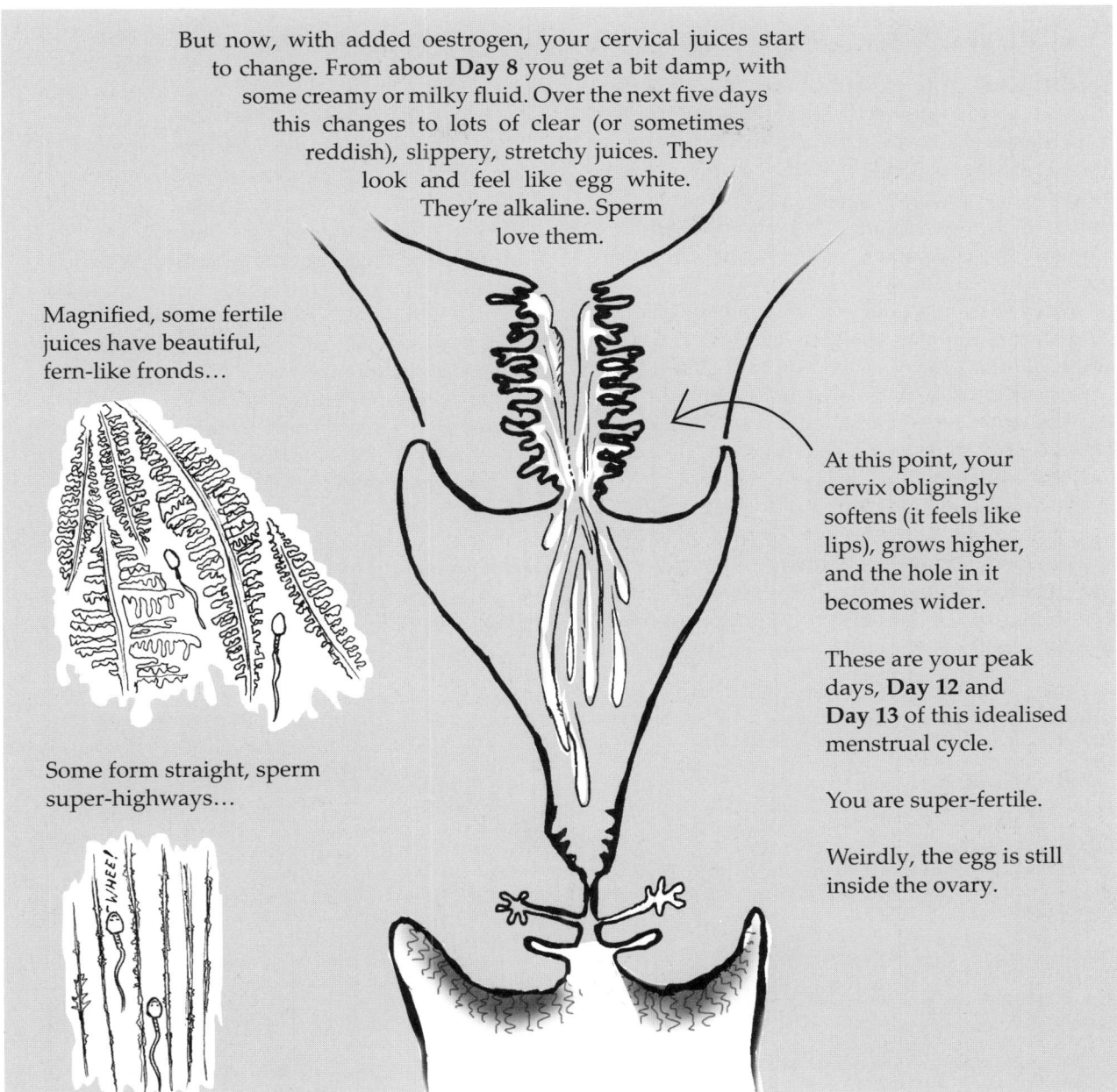

But now, with added oestrogen, your cervical juices start to change. From about **Day 8** you get a bit damp, with some creamy or milky fluid. Over the next five days this changes to lots of clear (or sometimes reddish), slippery, stretchy juices. They look and feel like egg white. They're alkaline. Sperm love them.

Magnified, some fertile juices have beautiful, fern-like fronds…

Some form straight, sperm super-highways…

At this point, your cervix obligingly softens (it feels like lips), grows higher, and the hole in it becomes wider.

These are your peak days, **Day 12** and **Day 13** of this idealised menstrual cycle.

You are super-fertile.

Weirdly, the egg is still inside the ovary.

17

Feeling fruity?

That is not all. Women change in more profound ways under the influence of oestrogen ('oestrogen' from the Greek *'oistros'* meaning 'sexiness', and 'gen', meaning 'producer'). In fact, a minor cottage industry has sprung up among psychologists testing all aspects of human behaviour on fertile women. (I've cited all my references here because the titles are hilarious.)

When you are fertile, you smell nicer,[1] your voice becomes higher and sounds sweeter,[2] and you walk more sexily.[3] Your skin feels softer. Unsurprisingly, in all these aspects, men rate fertile women as more attractive: researchers have found that lap dancers make more money when they are ovulating.[4]

Heterosexual women are more interested in men when they are ovulating. They are more likely to look at other men besides their partners[5] and they report that their partners are more possessive and jealous (I wonder why).[6] Fertile women find it easier to tell whether men are straight or gay.[7]

The one man a fertile woman is not interested in, however, is her dad. He's not a good potential mate, so she's statistically less likely to phone him when she's about to ovulate.[8]

You are more easily sexually aroused when you're fertile (it all feels more lush down there).[9] You might have more sexual fantasies, potentially featuring more sexual partners (blush!).[10] You'll want to spend more money on beauty products,[11] wear sexier and more revealing clothes,[12] and then go dancing in them.[13] You're less hungry when you're fertile, so you eat less (but you make up for that later in the month).[14]

This is important information! We should be told this stuff. Our education about the menstrual cycle should be more meaningful than the talk that the Tampax lady gave us at school. This makes sense of the wild swings in sexual desire that can mean that you fancy the pants off someone one (fertile) week, yet feel distinctly unthrilled when you get a date with them a week later. It explains the following cyclical variation in my relationship with my knickers…

(1) 'Body odor attractiveness as a cue of impending ovulation in women', Gildersleeve *et al*, *Hormones and Behaviour*, Vol 61, pp.157–66, February 2012.
(2) 'The unique impact of menstruation on the female voice: implications for the evolution of menstrual cycle cues', Pipitone and Gallup, *Ethology*, Vol 118, pp.281–91, March 2012.
(3) 'Differences in gait across the menstrual cycle and their attractiveness to men', Provost *et al.*, *Archives of Sexual Behaviour*, Vol 37, pp.598–604, August 2008.
(4) 'Ovulatory cycle effects on tip earnings by lap dancers: economic evidence for human estrus?', Miller *et al.*, *Evolution and Human Behavior*, Vol 28, pp.375–81, 2007.
(5) 'Fertility in the cycle predicts women's interest in sexual opportunism', Gangestad *et al.*, *Evolution and Human Behaviour*, Vol 31, pp.400–11, November 2010.
(6) 'Conditional expression of women's desires and men's mate guarding across the ovulatory cycle', Haselton, MG, & Gangestad, SW, *Hormones and Behavior*, Vol 49, pp.509–18, 2006.
(7) 'Mating interest improves women's accuracy in judging male sexual orientation', Rule *et al.*, *Psychological Science*, Vol 22, pp.881–6, July 2011.

(8) 'Kin affiliation across the ovulatory cycle: females avoid fathers when fertile', Leiberman, D *et al.*, *Psychological Science*, Vol 22, pp.13–18, January 2011.
(9) 'Women's sexual experience during the menstrual cycle: identification of the sexual phase by noninvasive measurement of lutenizing hormone', Bullivant *et al.*, *The Journal of Sex Research*, February 2004.
(10) 'Sexual fantasies and viewing times across the menstrual cycle: a diary study', Dawson, SJ *et al.*, *Archives of Sexual Behaviour*, Vol 41, pp.173–83.
(11) 'Do women feel worse to look their best? Testing the relationship between self-esteem and fertility status across the menstrual cycle', Hill, SE and Durante, KM, *Personality and Social Psychology*, Vol 35, pp.1592–601.
(12) 'Changes in women's choice of dress across the ovulatory cycle: Naturalistic and laboratory task–based evidence', Durante, KM *et al.*, *Personality and Social Psychology Bulletin*, Vol 34, pp.1451–60.
(13) 'Conditional expression of women's desires and men's mate guarding across the ovulatory cycle', Haselton, MG and Gangestad, SW, *Hormones and Behavior*, Vol 49, pp.509–18, 2006.
(14) 'The right time for a woman to diet?', *New Scientist*, 25 April 1992.

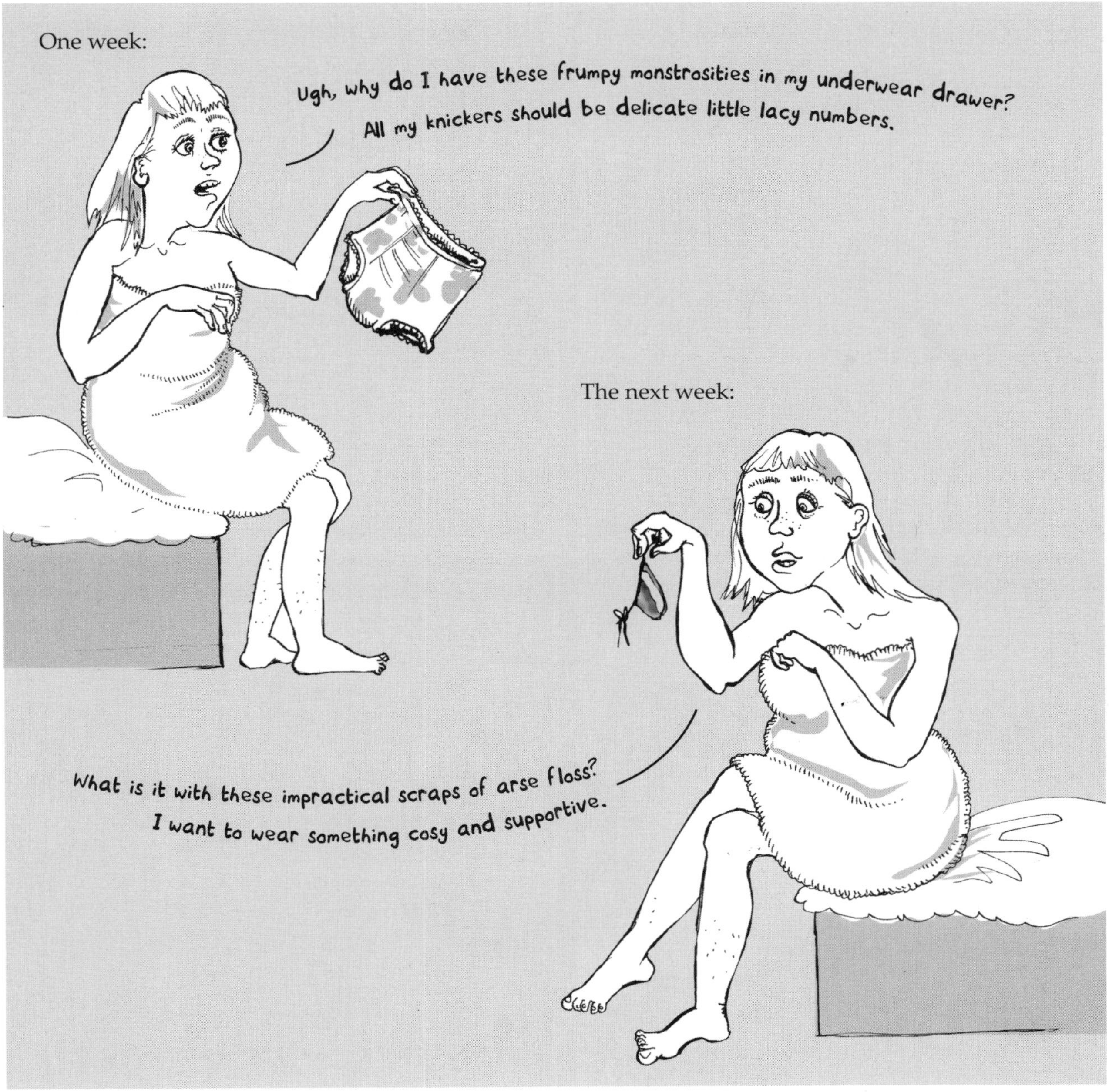
One week:
Ugh, why do I have these frumpy monstrosities in my underwear drawer?
All my knickers should be delicate little lacy numbers.
The next week:
What is it with these impractical scraps of arse floss?
I want to wear something cosy and supportive.

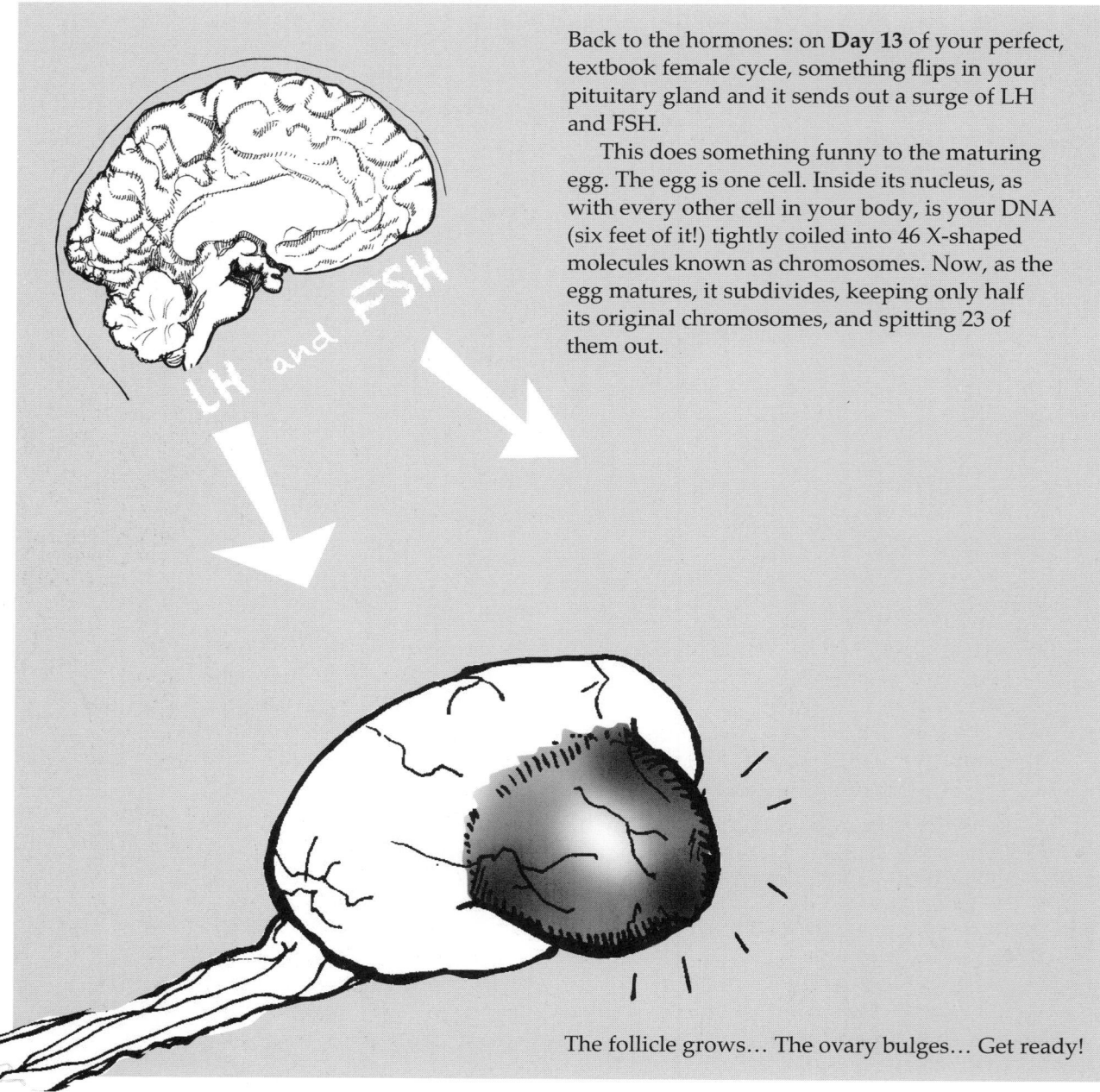

Back to the hormones: on **Day 13** of your perfect, textbook female cycle, something flips in your pituitary gland and it sends out a surge of LH and FSH.

This does something funny to the maturing egg. The egg is one cell. Inside its nucleus, as with every other cell in your body, is your DNA (six feet of it!) tightly coiled into 46 X-shaped molecules known as chromosomes. Now, as the egg matures, it subdivides, keeping only half its original chromosomes, and spitting 23 of them out.

The follicle grows… The ovary bulges… Get ready!

The Egg

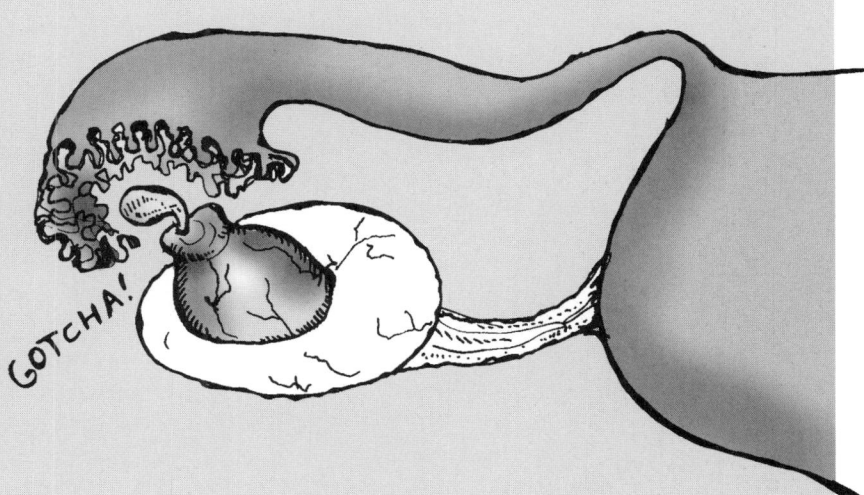

On the morning of **Day 14** out gushes the egg, in a protective covering of sticky granulosa cells, with a burst of follicular fluid. It's very small. It's smaller than this $\longrightarrow$.

Despite its tininess, the oviduct swoops round to find it and with its crazy fingery things, the fimbria, it swooshes it gently into the tube.

Some women can tell! Watch out for a twingeing pain, or a dull ache, low down in your belly on one side or the other. You can also tell which side ovulation occurs because the lymph gland at the top of that leg will be slightly swollen. Apparently, the lips of your vulva swell slightly more on that side too.

(I suppose it's a good excuse to get your partner to spend some time down there, investigating.) Some women bleed when they ovulate, just a spot, or quite a bit, so a very light, very short period could be ovulation, not menstruation.

What's going to happen to this egg? Er, nothing. There's no sperm around. We get to the fish part of our story later.

The egg disappears off into your oviduct and disintegrates within the next 24 hours. But! Your ovary isn't finished yet! Oh, no, that follicle is still busy. It collapses down, turns yellow, acquires the name 'corpus luteum', and starts pumping out progesterone.

Days 15 to 27

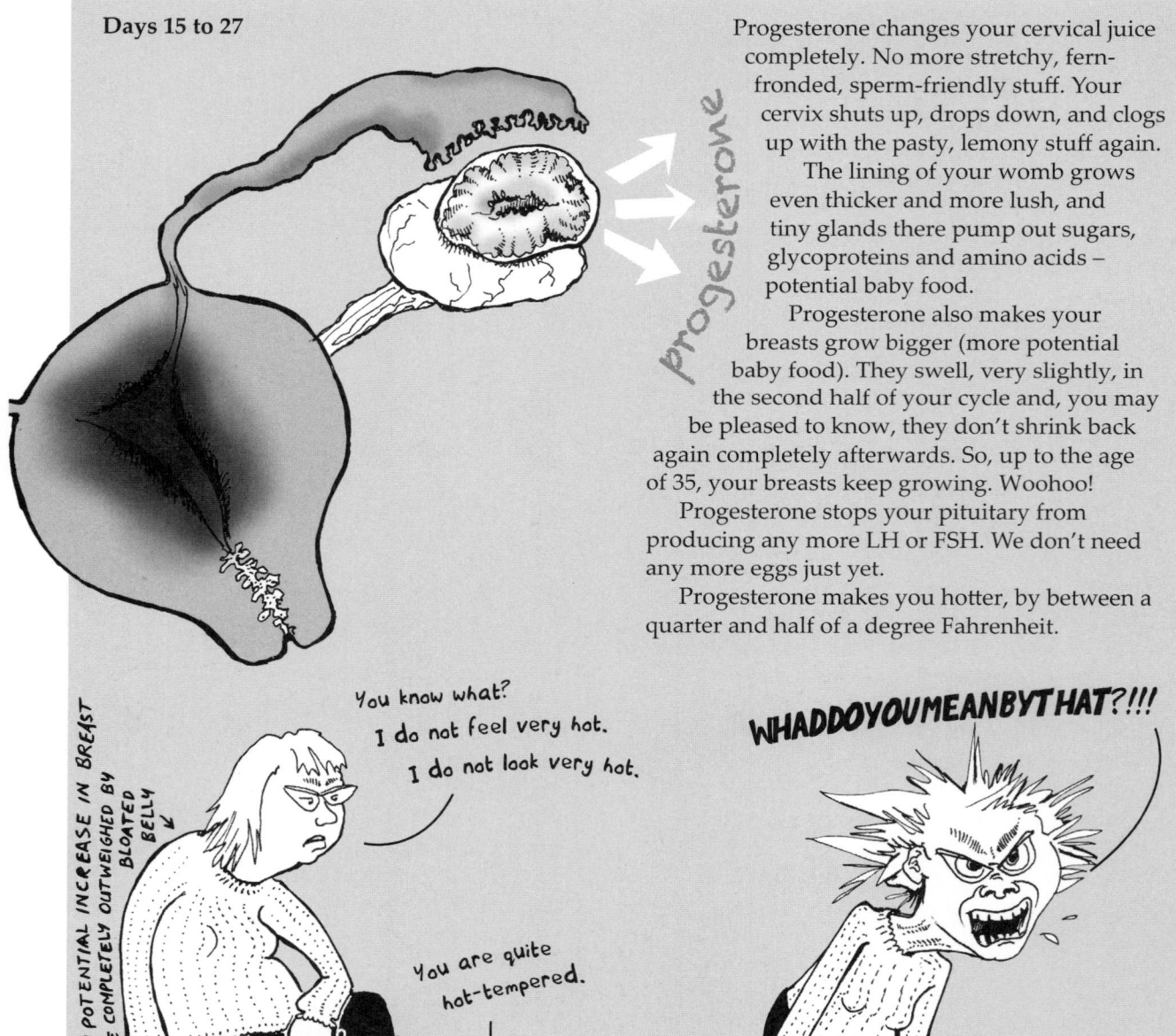

Progesterone changes your cervical juice completely. No more stretchy, fern-fronded, sperm-friendly stuff. Your cervix shuts up, drops down, and clogs up with the pasty, lemony stuff again.

The lining of your womb grows even thicker and more lush, and tiny glands there pump out sugars, glycoproteins and amino acids – potential baby food.

Progesterone also makes your breasts grow bigger (more potential baby food). They swell, very slightly, in the second half of your cycle and, you may be pleased to know, they don't shrink back again completely afterwards. So, up to the age of 35, your breasts keep growing. Woohoo!

Progesterone stops your pituitary from producing any more LH or FSH. We don't need any more eggs just yet.

Progesterone makes you hotter, by between a quarter and half of a degree Fahrenheit.

Feeling fractious?

Not everyone will find this to be true, but, statistically, you are more likely to experience reduced sex drive, constipation, bloating, insomnia, increased appetite and acne in the post-ovulatory part of your cycle. You're also more likely to be depressed.

And you just might be more irritable.

WELL! Maybe that's because I'm fat, spotty, can't sleep and I can't shit!

Huh, Sherlock?

HAVE YOU CONSIDERED THAT ?!!!!

Some people call this PMS.

I call it **SPEAKING THE TRUTH!**

Let's get one thing straight. If, while reading this book, you get the impression that women are a bunch of violent, unstable lunatics, enslaved to their hormones, let me remind you that it is now, and has historically been, **MEN** who go around raping people, starting wars and building concentration camps.

Men suffer from extreme hormonal mood-swings too, and theirs are far more unpredictable.

At least I can tell you, with scientific certainty, that, if you want me to be nice to you, you'll have to come back next week.

Premenstrual symptoms can be no laughing matter. If you're suffering, keep a diary of your menstrual cycles and moods to show to your GP. Reflexology and acupuncture claim success for alleviating the symptoms of PMS. The herbal supplement Vitex agnus castus has been proven to help[15]: the dosage is 40mg daily, first thing in the morning, so you need to source 20mg tablets, not 5mg ones.

Try less caffeine and alcohol and more exercise, wholefoods, fresh fruits and vegetables.

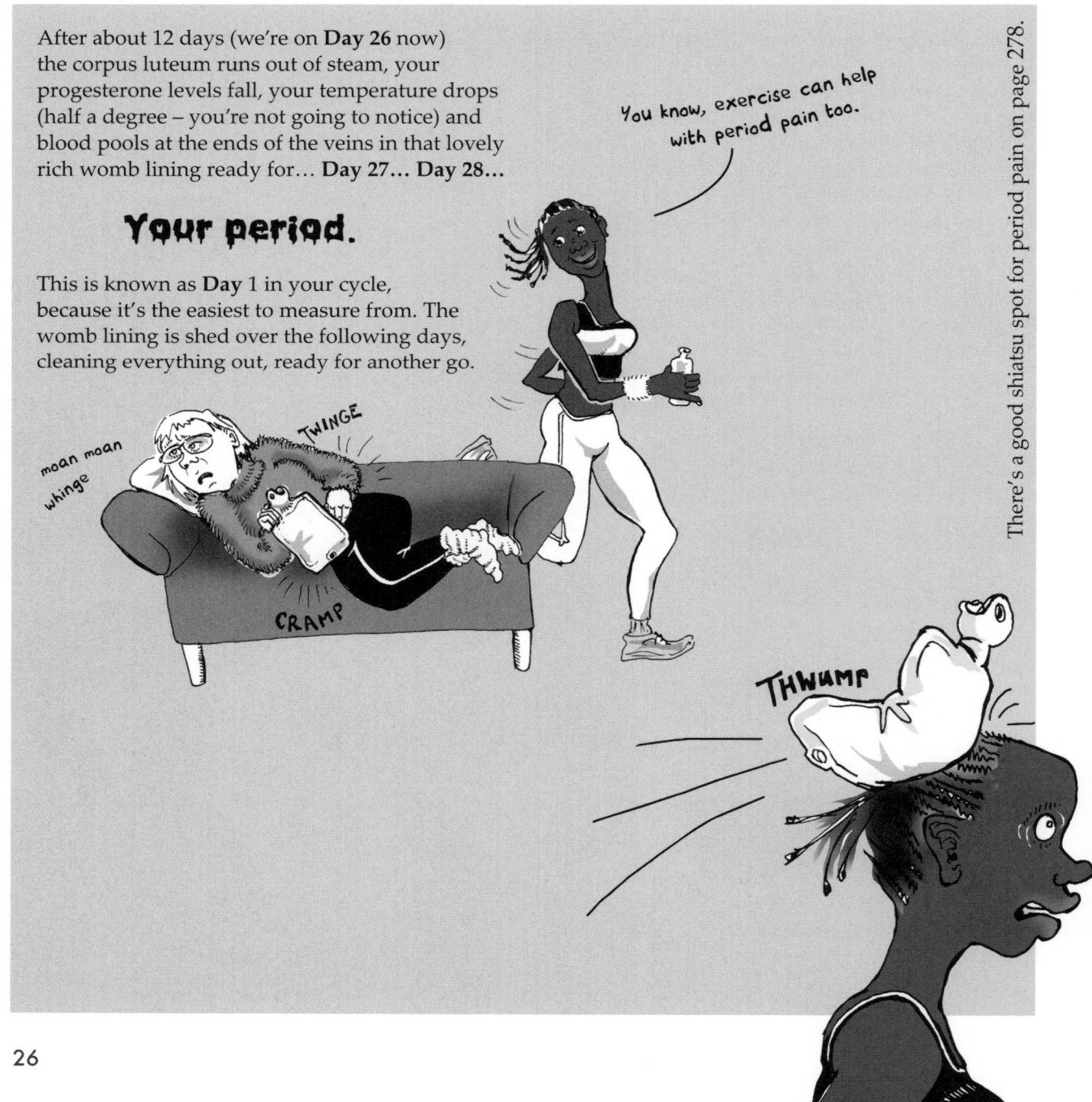

After about 12 days (we're on **Day 26** now) the corpus luteum runs out of steam, your progesterone levels fall, your temperature drops (half a degree – you're not going to notice) and blood pools at the ends of the veins in that lovely rich womb lining ready for... **Day 27... Day 28...**

Your period.

This is known as **Day** 1 in your cycle, because it's the easiest to measure from. The womb lining is shed over the following days, cleaning everything out, ready for another go.

You know, exercise can help with period pain too.

There's a good shiatsu spot for period pain on page 278.

moan moan whinge

TWINGE

CRAMP

THWUMP

The Fish

Sperm are amazing.[16]

Have a look. Each one is five and a half hundredths of a millimetre long, so you'll need a microscope. Fortunately. It would be a bit freaky if you could see them with the naked eye.

Acrosome 'depth charge' to bust through the female eggshell.

Glycosyn 'invisibility cloak' to evade female immune defences.

Mitochondria 'power-pack' with stored-up energy for swimming.

Tail flicks round in a cone-shaped spiral, to propel it forward.

A 'nose' for sniffing out the female egg.

The most densely packed DNA of any human cell. Each sperm carries either an X or a Y chromosome that determines the sex of the baby.

Two swim modes – a straight-ahead gentle jog speed for swimming up the vagina and womb, and a crazy-fast-twisty mode for navigating the fallopian tube and racing to the egg.

When they were discovered, in 1677, sperm were originally named 'animalcules'. How cute!

Men produce sperm in truly astonishing quantities – between a quarter to half a billion in each ejaculation. Sperm-production continues day and night, from puberty until death, at the rate of a thousand sperm per heartbeat. It's a wonder that men have any energy left for maintaining glass ceilings.

This is what a thousand sperm looks like:

Our potential dad has favoured quantity over quality when boshing this lot out. Some sperm have two heads, some have two tails, some can't swim straight, some are already dead.

We don't actually need five hundred million sperm to fertilise our egg. We only need one. So the female body operates a very selective entry system, to let in only the best sperm, while ruthlessly eliminating any unwanted intruders.

PICK YOUR OWN ADVENTURE MOMENT!

You have some sperm. You could have obtained it in any number of ways. For example:

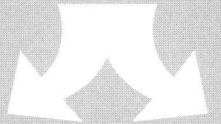

Sex with a loving partner and devoted father to your children

Sex with someone who is not biologically equipped to be the father of children, so you're improvising with a turkey baster and some donor sperm

Sex with someone you were under the erroneous impression was a loving partner and devoted father to your children

Just the turkey baster and donor sperm

A contraceptive failure with someone you had no intention would be the father of your children

Non-consensual sex

X-RATED PAGE

Let's hope that this encounter with sperm is taking place in a romantic atmosphere, because sexual excitement is going to help the sperm survive.[17]

Your vagina is naturally, anti-bacterially, slightly acidic, and remember, acid kills sperm. Leucocytes (white blood cells) there kill foreign invaders – germs, but also sperm. But when you become aroused, your sexy juices give your vagina a sperm-friendly protective coating. And orgasm then helps suck friendly juices and sperm out of the vagina and into the womb.*

Unfortunately, we live in a sexist world, and although there are a lot of depictions of heterosexual sex around, very few of them do justice to female sexuality. You would think, from watching the movies or surfing the net, that…

- Women are extremely skinny, yet have massive, bouncy breasts, and are entirely hairless.
- Frantic deep thrusting is the correct way to have sex.
- Women gain the most pleasure and fulfilment from giving men oral sex.
- Having sex when drunk is a good idea.
- Sex is a performance, not an experience.

If you reverse these assumptions, I predict a lot more orgasms.

I also think that expecting a male partner to provide all the clitoral stimulation during sex is an unreasonable amount of multi-tasking for a man to handle.

We refer to a man 'penetrating' a woman's vagina. Ouch! The word 'vagina' actually comes from the Latin for 'scabbard', the thing you put your sword in. There are not meant to be swords involved! It's just as accurate to say that the woman 'engulfs' the man's penis. Just a thought.

We don't even have a proper name for our genitalia.** 'Vagina' refers to the inside part, 'clitoris' to the sensitive button at the front, and 'vulva' to the lips at each side. But what we think of as a clit is just the tip of an iceberg: an amazing, hidden, wishbone-shaped network of erectile tissue that extends through the lips of your vulva, outer and inner, and around the walls of your vagina. Just the little tip that you can feel with your finger has 8,000 nerve-endings. That's twice as many as a penis.

Yes, you read that right, we have erectile tissue too! It's not just a hole. It swells and stretches. It can shift shape just as much as a man's bits can. It'll do some amazing transformations by the end of this book! So explore and have fun. And it's not only women who benefit from good quality lovemaking. When a man has more prolonged, tantalising and loving sex, he draws sperm from further back in the testicles; he ejaculates healthier sperm, and more of them.[18]

Just in case 250,000,000 wasn't enough.

---

* There was an insane assertion made in the 2012 US presidential race that women cannot become pregnant as a result of rape. Obviously, they can. I'm not saying that women have to enjoy sex in order for conception to occur. I'm describing how sexual response optimises fertility.

** The word 'c*nt' is more accurate, as it refers to the whole thing, but the word is now unprintably rude, which says something about how scared our society is of the power of women's parts.

What you can see:

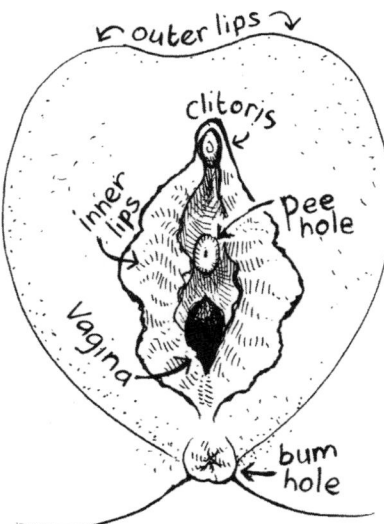

And what you can't see:

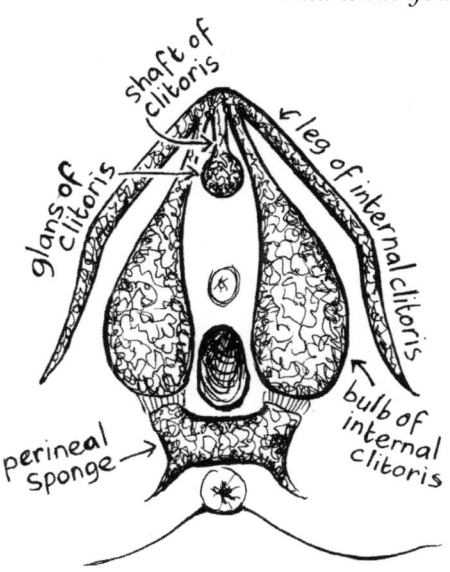

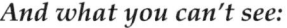

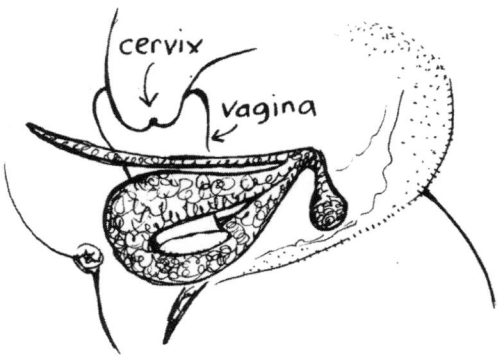

The erectile tissue of the internal clitoris and perineum swells around the vagina and makes it feel lush.

Man has evolved a delivery system that deposits the sperm as close to the cervix as it can get. (Although, as mentioned earlier, you can substitute a turkey baster or an oral medicine syringe.)

But that's not all he deposits…

Sperm arrive in a gel of semen. On a very simple level, semen forms a soft jelly that helps stop the sperm from falling out of the vagina immediately. But, take a closer look!

Semen is a potent love potion containing a whole bunch of feel-good chemicals: serotonin, prolactin, estrone, thyrotropin-releasing hormone and oxytocin, all rounded off with the sleep hormone melatonin. There is evidence that women who are regularly (and willingly!) exposed to human semen tend to suffer from depression less than women who aren't. Semen gets you hooked on your man![19]

Semen is sneakily multi-functional. It contains LH and FSH to help ripen your eggs and trigger ovulation. It's a conspiracy! It is actually trying to get you pregnant! And, in case you're already pregnant, it also contains the hormones human chorionic gonadotropin and human placental lactogen, to help maintain the pregnancy.[20]

Semen, being alkaline, also counteracts the acidity of the vagina. And although the anti-microbial agents in the vagina will kill sperm, with several hundred million sperm there, some of them are going to make it.

What happens next depends on the quality of your cervical juices. If you have infertile juice, as previously stated, nothing gets in that cervix. Game over.

Fertile juice changes everything. It's kinda gloopy, but semen contains a special chemical that breaks the surface tension. And off they go![21]

The fern-like branches in the juices trap malformed sperm that can't swim in a straight line. The straight super-highways speed only the correctly sized sperm up through the cervix, into the womb.

Aaaagh! The womb has a lot of leucocytes in it. The sperm use their glycosyn invisibility cloaks, to help them dodge your body's immune defences.

Waves in the muscle in the wall of the womb help propel the sperm towards the correct oviduct, the one with the ripening egg follicle at the top.[22] Orgasm will also give them a helping hand, by sucking cervical juices up into the inside of your womb to protect the sperm.

The entrance to the oviduct is very tiny. It has a strict door policy, responding to particular sperm proteins, and not letting anything else in.

Once inside, the sperm have made it! There are no leucocytes here. The oviduct is filled with sperm-nourishing fluid, and little pillows for them to rest on. Remember, the egg is still inside the ovary. The fertile cervical fluid gets the sperm in place *ahead of time*, lined up in the tube ready for the release of the egg.

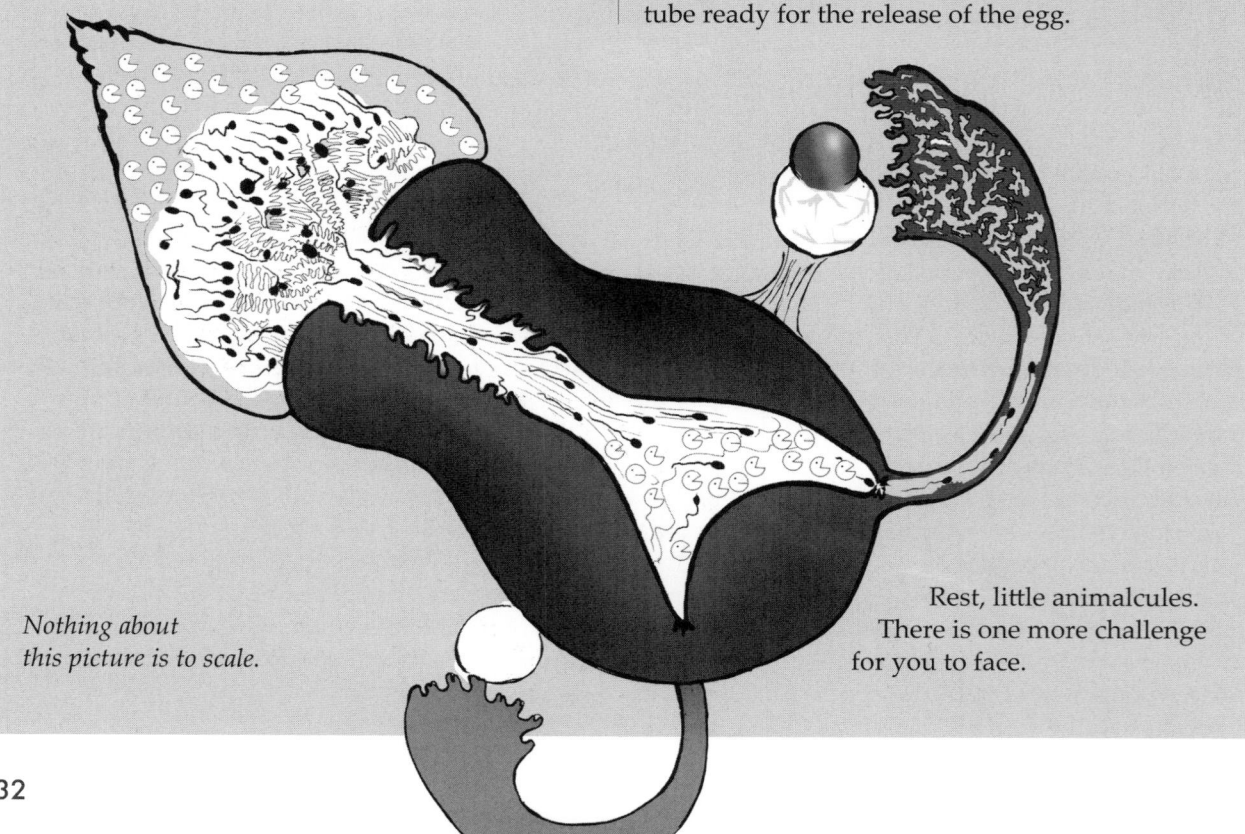

*Nothing about
this picture is to scale.*

Rest, little animalcules.
There is one more challenge
for you to face.

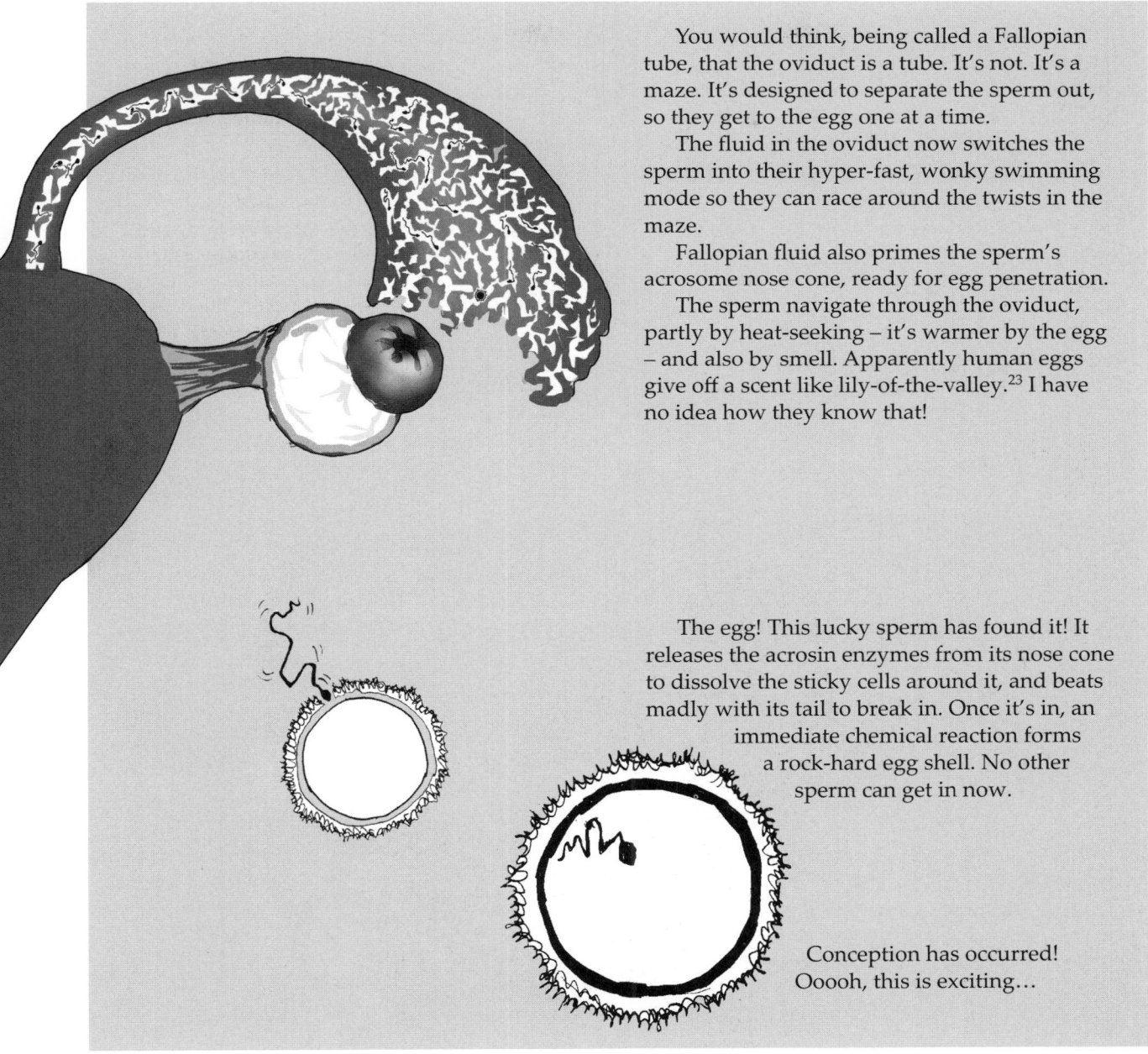

You would think, being called a Fallopian tube, that the oviduct is a tube. It's not. It's a maze. It's designed to separate the sperm out, so they get to the egg one at a time.

The fluid in the oviduct now switches the sperm into their hyper-fast, wonky swimming mode so they can race around the twists in the maze.

Fallopian fluid also primes the sperm's acrosome nose cone, ready for egg penetration.

The sperm navigate through the oviduct, partly by heat-seeking – it's warmer by the egg – and also by smell. Apparently human eggs give off a scent like lily-of-the-valley.[23] I have no idea how they know that!

The egg! This lucky sperm has found it! It releases the acrosin enzymes from its nose cone to dissolve the sticky cells around it, and beats madly with its tail to break in. Once it's in, an immediate chemical reaction forms a rock-hard egg shell. No other sperm can get in now.

Conception has occurred! Ooooh, this is exciting…

The sperm dissolves. The egg absorbs its packet of DNA. Within four to seven hours, the chromosomes of the new baby form. The cell splits, then splits again, about every 12 hours.

The cilla in the oviduct gently wave it towards the womb. The cell continues to split, looking increasingly like a mulberry. Seriously, it has the scientific name *morula*, which is Latin for mulberry.

Safely protected inside its hard eggshell, the egg/mulberry/baby takes about a week to float down the tube. Once it gets to the womb, the egg hatches out of its shell and the tiny baby/ speck floats off to find a good spot

on the wall of the womb. It buries right in. It starts to secrete the pregnancy hormone human chorionic gonadotrophin (hCG), which tells the corpus luteum (remember him?) to bump up progesterone and oestrogen production.

The outer cells of the mulberry-lump form a sac for a streak of baby to grow inside. It doesn't need much oxygen – glycoproteins and sugars in the womb keep mulberry-baby fed and happy.[24]

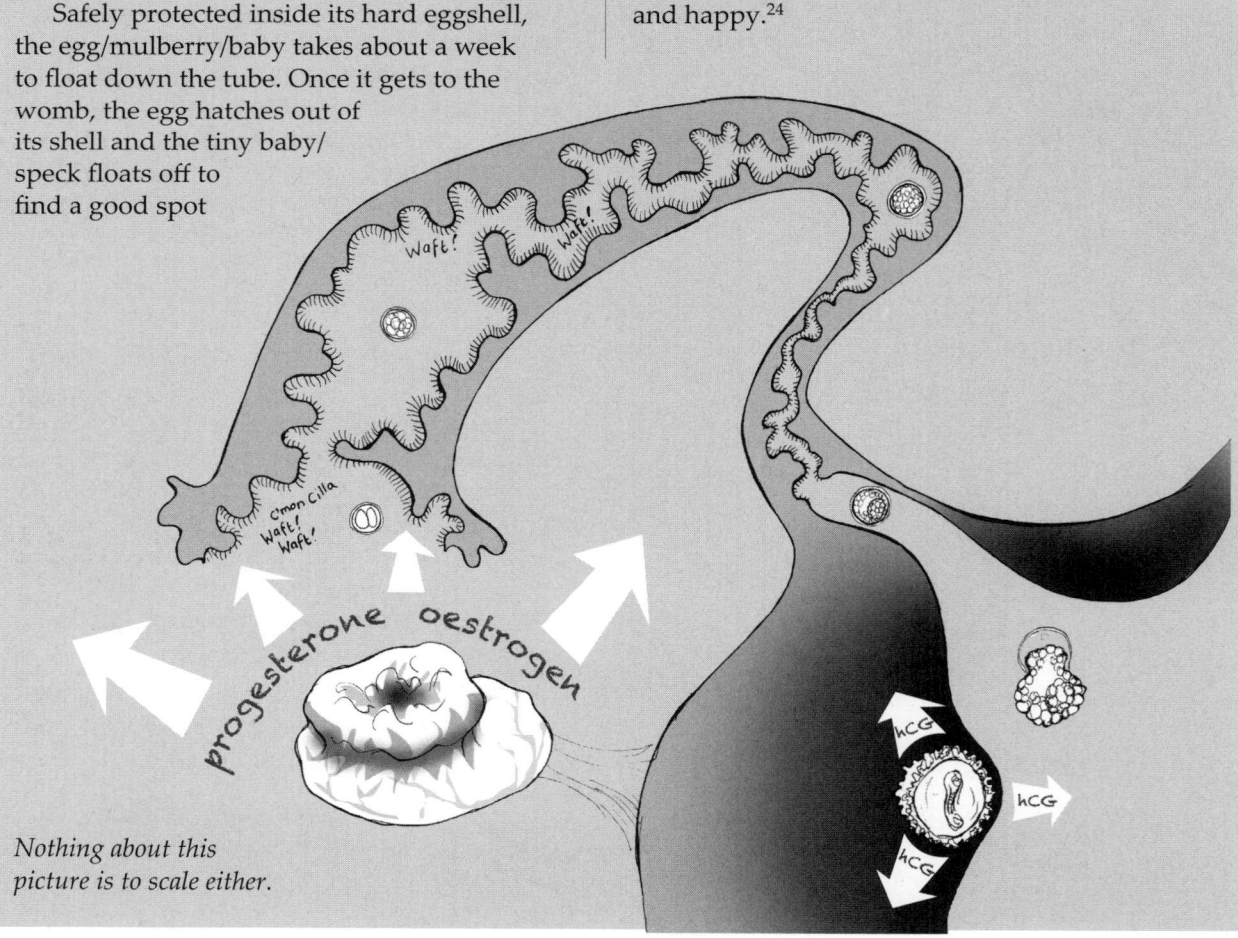

Nothing about this picture is to scale either.

What happens next?

Well, a lot of the time, nothing at all. We're sold a very simplistic narrative of human conception: one egg + one sperm = a guaranteed new baby. But that's just a story. Reality is more random than that. Not all fertile couples will conceive every cycle. Not all pregnancies are viable. Either your next period arrives, or it doesn't.

PICK YOUR OWN ADVENTURE MOMENT!

We have four options.

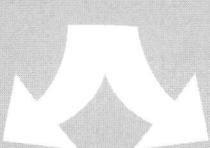

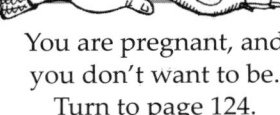

YES!

You are not pregnant, and you don't want to be. Turn to page 36.

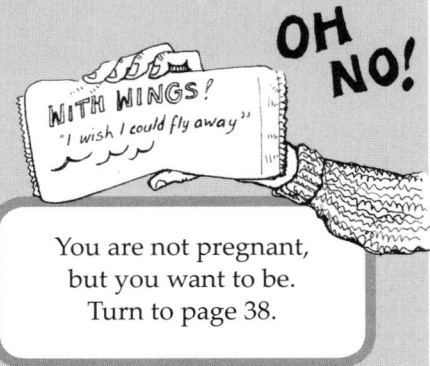

OH NO!

You are not pregnant, but you want to be. Turn to page 38.

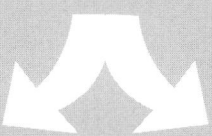

OH NO!!!

You are pregnant, and you don't want to be. Turn to page 124.

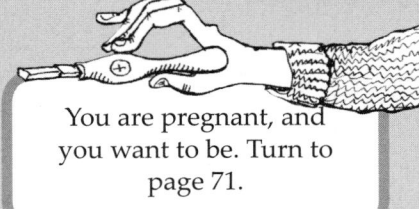

YESSS!

You are pregnant, and you want to be. Turn to page 71.

(It is possible to feel more than one of the emotions on this page.)

2 Breeders versus non-breeders

This may seem like a slight digression in a book about fertility and pregnancy, but it is worth pointing out that there are women in the world who don't want children. It would be nice if the rest of the human race respected their ability to make a decision on this issue.

A typical conversation tends to go like this:

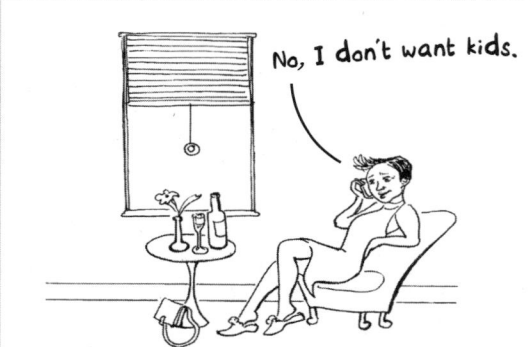

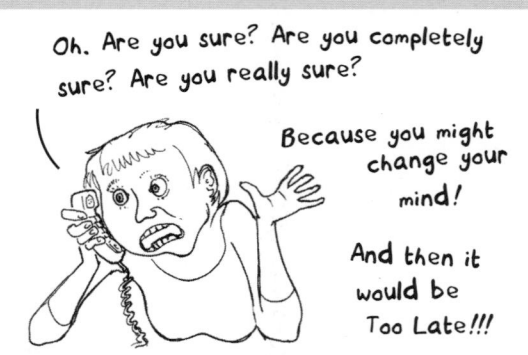

This is faulty logic, and could be applied to any major life decision.

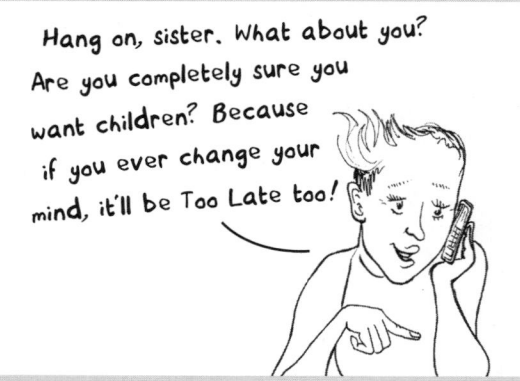

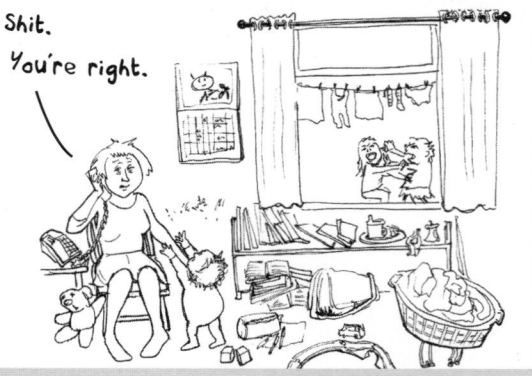

Anyway, non-breeders read on, because this book (despite being about pregnancy and birth) may still have some relevant information for you.

PICK YOUR OWN ADVENTURE MOMENT!

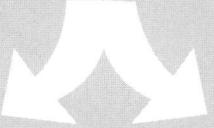

| Are you gay? | Are you straight or bi? |

There's not much chance of you accidentally falling pregnant. You can stop reading now.

Or you could flick through the rest of the book to find out what other women go through, perhaps with a mounting sense of shock and awe.

Read the next chapter, because it will explain how to avoid getting pregnant from heterosexual sex.

3 *You and your cycle*

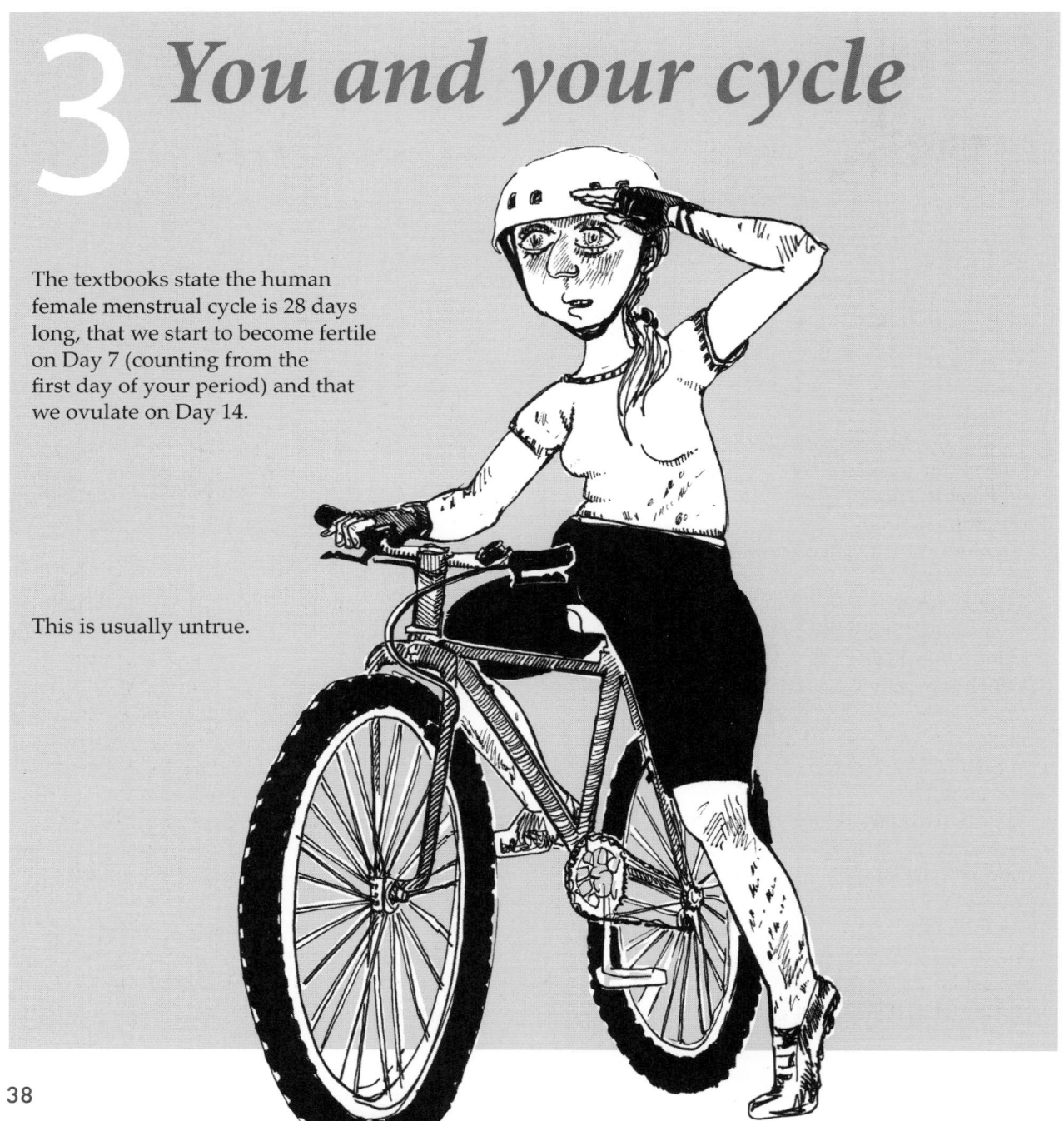

The textbooks state the human female menstrual cycle is 28 days long, that we start to become fertile on Day 7 (counting from the first day of your period) and that we ovulate on Day 14.

This is usually untrue.

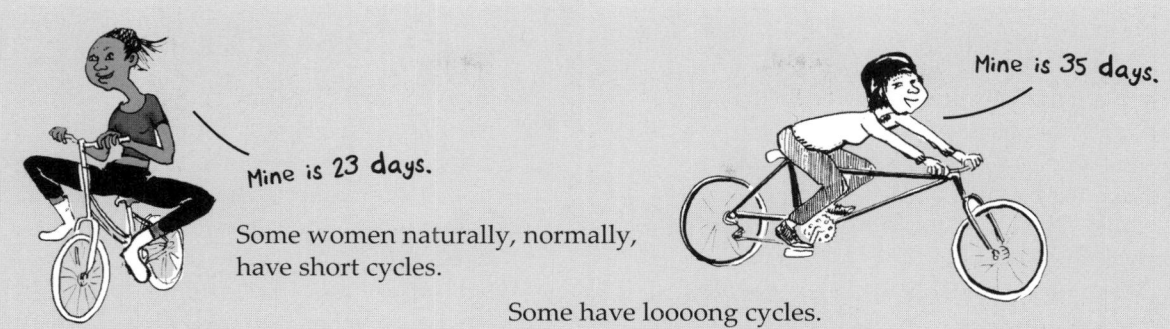

Mine is 23 days.

Some women naturally, normally, have short cycles.

Mine is 35 days.

Some have loooong cycles.

Some have irregular cycles, and they never know when their period is due.

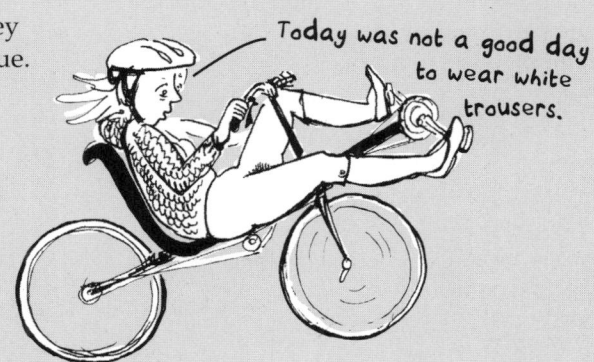

Today was not a good day to wear white trousers.

Even for women whose cycles are usually predictable, shock or stress can delay ovulation from time to time.

Only 15% of women bleed every 28 days, and, of them, only a proportion ovulate exactly halfway through.[1]

The mean average length of the menstrual cycle isn't even 28 days, it's actually 29.5 days. (Which is exactly the same length as the lunar cycle! This is so hippy – yet so scientifically precise! It's as if we're part of the moon's gravitational pull on the earth – we have tides!)

So what?

Well, if you want to get pregnant, you need to know how to identify your own personal 'fertile window', which won't necessarily be from Day 7 to Day 14.

Once you get pregnant, the medical establishment will date your pregnancy from your last period *on the assumption that you ovulated 14 days later*. If you didn't, you will be given the wrong due date. So it's very useful to know exactly when you conceived your baby.

And if you have no current plans to get pregnant you can also use fertility awareness for contraception. Fertility awareness is often confused with 'the rhythm method'. The rhythm method doesn't work, because it uses a calendar to determine when you are fertile. Fertility awareness does work, because it uses information from your body.

Also, if you often have irregular cycles, this chapter will teach you how to predict when you'll get your period, which is very useful information.

So, how does it work?

There are three indicators of fertility that you can track: the position of your cervix, the quality of your cervical juices, and your basal body temperature.

Here's how. Let's start on the first day after your period finishes.

Wash your hands thoroughly and dry them well. Squat down, and pop two fingers into your vagina.

Yuk! No! I couldn't do that!

Why not? You'd let your boyfriend!* There's nothing inherently more hygienic about men than women. If you end up having a baby, you'll probably let perfect strangers assess your cervix when you're in labour.** Go on. Have a feel.

Do this every day, throughout your cycle. Squat in the same position each time, so you can feel how your cervix changes in height.

Your cervix is a nose-like projection that's probably on the front wall of your vagina. Very rarely, women have two cervixes, leading to two wombs.

* I'm assuming that no lesbian would be this uptight.
** But you don't have to. See page 250.

During the infertile early days of your cycle, your cervix is low-slung, it feels firm, and the hole or dimple in the end of it feels small. Put your fingers either side of it, then close them together over it. Pull them out, have a look at them, and spread them apart.

What have you got? Juice.

Infertile juice is white, thick and pasty. It tastes lemony. (Why not? You'd let your boyfriend!) There isn't very much of it.

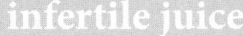
infertile juice

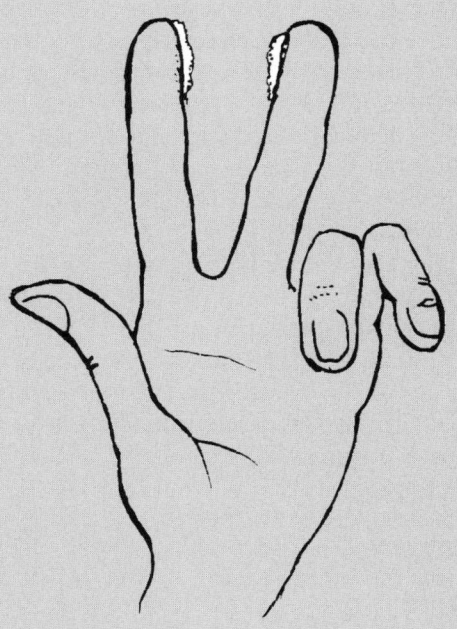

infertile cervix
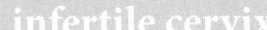
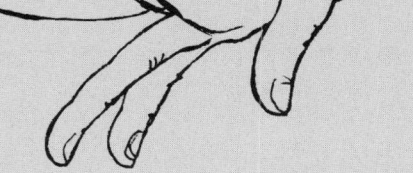

Over the following days or weeks, as you start to become fertile, you will notice more juice. It may turn creamy or start to form clear blobs. Your cervix will feel wider, and the dimple in it will feel a bit bigger.

When you reach peak fertility – on whatever day that is for you – the cervix will rise right up. Some women find that it's too high to reach. It feels soft, like your lips, and slippery with juice.

Fertile juice is usually clear, but it may be pink or brownish, and it stretches like egg white between your fingers.

Once you have ovulated, the cervix drops back down and closes up. The juice changes back to the infertile-type paste.

This is the basic information you need to help you conceive a baby: *have lots of sex in the part of your cycle when you have stretchy juice, and a soft, high cervix.*

It's not rocket science.

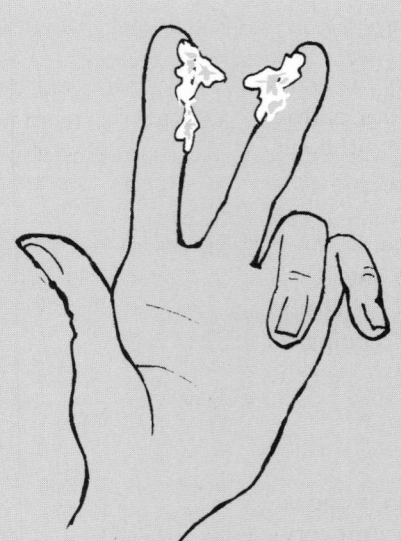

fertile juices

fertile cervix

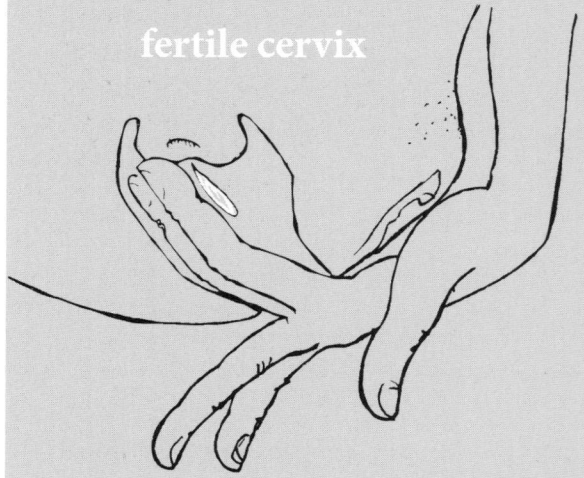

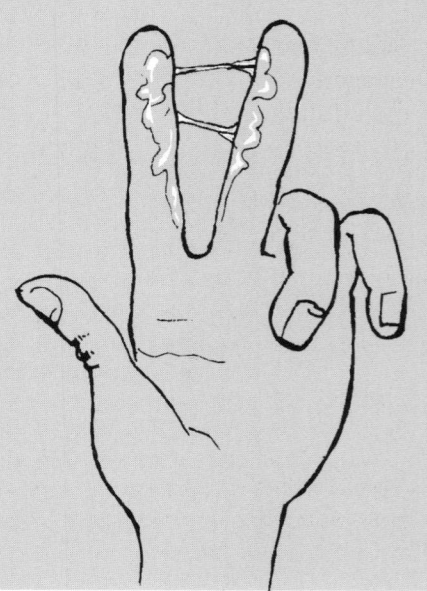

Yes, but…

Not everyone is mobile enough to feel their own cervix. Your partner could check.* In this case, lying on your back in bed would probably be the easiest position. Use the same position every day.

Another option is to use a vaginal speculum (buy one online), position a mirror between your legs, and shine a bright torch on it. Then you can see what's going on.

You can also check your juices as they come out onto your panties. Fertile juice makes round wet patches, and infertile juice makes dry white streaks.

Semen in the vagina makes it harder to evaluate your cervical juices. If you're trying for a baby, I'm not suggesting that you stop, because that would be silly. If you aren't, though, then using condoms or abstaining from vaginal sex for a couple of cycles will help you to learn about your body. Ideally we'd be taught all this when we were teenagers, and we'd know about our bodies all our adult life.

If you don't see the types of juice described here, if your cervical fluid smells unpleasant, if you're sore or itchy or if you get bleeding which is not part of your natural cycle, then see your GP in case you have an infection. Also ask them if

any medication you are taking could affect your cervical fluid.

If your period lasts for longer than five days, your fertile juices could start when you are still menstruating. Yes, it is possible to get pregnant when you are on your period! It can be a bit more confusing to interpret what's going on with cycles like this, but with regular observations for a few months you will learn your fertile signs.

If you have long or irregular cycles, then the long part is in the first, fertile half of your cycle. Once you have ovulated, then there will always be the same number of days until you menstruate. Find out how many days that is for you – it will probably be between 12 and 16 days. Bingo! From now on, you will be able to predict, once you ovulate, when your period will arrive. Feel smug.

Your body does, however, have an unpredictable trick up its sleeve. From time to time, you can start gearing up to produce an egg, then some kind of shock or stress (accident? exams? mother coming to visit?) will make everything shut down. When your hormonal/limbic system decides that the danger has passed, it will unexpectedly then start back up again. So, while your cervix gives you good information about when you are potentially fertile, it can't tell you definitively whether you have ovulated or not.**

For that, you have to take your temperature…

* In fact, guys, you could be totally pro-active here. Consider how useful this information is. If you examine your lady friend right, you'll be able to tell whether she is fertile, fruity and lovely, or post-ovulatory and potentially suffering PMT hell. Remember, premenstrual women need extra love, flowers and niceness.

Or else.

** If you get unmissable ovulation signs such as cramps or blood spotting, you can also use these to confirm that you have ovulated.

Taking your temperature

Progesterone raises your temperature, but to such a minute degree that you need to be very specific about how you take it. Your underlying body temperature rises and falls very slightly throughout the day, so you have to take it at the same time every day. Exercise also raises your temperature, even very mild exercise, so take it after you have been resting completely for at least four hours. That means first thing in the morning, when you wake up.

You will need: a digital thermometer that is accurate to two decimal places Celsius, or a glass 'basal body thermometer' (ask your pharmacist) which has extra-fine gradings. A normal glass fever thermometer that you use when you're sick won't be accurate enough. Use the same thermometer every day, because different thermometers can vary slightly in the readings they give.

You will also need an alarm clock (though these days we have phones for that), a pen and some paper. Put all these items right next to your bed. If you're using a glass thermometer, shake the line down before you go to sleep.

As soon as your alarm goes off, take your temperature. Do not get up. Do not sit up. Do not have a cup of tea. Do not have a drink of water. Do nothing except turn the thermometer on, stick it in your mouth and wait. Try not to fall back asleep until it's done! Scribble down your temperature reading on the pad – you can go back to sleep now.

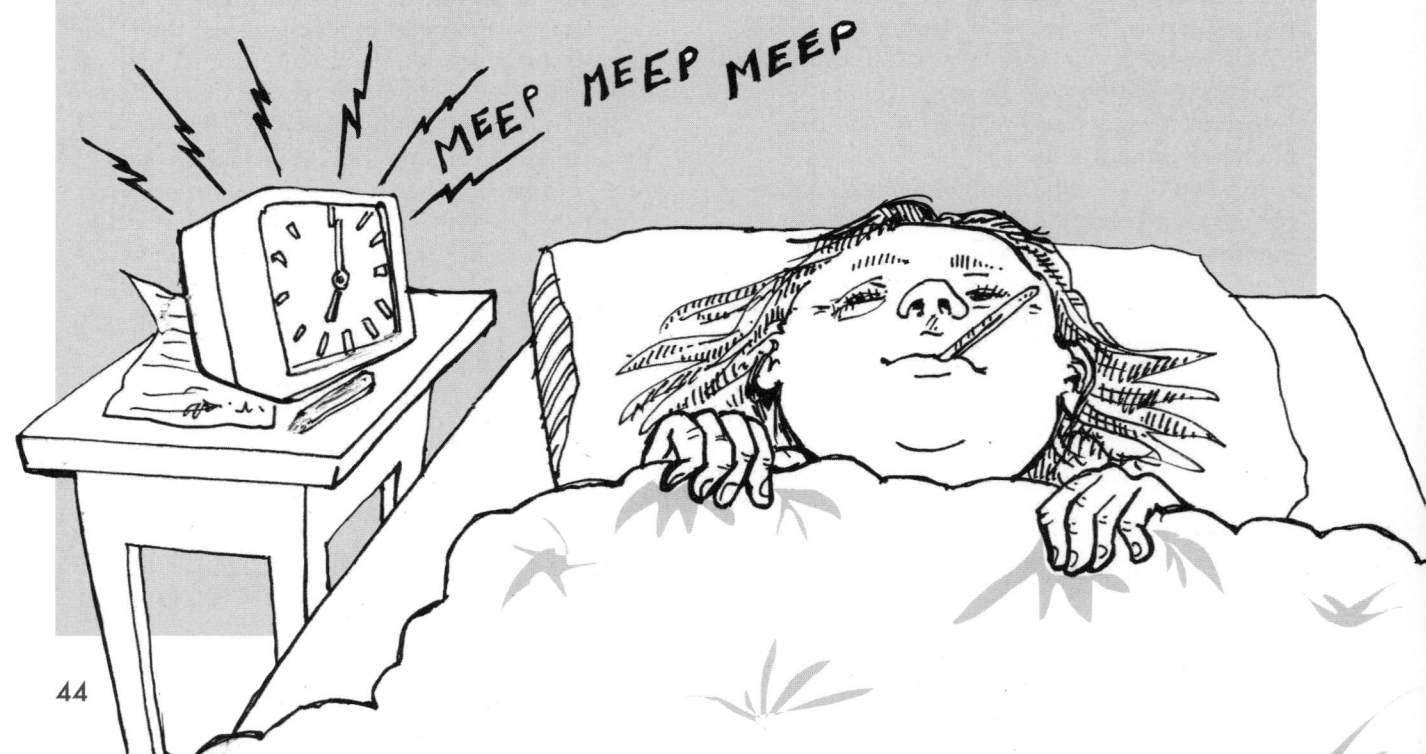

MEEP MEEP MEEP

Charting your temperature

Later on, when you're a bit more awake, enter your temperature on your fertility chart. You can photocopy the one on page 49, or make your own. If your cycle is very long, tape some charts together. Keep all your old charts, to help you get to know your body.

Hangovers, really late nights, working night shifts and illness can all give you freak high temperatures. Sometimes you have to ignore one weird temperature, and draw a dotted line between the ones on either side.

You will potentially end up with something that looks a bit like this:

fertility awareness chart for Bonnie Lagg — start date April 14th 2014

Some low temperatures… …and some higher temperatures.

The picture becomes clearer if you draw a line to separate the low and high temperatures…

fertility awareness chart for …… Bonnie Lagg …… start date April 14th 2014

You sometimes get higher temperatures on the first three days of your period. You can ignore these.

This is the shift up from oestrogen to progesterone in your system, so this would be when you ovulated.

See how the temperatures head back downwards again at the end of the chart? That means you're about to get your period. Carry some sanitary protection today, girl!

You can tell a lot more about your cycle if you compare this temperature shift with other information from your body:

Charting your cervix

Start monitoring your cervix after your period ends. Use a dot to represent a low, firm cervix, and bigger, higher circles for a higher, open one.

cycle day	1	2	3	4	5	6	7	8	9	10	11	12	13	14	15	16	17	18	19	20	21	22	23	24	25	26	27	28	29	30	31	32	33	34	35	36
cervix							·	,	,	·	◦	●	●	◉	◍	◌	▢	◘	·	·	·	·	·	·	·	·	·	·	·	·	·	·	·	·	·	·

Charting your juices

Start monitoring your juices after your period ends. You can use these symbols for your juices, or invent your own. Use any words you like. You can't check your juice when you've had unprotected heterosexual sex, hence the blanks.

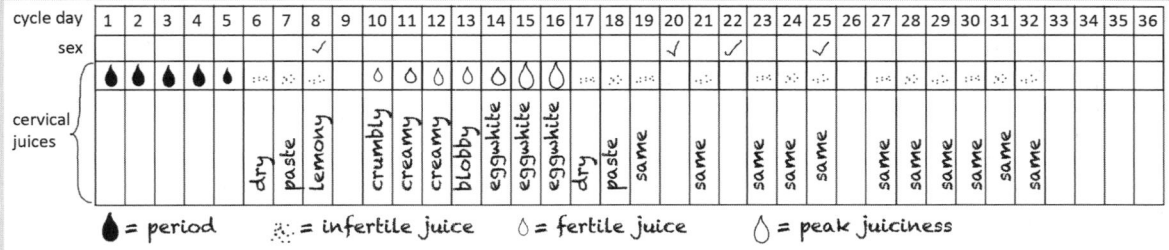

cycle day	1	2	3	4	5	6	7	8	9	10	11	12	13	14	15	16	17	18	19	20	21	22	23	24	25	26	27	28	29	30	31	32	33	34	35	36
sex								✓												✓		✓			✓											
cervical juices	●	●	●	●	●	dry	paste	lemony		crumbly	creamy	creamy	blobby	eggwhite	eggwhite	eggwhite	dry	paste	same		same		same	same	same		same	same	same	same	same	same				

● = period   ∴ = infertile juice   ◊ = fertile juice   ◊ = peak juiciness

Charting other signs

If you have clear ovulation signs, like cramps or twinges, mark them down. Bonus! Lustful urges? Moody strops? This can be part of your cycle, so write them in too. Stressful events or holiday travel can delay your ovulation. Put it on the chart.

cycle day	1	2	3	4	5	6	7	8	9	10	11	12	13	14	15	16	17	18	19	20	21	22	23	24	25	26	27	28	29	30	31	32	33	34	35	36
ovulation pain																✗																				
emotions stress travel illness hangover no sleep	whinge	moan								Sandy's party	overslept				feel lush!	fancy everyone													Grrrr!		snappy	panicky				

Putting it all together

fertility awareness chart for ...... Bonnie Lagg ......   start date... April 14th 2014

date	14/4	15/4	16/4	17/4	18/4	19/4	20/4	21/4	22/4	23/4		26/4	27/4	28/4	29/4	30/4	1/5	2/5	03/5	04/5	05/5	06/5	07	08/5		09/5	10/5	11/5	12/5	13/5	14/5	15/5	16/5		

waking temperature (scale from .05 up through 36 / 37 °C range)

| cycle day | 1 | 2 | 3 | 4 | 5 | 6 | 7 | 8 | 9 | 10 | 11 | 12 | 13 | 14 | 15 | 16 | 17 | 18 | 19 | 20 | 21 | 22 | 23 | 24 | 25 | 26 | 27 | 28 | 29 | 30 | 31 | 32 | 33 | 34 | 35 | 36 |

sex — ✓ (day 8), ✓ (day 20), ✓ (day 22), ✓ (day 25)

cervix (symbols across days)

cervical juices: dry, paste, lemony, crumbly, creamy, creamy, blobby, eggwhite, eggwhite, eggwhite, dry, paste, same, same, same, same, same, same, same, same, same, same

ovulation pain: X (day 16)

emotions / stress / travel / illness / hangover / no sleep: whinge, moan, Sandy's party, overslept, feel lush!, fancy everyone, Grrrr!, snappy, panicky

It only takes five minutes a day to chart your cycle. It's a lot less complicated than it looks. Try it. Photocopy this blank chart and fill it in…

fertility awareness chart for .... start date..

date																																				
waking temperature	.10	.10	.10	.10	.10	.10	.10	.10	.10	.10	.10	.10	.10	.10	.10	.10	.10	.10	.10	.10	.10	.10	.10	.10	.10	.10	.10	.10	.10	.10	.10	.10	.10	.10	.10	.10
	.05	.05	.05	.05	.05	.05	.05	.05	.05	.05	.05	.05	.05	.05	.05	.05	.05	.05	.05	.05	.05	.05	.05	.05	.05	.05	.05	.05	.05	.05	.05	.05	.05	.05	.05	.05
	37	**37**	**37**	**37**	**37**	**37**	**37**	**37**	**37**	**37**	**37**	**37**	**37**	**37**	**37**	**37**	**37**	**37**	**37**	**37**	**37**	**37**	**37**	**37**	**37**	**37**	**37**	**37**	**37**	**37**	**37**	**37**	**37**	**37**	**37**	**37**
	.95	.95	.95	.95	.95	.95	.95	.95	.95	.95	.95	.95	.95	.95	.95	.95	.95	.95	.95	.95	.95	.95	.95	.95	.95	.95	.95	.95	.95	.95	.95	.95	.95	.95	.95	.95
	.90	.90	.90	.90	.90	.90	.90	.90	.90	.90	.90	.90	.90	.90	.90	.90	.90	.90	.90	.90	.90	.90	.90	.90	.90	.90	.90	.90	.90	.90	.90	.90	.90	.90	.90	.90
	.85	.85	.85	.85	.85	.85	.85	.85	.85	.85	.85	.85	.85	.85	.85	.85	.85	.85	.85	.85	.85	.85	.85	.85	.85	.85	.85	.85	.85	.85	.85	.85	.85	.85	.85	.85
	.80	.80	.80	.80	.80	.80	.80	.80	.80	.80	.80	.80	.80	.80	.80	.80	.80	.80	.80	.80	.80	.80	.80	.80	.80	.80	.80	.80	.80	.80	.80	.80	.80	.80	.80	.80
	.75	.75	.75	.75	.75	.75	.75	.75	.75	.75	.75	.75	.75	.75	.75	.75	.75	.75	.75	.75	.75	.75	.75	.75	.75	.75	.75	.75	.75	.75	.75	.75	.75	.75	.75	.75
	.70	.70	.70	.70	.70	.70	.70	.70	.70	.70	.70	.70	.70	.70	.70	.70	.70	.70	.70	.70	.70	.70	.70	.70	.70	.70	.70	.70	.70	.70	.70	.70	.70	.70	.70	.70
	.65	.65	.65	.65	.65	.65	.65	.65	.65	.65	.65	.65	.65	.65	.65	.65	.65	.65	.65	.65	.65	.65	.65	.65	.65	.65	.65	.65	.65	.65	.65	.65	.65	.65	.65	.65
	.60	.60	.60	.60	.60	.60	.60	.60	.60	.60	.60	.60	.60	.60	.60	.60	.60	.60	.60	.60	.60	.60	.60	.60	.60	.60	.60	.60	.60	.60	.60	.60	.60	.60	.60	.60
	.55	.55	.55	.55	.55	.55	.55	.55	.55	.55	.55	.55	.55	.55	.55	.55	.55	.55	.55	.55	.55	.55	.55	.55	.55	.55	.55	.55	.55	.55	.55	.55	.55	.55	.55	.55
	.50	.50	.50	.50	.50	.50	.50	.50	.50	.50	.50	.50	.50	.50	.50	.50	.50	.50	.50	.50	.50	.50	.50	.50	.50	.50	.50	.50	.50	.50	.50	.50	.50	.50	.50	.50
	.45	.45	.45	.45	.45	.45	.45	.45	.45	.45	.45	.45	.45	.45	.45	.45	.45	.45	.45	.45	.45	.45	.45	.45	.45	.45	.45	.45	.45	.45	.45	.45	.45	.45	.45	.45
	.40	.40	.40	.40	.40	.40	.40	.40	.40	.40	.40	.40	.40	.40	.40	.40	.40	.40	.40	.40	.40	.40	.40	.40	.40	.40	.40	.40	.40	.40	.40	.40	.40	.40	.40	.40
	.35	.35	.35	.35	.35	.35	.35	.35	.35	.35	.35	.35	.35	.35	.35	.35	.35	.35	.35	.35	.35	.35	.35	.35	.35	.35	.35	.35	.35	.35	.35	.35	.35	.35	.35	.35
	.30	.30	.30	.30	.30	.30	.30	.30	.30	.30	.30	.30	.30	.30	.30	.30	.30	.30	.30	.30	.30	.30	.30	.30	.30	.30	.30	.30	.30	.30	.30	.30	.30	.30	.30	.30
	.25	.25	.25	.25	.25	.25	.25	.25	.25	.25	.25	.25	.25	.25	.25	.25	.25	.25	.25	.25	.25	.25	.25	.25	.25	.25	.25	.25	.25	.25	.25	.25	.25	.25	.25	.25
	.20	.20	.20	.20	.20	.20	.20	.20	.20	.20	.20	.20	.20	.20	.20	.20	.20	.20	.20	.20	.20	.20	.20	.20	.20	.20	.20	.20	.20	.20	.20	.20	.20	.20	.20	.20
	.15	.15	.15	.15	.15	.15	.15	.15	.15	.15	.15	.15	.15	.15	.15	.15	.15	.15	.15	.15	.15	.15	.15	.15	.15	.15	.15	.15	.15	.15	.15	.15	.15	.15	.15	.15
	.10	.10	.10	.10	.10	.10	.10	.10	.10	.10	.10	.10	.10	.10	.10	.10	.10	.10	.10	.10	.10	.10	.10	.10	.10	.10	.10	.10	.10	.10	.10	.10	.10	.10	.10	.10
	.05	.05	.05	.05	.05	.05	.05	.05	.05	.05	.05	.05	.05	.05	.05	.05	.05	.05	.05	.05	.05	.05	.05	.05	.05	.05	.05	.05	.05	.05	.05	.05	.05	.05	.05	.05
	36	**36**	**36**	**36**	**36**	**36**	**36**	**36**	**36**	**36**	**36**	**36**	**36**	**36**	**36**	**36**	**36**	**36**	**36**	**36**	**36**	**36**	**36**	**36**	**36**	**36**	**36**	**36**	**36**	**36**	**36**	**36**	**36**	**36**	**36**	**36**
cycle day	1	2	3	4	5	6	7	8	9	10	11	12	13	14	15	16	17	18	19	20	21	22	23	24	25	26	27	28	29	30	31	32	33	34	35	36
sex																																				
cervix																																				
cervical juices																																				
ovulation pain																																				
emotions stress travel illness hangover no sleep																																				

How to not get pregnant

The egg is released on the day that your temperature rises, which is usually the day after your most slippery, lush juices. This egg lives for about 24 hours without any sperm around, then it dies. Very occasionally, you might release another egg in that cycle (think 'twins') but, if you do, it will be within 24 hours of the first. To make sure both those eggs are out of the picture, you need to wait for a few days after you have ovulated.

Wait until the evening of the *third* day of higher temperatures, and the *fourth* day after your peak fertile juices before having unprotected sex.

That should give you some fun time at the end of your cycle. What about the first part? If you have long cycles, you could be waiting for weeks or months for the post-ovulatory phase.

The first five days of a period is safe. It's a real period – not some weird other sort of blood – if you ovulated between 12 and 16 days before it started. Check that by looking for a temperature shift on last month's chart.

After Day 5, it gets a bit tricky. As long as your cervix remains low and tightly shut, and your juice is a scanty, lemony paste, you're still infertile. *As soon as you see any increase in your juices at all, you're potentially fertile.* You can't tell what your juices are doing if you have semen or menstrual blood in your vagina, so the rule is:

Is your cervix dry, low, and firm? Are you *sure*? OK, you can have unprotected sex. Next day either abstain, or use a condom. The day after that, check your cervix again. Are you sure, I mean *really sure* that you're not starting to get juicier? OK… repeat as long as appropriate.

How to NOT not get pregnant

Some people make a half-hearted pretence at using fertility awareness, because they're not happy with other methods of birth control and/or they really like to have unprotected sex.

Wise up! If you can't get it together to check your cervix every day then you can't assess whether you are fertile. And the safest way to know that you're post-ovulatory is to chart your temperature too (although if you always get secondary ovulation signs like spotting or cramps you could also rely on these).

Stick to the rules on this page.

Don't mess about with them.

If your cycle is confusing, and you can't tell what's going on, see a Fertility Awareness Method instructor, and ask her for help to interpret your results. You could also consult Toni Weschler's excellent book *Taking Charge of Your Fertility*.[2]

If you are going to have *any contact at all* between your lady parts and a man's bits when you are fertile, then use a barrier method of contraception. Condoms are the safest. Use them properly. No 'Oh, just be inside me for a bit and then put a condom on in a minute.' No 'Oh, you should pull out now you've come, but you feel so nice, just stay there.' None of that!

Not wanting to use contraception properly is not the same as wanting to have a baby. If you don't know what you want, and you don't know what your partner wants, then have a conversation about this. Not during sex! You both might not be thinking straight!

4 *Trying for a baby*

It's not fair! You've found your perfect partner,* you've fallen in love, you may have got married… The fairy stories said you get to live Happily Ever After now.

The fairy story lied. Some people become pregnant very quickly (and this can be a blessing, or a curse!) For others, the path to parenthood is long, and potentially difficult.

On average, 70% of couples won't conceive the first month that they 'try'; for a quarter of couples it takes longer than six months; 10% still haven't conceived after a year, and half of them are still 'trying' after two years.

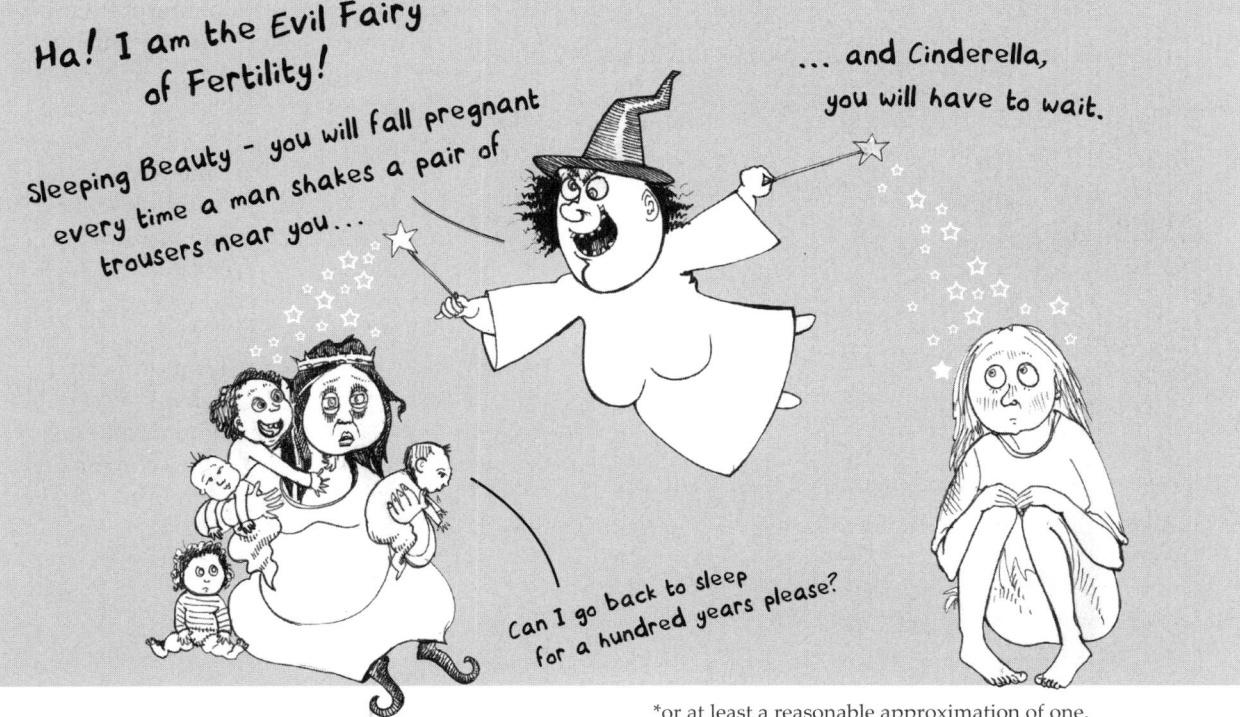

Ha! I am the Evil Fairy of Fertility!

Sleeping Beauty - you will fall pregnant every time a man shakes a pair of trousers near you…

Can I go back to sleep for a hundred years please?

… and Cinderella, you will have to wait.

*or at least a reasonable approximation of one.

51

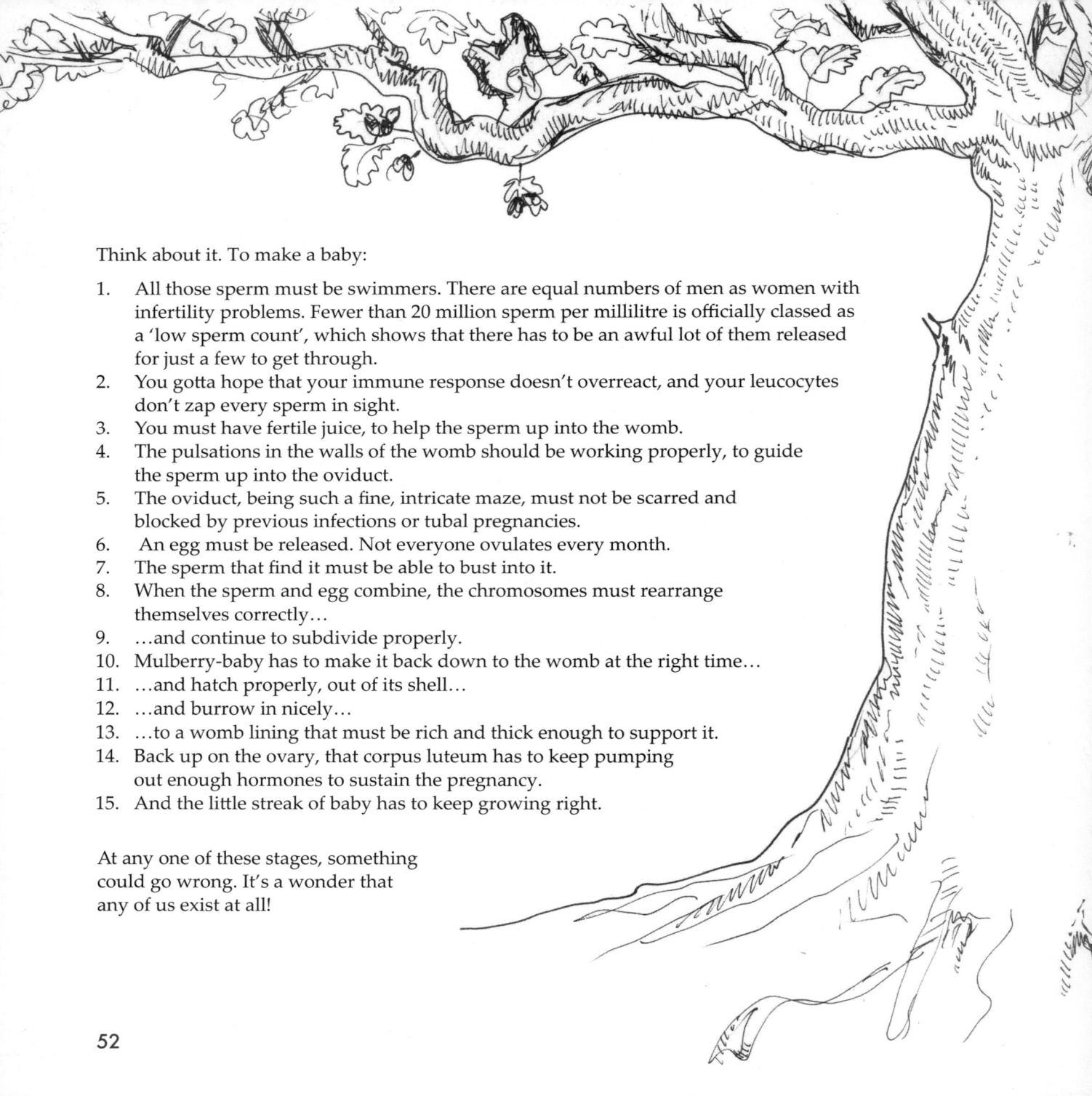

Think about it. To make a baby:

1. All those sperm must be swimmers. There are equal numbers of men as women with infertility problems. Fewer than 20 million sperm per millilitre is officially classed as a 'low sperm count', which shows that there has to be an awful lot of them released for just a few to get through.
2. You gotta hope that your immune response doesn't overreact, and your leucocytes don't zap every sperm in sight.
3. You must have fertile juice, to help the sperm up into the womb.
4. The pulsations in the walls of the womb should be working properly, to guide the sperm up into the oviduct.
5. The oviduct, being such a fine, intricate maze, must not be scarred and blocked by previous infections or tubal pregnancies.
6. An egg must be released. Not everyone ovulates every month.
7. The sperm that find it must be able to bust into it.
8. When the sperm and egg combine, the chromosomes must rearrange themselves correctly…
9. …and continue to subdivide properly.
10. Mulberry-baby has to make it back down to the womb at the right time…
11. …and hatch properly, out of its shell…
12. …and burrow in nicely…
13. …to a womb lining that must be rich and thick enough to support it.
14. Back up on the ovary, that corpus luteum has to keep pumping out enough hormones to sustain the pregnancy.
15. And the little streak of baby has to keep growing right.

At any one of these stages, something could go wrong. It's a wonder that any of us exist at all!

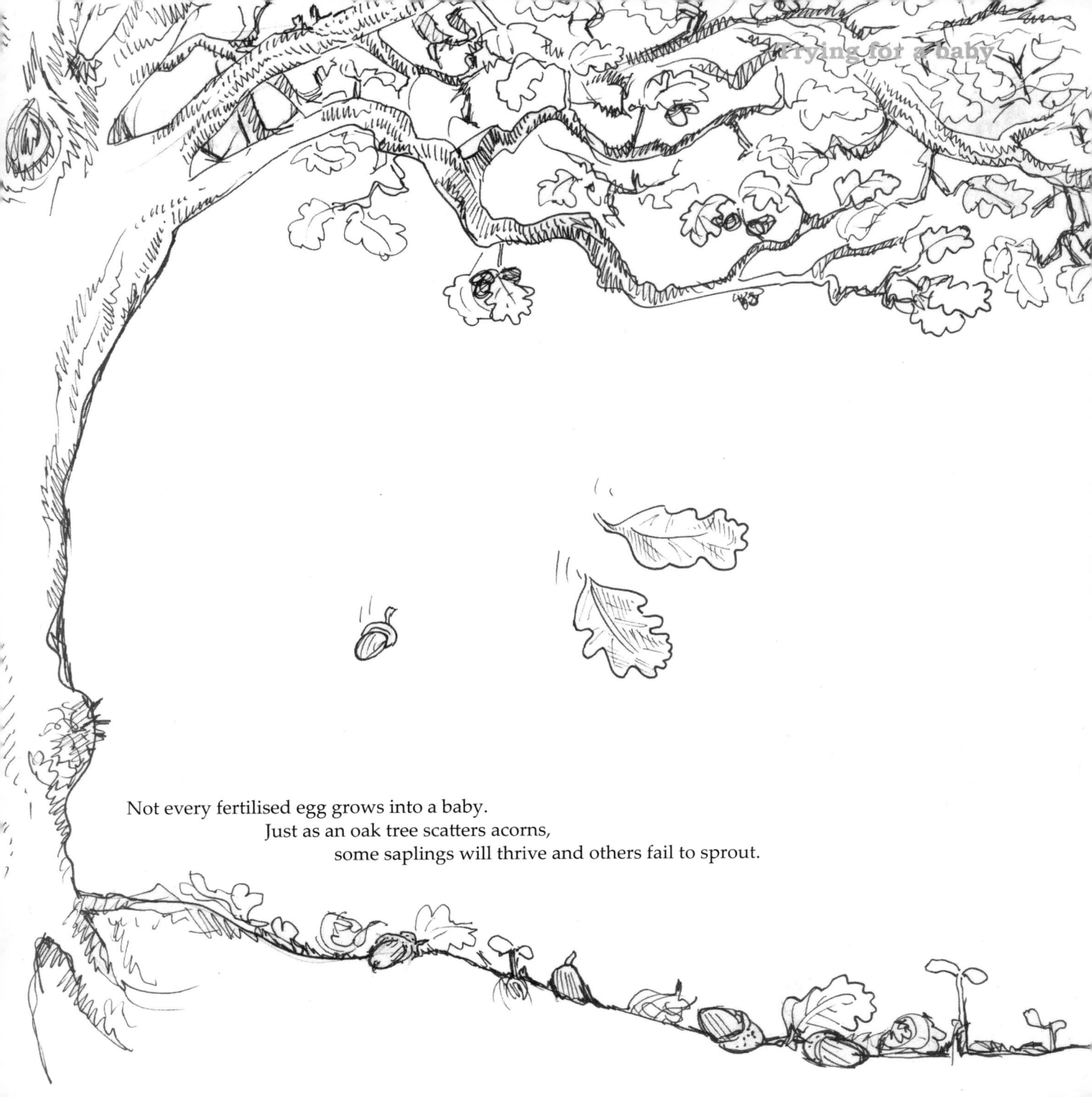

Not every fertilised egg grows into a baby.
Just as an oak tree scatters acorns,
some saplings will thrive and others fail to sprout.

This is what life can feel like on the gynaecological rollercoaster:

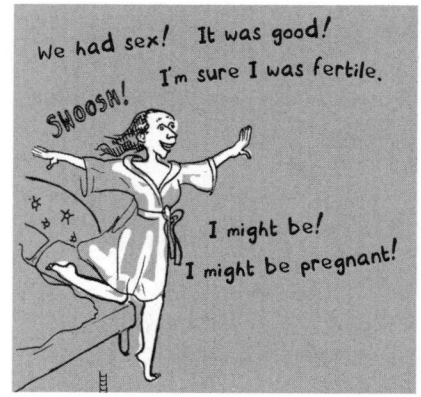
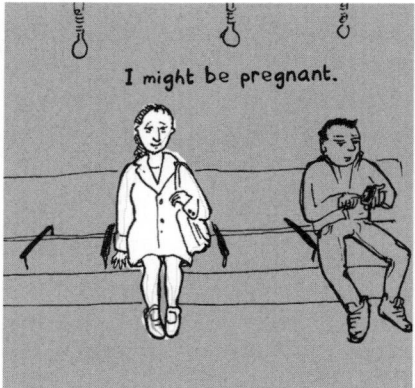
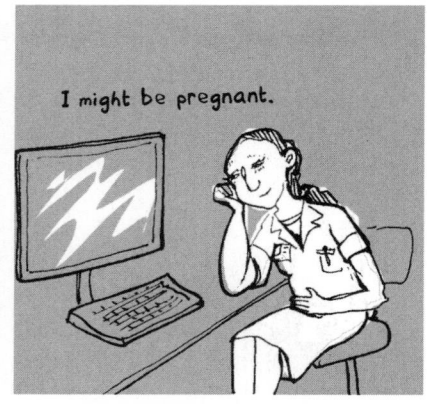
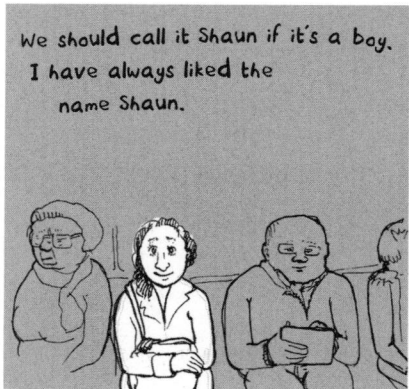
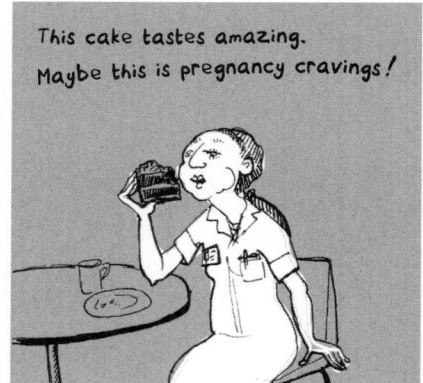
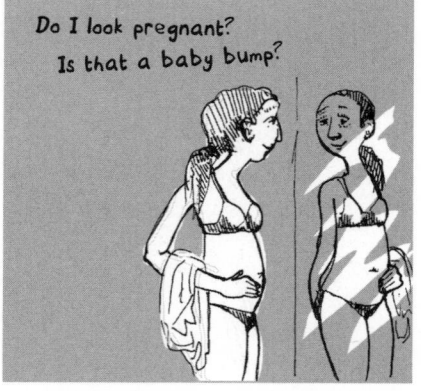
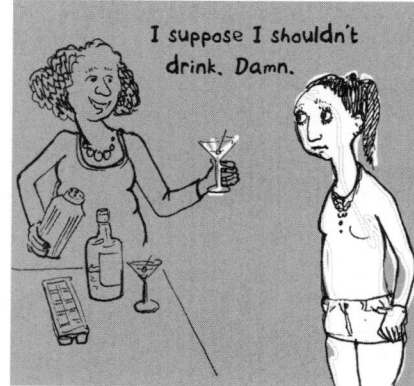
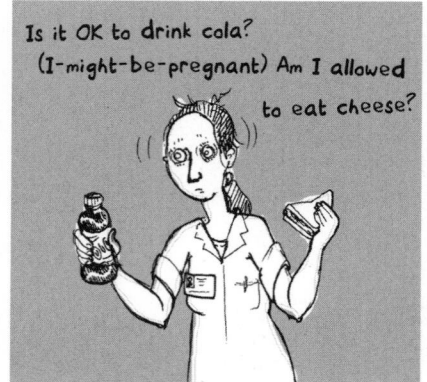
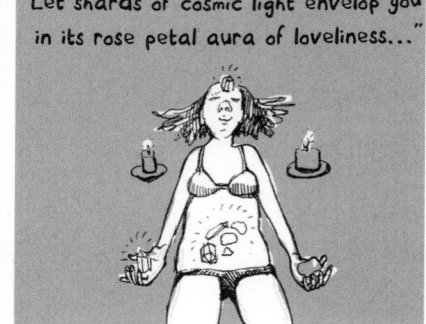

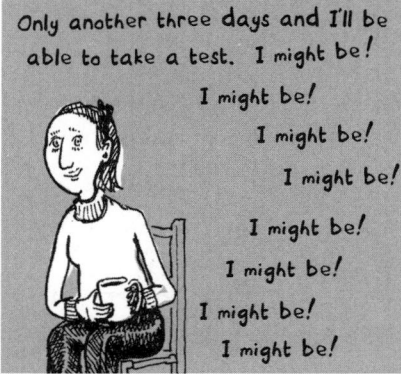

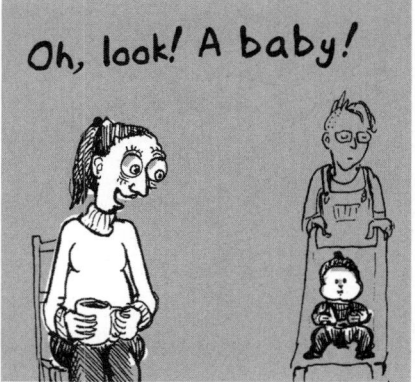

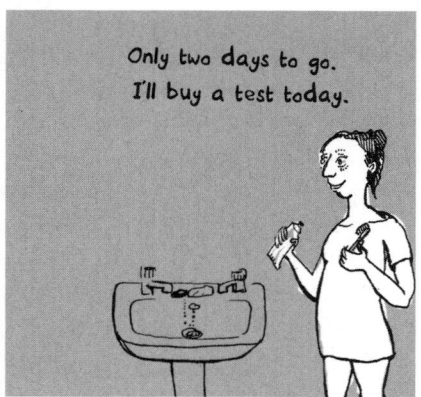

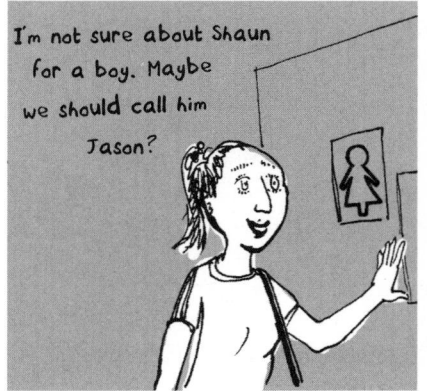

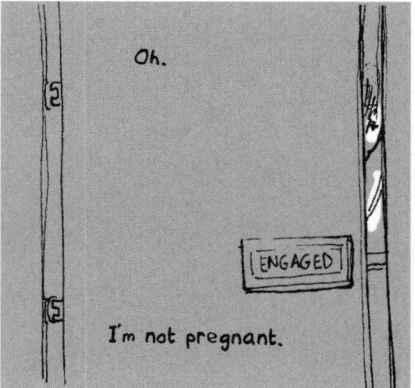

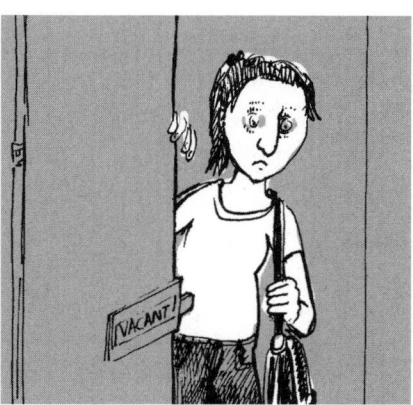

Repeat, for at least two weeks per month, for as long as it takes you to conceive.

After a while you can add some of these kinds of thoughts too:

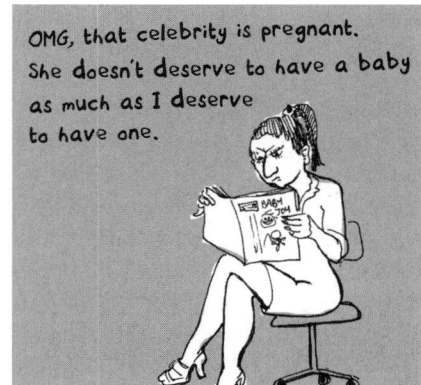

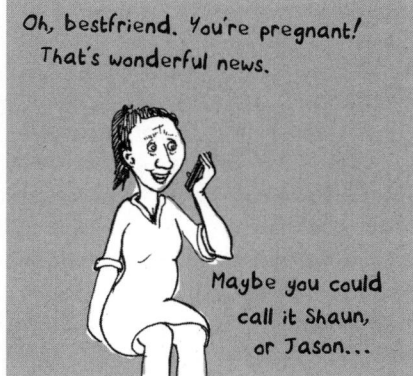

Wanting a baby

For most sufferers, fertility problems come as a complete shock. The unconscious logic is that your parents conceived you, and therefore, naturally, you will go on to conceive a child in turn. You watch friends and colleagues become pregnant – some by accident, some by design – and you assume that you will do the same. You may even have been pregnant before, perhaps when you didn't want to be. So why the hell can't you conceive now?

Infertility (which includes recurrent miscarriage) is a hidden grief in our society. It *hurts* to want a baby. It teaches you the double meaning of 'want' – the verb: to 'desire', and the noun: 'to lack'. It's a trauma that becomes more profound, the longer it continues, yet you may feel less and less able to appeal to friends for sympathy. (Hey, friends! Offer some sympathy! Learn how on pages 121 and 138!)

It doesn't help that we're kept in ignorance of the biological processes involved, something the two previous chapters have attempted to redress. Have you read them? Good. You now know more about human fertility than most of the population, including many members of the medical profession.

The overwhelming majority of research into human fertility is focused upon improving techniques for IVF. *In vitro* fertilisation is an incredible technological advance, which has enabled millions of people to become parents. It's a good thing. When you take the egg from a woman and the sperm from a man and mix them in a petri dish, you bypass many of the complexities of reproductive anatomy. If you look back at the list of things that can go wrong on page 52, with IVF you can skip the first ten steps. But scientific endeavour has become skewed towards formulating newer, more expensive IVF drug protocols. Where research does exist into how babies are actually made *inside women*, the final paragraph is inevitably entitled 'Implications for assisted conception'. Doh! If we had more research into *natural* conception, fewer people would need IVF at all!

There is very little evidence-based research on techniques for women to get pregnant naturally. And while there's money in IVF – people are prepared to bankrupt themselves to become parents – there's no profit in helping women to help themselves.

If you are under 35 years of age, and you have been 'trying' for a baby for more than a year, or older and 'trying' for longer than six months (it can be very trying – indeed it can) then see your GP and ask to be referred for medical investigation. There's a lot that can be done to help. You'll be stepping into a complicated and medicalised world, which will probably involve lots of late night Google searches about obscure scientific tests and techniques.

Seek out the friendship of other people on the gynaecological rollercoaster. Infertility is incredibly stressful, and the company of other people who know what you're going through will really help. Subfertile heterosexual couples can find that their gay friends are good to turn to, as they know what it's like to have to work to get a baby.

And this book will help you to maximise your fertility, with suggestions that are supported by medical research, where it exists.

Have you left it Too Late?

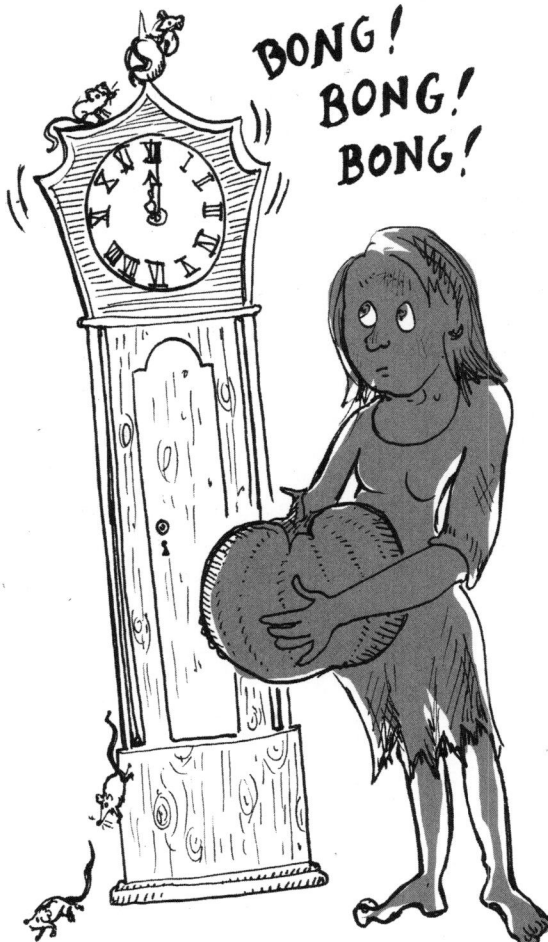

BONG! BONG! BONG!

Women are, on average, embarking upon motherhood slightly later in life these days. This trend tends to be reported in the media as 'Women put off having children because they are putting their career first!' The subtext is: 'Those selfish feminists are pursuing their own interests, to the detriment of the survival of the species.'

What rubbish. The majority of women 'put off' having children because easy access to contraception means they aren't trapped into motherhood with the first emotionally incompatible and immature man they sleep with. It takes a while to find a decent father.

This is not feminism's fault. In fact, more feminism is only going to help this situation.

I'm not going to repeat the statistics here about to what extent women in their late thirties are less fertile than women in their early twenties. If you have been living with a ticking biological clock for some years, you will already have read those statistics, and they will put the Fear into you. Whatever the statistics say, you are not an average – you are an individual.

There is some good news. We used to think that women were born with their lifetime's supply of eggs stored in their ovaries, which they steadily used up until they reached menopause. Now we know that's not true. Every month, some of the oocytes (primordial egg cells) in your ovaries die off, and others are created, by stem cells in your ovaries. You are continually growing new eggs![1]

It takes about 120 days for an early-stage oocyte to grow into a fertile egg, and around 70 days for sperm to develop to maturity. So, have a look at your lifestyle and institute some changes, and in three months you could have healthier eggs or sperm, which would increase your chances of conception.

Nothing about this is guaranteed, but then, everything that this book is about to suggest is worth doing *in its own right*, because it will make your life better, whether or not it results in a pregnancy.

Lifestyle changes

Make love…

Once you've been in a relationship for a while, sex can get a bit repetitive. You both know what you like, and you're tired, and it's late, so you do it the way you know works, and there's nothing wrong with that. Feeling under pressure to conceive can exacerbate this situation: sex becomes mechanistic, frustrating and ultimately, a source of disappointment. Take this opportunity to revitalise your sex life. Do some loving touching that doesn't involve trying to conceive. Try tantric sex techniques. Spice it up. Live your fantasies. Stop making babies and start making love.

From a fertility perspective, better sex could improve the blood flow to your genitalia and might help you to ovulate. Chemicals in semen help to trigger ovulation, and also to preserve pregnancy.[2] If low sperm count is an issue, daily ejaculation (yes, that's a lot of sex!) during your most fertile time improves the quality of sperm,[3] and really good sex can improve the quantity.[4]

But the main reason for having lovely, interesting, fun sex is because… you can! You don't have to bother with contraception! And you don't yet have a baby who wakes up every time you try to get fruity.

(but don't use lubricant)

Lubricants damage sperm, so only use one that is specifically designed to help you conceive, such as 'Pre-Seed' (order it online). You can use raw egg white as a lubricant, which is cheap and easy to buy, but carries a one in 20,000 risk of exposure to salmonella. Your choice. If you use egg white, an oral medicine syringe helps apply it, and take it out of the fridge well in advance.

…at the right time

When is the right time to have sex? Well, spring is a good time to conceive. Seriously, birth rates in the northern hemisphere peak in March, because conception occurs most easily in the late spring and summer. (In Scotland there is also a small surge in October, which might have something to do with Hogmanay). It's worth bearing this timing in mind if you only have one shot at IVF.

If you're wondering when to conceive on a monthly rather than an annual basis, then try when you have a soft, high, open, slippery cervix. You don't have to take your temperature to determine when you are fertile; in fact, once the temperature shift has occurred, it's probably too late to conceive in that cycle. Commercial ovulation kits can be unhelpful for the same reason – they tell you when you have ovulated, and by then it's too late. Directly checking your cervix is more reliable, easier and cheaper than any other method there is.[5]

Having said that, temperature charting will build a fuller picture of your fertility, so, once you have been trying for a few months, it's worth taking your temperature too.

Check that the second part of the cycle, from the temperature shift until your period, lasts for 11 days or more. If it's shorter, this could indicate that your body is not producing enough progesterone to grow a thick womb lining and nurture a growing embryo. This condition is unhelpfully known as 'luteal phase defect'. (Men don't get their reproductive systems labelled as 'defective'!) It is associated with your body producing too much prolactin, the hormone that suppresses your fertility when you are breastfeeding. Inform your doctor.

Are you seeing a clear pattern of low temperatures in the first half of your cycle, shifting to higher temperatures for the second part? If the temperatures on your chart dance about all over the place (and you're taking a resting temperature, at the same time each day, using the same thermometer) then you probably didn't ovulate in that cycle.

But just because you didn't ovulate one month, that doesn't mean you never will. There can be a terrible finality to medical investigations into infertility: the result of one test can leave you labelled as 'anovulatory' or 'high FSH' or 'low sperm count'. We are complex living systems, with the capability for change.

If you keep charting your temperature, and you see a thermal shift another month, you will know you ovulated, whether or not you got pregnant. This is useful feedback. Knowledge is empowering.

No clear temperature shift because no egg was released

Temperature charting can also tell you if you're pregnant. If you have 18 consecutive days of higher temperatures (and you're taking your temperature correctly, and you don't have a fever, or a hangover) then you're pregnant.

Sometimes you can see a second shift, to a set of even higher temperatures, as pregnancy hormones kick in, though not all charts show this clear three-stage pattern.

If you then go on to bleed, that's not a period, it's an early miscarriage. This can be an upsetting discovery, but it does mean that you are able to conceive. If you're worried about threatened miscarriage in early pregnancy, keep taking your temperature. A dive back down to pre-ovulatory levels is an indicator that you may be about to lose the baby. On the other hand, continued higher temperatures may put your mind at rest. A bit. For a while.

18th higher temperature means you're pregnant!

Women – stay warm

Keep your tummy covered, and wear snuggly socks and boots. Carry a hot water bottle around in winter, and have comfortably warm baths and saunas. Eat warming soups and stews in the colder months, with root vegetables in. This advice is based on the principles of Chinese rather than Western medicine, but it's not going to do you any harm.

Men – let it all hang out

Guys, you're meant to hang low. The testicles dangle outside the body because the slightly lower temperatures there are optimum for sperm production. Wear boxer shorts not briefs or tights or spandex. If your job involves sitting down for long periods, especially on hot truck seats, then work out if there is any way to cool yourself that won't get you arrested for indecent exposure.

Everyone – just chill

Your hormone system is controlled by the same region of your brain that regulates stress and fear. So pay attention to major stresses in your life, and make positive changes where you can.

Do you hate going to work every morning? Incompetent, abusive managers, manipulative colleagues, budget cuts, increased workloads… sound familiar? This is not about whether your job is challenging or difficult – stress in the workplace is related to the amount of control you have over events at work, the support you receive to do your job well, and the recognition you get for giving it your best efforts. If you don't, haven't and aren't, is there any way you can change what you do?

While we're on the subject of employment, you should know that working night shifts,[6] or occupational exposure to radiation, pesticides, dry-cleaning fluids, printing inks, lead, cadmium, arsenic, mercury, traffic fumes or industrial microwaves can all reduce your fertility.[7]

Unemployment brings its own stresses, including poverty, frustration, lack of direction in life, and coping with Jobcentre bureaucrats. Try volunteering? There are people out there you can help, which will in turn help you.

You need a safe home to have a baby. It doesn't have to be very big, though – babies are small and don't take up much room. So if you need to move to find your home, then do. If you don't need to move but are, then stop. If you live in shared housing with people you don't like, then they need to leave or you do.

Is your partner the source of the stress? Read more about abusive relationships on page 122. Are you trying not to think about traumatic past events? How unhelpful is your family? How is your relationship with your mother? How do you feel about becoming a mother yourself? There's nothing in human experience that can't be helped by talking about it to the right person.

Infertility itself is incredibly stressful, especially when you are dealing with invasive and expensive medical procedures. You can't control this, you have to just accept it, but be honest with yourself and your partner about how you feel.

Don't stress about being stressed! There are things you can do to relax: yoga, massage, meditation, hypnotherapy, walking, singing, dancing. These are nice things to do, so do them. Enjoy!

Eat well

If your body mass index (BMI) is lower than 19, then you are four times as likely to be infertile than if you maintain a healthy weight,[8] and when you do get pregnant you are at increased risk of miscarriage. This is because body fat has a function: it converts the hormone androgen in the body into oestrogen. You need it to balance your hormones.

It really is wrong that the ideal of female beauty that we're surrounded with from childhood on, and that many women work so hard to achieve, is incompatible with human reproduction. It's really not very womanly!

At the other end of the scale, a BMI of over 29 is associated with slightly reduced fertility, and if your BMI is over 35 then you are twice as likely to be infertile.[9] This applies to men too.[10] Losing as little as 5% of your body weight may be enough to kick-start your reproductive system.

There is a link between obesity and polycystic ovary syndrome (PCOS). Change your diet to one based on five small meals of savoury wholefoods every day, to stop the wild swings in your blood sugar levels and help your body to process insulin more effectively. PCOS is a strong predictor of Type 2 diabetes, so tackle any addiction to starchy, sugary foods now, before your health really suffers as a result.[11]

Turn to page 92 to learn more about healthy eating, body image, and renegotiating your relationship with food.

Exercise, in moderation

Get fit, because your body works better when you're fit. And it'll make you feel great. But don't overdo it. Exercising until you're completely exhausted stresses your body. Professional athletes are less likely to be able to conceive, either naturally, or through IVF. So, if you are already super-fit, then take it easy. If you always exercise hard for more than four hours a week, then reconsider your training programme.[12] Eat more. You need a bit of fat.

Stop smoking

Sorry. But if you got pregnant, you'd need to stop anyway.

Use every method available to help you stop, both because it will probably significantly improve your fertility, and also because you're currently paying a multinational company a large amount of money for the privilege of killing yourself slowly.

It has been estimated that smokers are 3.4 times more likely to take more than a year to conceive than non-smokers.[13] The less you smoke, the lower the effect, so if you can't stop completely, cut down the amount that you smoke. It seems likely (although this hasn't been proven) that e-cigarettes and nicotine replacement therapies are less harmful to your fertility, as most of the toxins in smoking are in the tobacco smoke, not the nicotine.[14] If you can't stop, switch.

If your partner smokes then he has to stop too, because smoking has an appreciable effect on sperm quality.[15] If your partner isn't the sperm donor, then he or she still isn't allowed to smoke near you. Primarily, this is because sidestream smoke also has an appreciable effect on your fertility.[16] Also, anyone who is insensitive enough to smoke in front of you, when you're giving up so that you can conceive and carry a child for the both of you, is a git.

Don't binge drink

The good news is that drinking alcohol up to the recommended number of units per week is probably OK.[17] That is, no more than 14 units per week, and no more than three units in any one day, with two alcohol-free days per week. Men are allowed 21 units per week, with up to four units per day, and two alcohol-free days, too.

The bad news is that most British people massively exceed this safe level. One pint of strong lager or one large glass of wine doesn't contain one unit of alcohol – it can contain three or four. So carefully monitor your alcohol intake.

Does the thought of being able to 'carefully monitor your alcohol intake' fill you with sarcastic hilarity? Do you find that, when you start drinking, there's no way you can stop? You could be alcoholic. If, when you drink, you or the people around you suffer unpleasant consequences, then you are abusing alcohol. If you keep doing this, despite the obvious ill effects, that's alcohol dependency.

Now is a good time to address your relationship with alcohol, before you have children who will suffer as a result.

If you need to scare your male partner into doing the same, inform him that 'alcoholic cirrhosis of the liver causes testicular atrophy'. That should sober him up.

Cut down on coffee

But three cups a day is OK.[18] Avoid strongly caffeinated 'energy drinks'.

Get tested…

… for sexually transmitted diseases.

What about other intoxicants?

Well, what do you think? You guessed it – no! The effect of street drugs isn't well researched, because they're illegal, but we do know that cannabis affects sperm production and can affect ovulation, heroin and methadone cause abnormal sperm function and interfere with the menstrual cycle,[19] and cocaine abusers have strange hormone levels.[20] Animal experiments show that ecstasy affects egg production,[21] and there is strong anecdotal evidence that it affects human menstrual cycles. There is a potential link between LSD and chromosomal abnormalities in the developing foetus.[22] Nobody has yet tested ketamine users for infertility, but really, just don't bother. Get an early night and have sex instead.

Take vitamins

Take a daily pregnancy multivitamin with folic acid, which will probably have an insufferably smug picture of a pregnant woman on the box. Floradix liquid iron supplement is excellent; it's not cheap, but it's much less expensive than IVF.

In conclusion…

These lifestyle changes are collectively known as preconceptual care. It could potentially amount to a lot all at once. Break this down into small, easy stages and make what changes you can, when you can. Don't beat yourself up if you backslide. Stay positive.

I'll say it again. It's not fair! Stick-thin, chain-smoking, night-shift-working, Red-Bull-swigging, drug- and booze-raddled couch potatoes get pregnant every day! Rage, rage, rage against the unfairness of it all!

And then get on with it.

The perils of preconceptual care

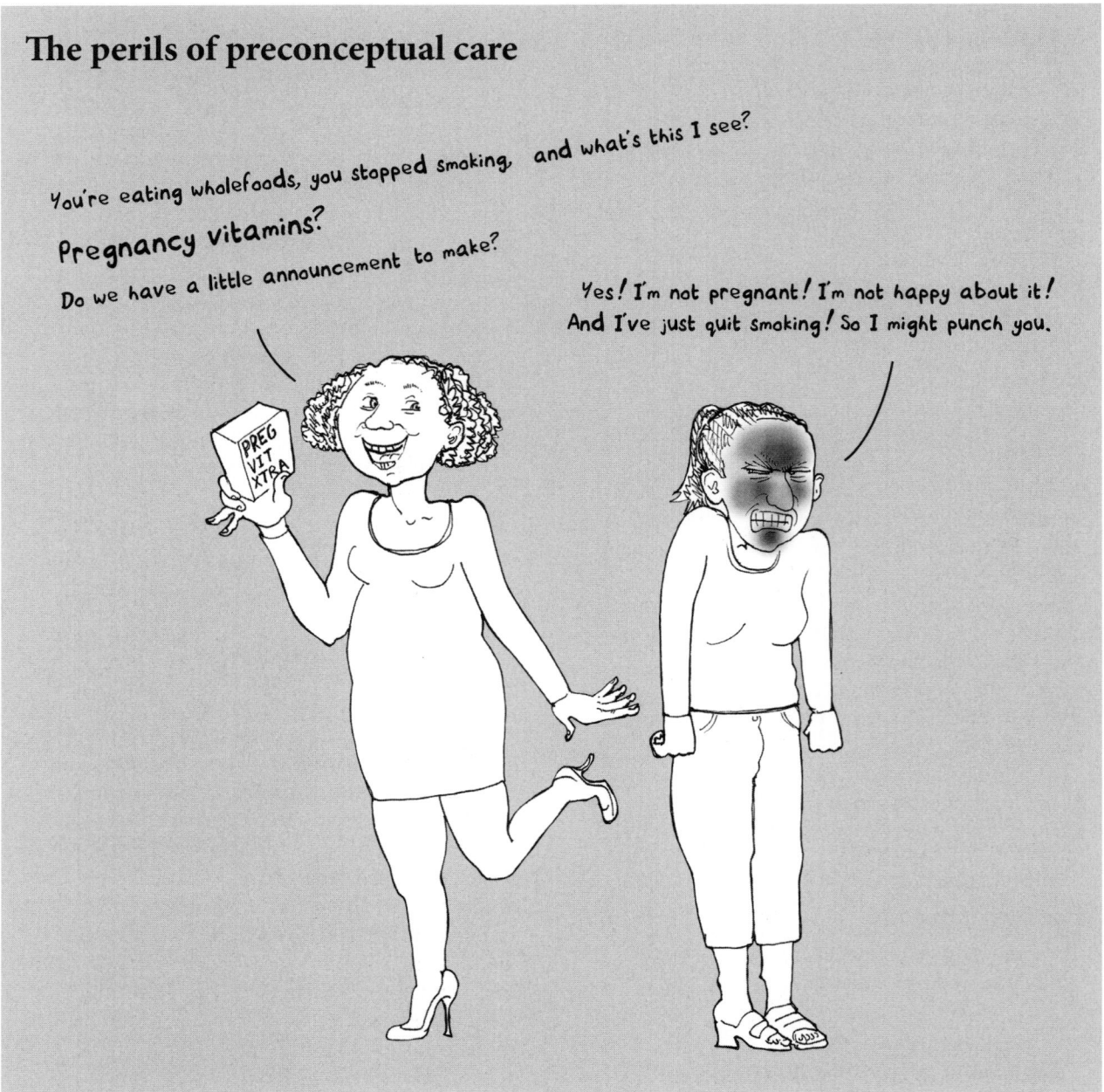

Alternatives

Western medicine can't solve all cases of infertility. The success rate for a single cycle of IVF for a 35-year-old woman in the US currently stands at 38%. This rises to around 80% for six cycles, but that still means that one in five couples who go through all that heartache and expense don't get a baby.[23] More than half of women suffering from recurrent miscarriage are given no medical reason for their condition, and current best clinical practice is to offer them TLC – that is, tender loving care.[24]

Let's see what alternative therapies can offer.

Acupuncture

Acupuncture has a good body of research to support claims that it can help with infertility. It has been proven to increase blood flow to the uterus and ovaries of women undergoing IVF[25] and increase the thickness of the lining of the womb.[26] One study suggests that acupuncture improves ovarian responsiveness to stimulating drugs, allowing more eggs to be harvested at lower dosages.[27] When women who had been classed as 'poor responders' were given acupuncture on the day that an IVF embryo was implanted, their pregnancy rates improved.[28] IVF patients who had acupuncture had lower levels of stress hormones, and were more likely to give birth to a baby.[29]

If acupuncture can do all that for women undergoing IVF, it would seem to make sense to try it as a first resort when you're considering getting pregnant. If it can support assisted conception, it is going to help with natural conception too. Choose a practitioner who has experience of treating pregnant women.

Western doctors can be suspicious of acupuncture, because the theories behind Traditional Chinese Medicine do not correspond to anything they learned in medical school. It is also difficult to conduct double-blind trials of the technique, although some of the studies cited here address this by comparing 'sham' acupuncture with the real thing.

Personally, I don't care how it works. It would seem that with three and half thousand years of refining a system of health care, the Chinese might be on to something. Acupuncture feels lovely; the needles are very fine and not painful, so try it, and see if you like it.

Reflexology and reiki

Reflexology also feels very nice, as does reiki. Neither of these therapies has been scientifically evaluated for effectiveness, but that doesn't necessarily mean that they don't work. And at the very least, an alternative therapist will give you an hour of undivided attention at a time when you really need it. You still might not get a baby, but you will be able to tell straight away if your chosen therapy helps your stress levels. If it does, that alone is a good enough reason to keep going.

Yoga

Take up yoga. Get your partner to do it too. It tones your internal organs more effectively than any other form of exercise, it's good for your sex life, and it will also give you a massive natural endorphin rush. Go to some classes, as a teacher can guide you more effectively than a book or DVD. When you suspect you could be pregnant, discuss this with your teacher so you can modify the poses.

Tai chi

Tai chi is another gentle form of exercise that can be very relaxing. Let's be honest: tai chi, yoga, reiki and the like all suffer from an image problem. There are millions of people in this country who would benefit from doing them but won't ever attempt to because they see them as the preserve of middle-class hippies. Take fire fighters, for example: they should do yoga, because it would keep them supple and help them de-stress after traumatic situations. But can you see the Fire Service setting up yoga sessions for their employees? No, I can't either. Maybe if we called yoga 'funky stretching' and tai chi 'feel-the-Force Jedi training', more people would sign up?

Once you get to a class, you might be surprised to find people there who are not middle-class hippies, or maybe just that middle-class hippies aren't so bad.*

Nutritional supplements

There is a huge market of very expensive supplements targeted at infertile couples. Some are accompanied by analyses of hair samples and blood tests, and claims that environmental toxins can be removed from the body by a three-month course of vitamins, eating organic food and drinking filtered water.

Are these claims true? Do observable levels of environmental toxins in your body fall if you eat organic papaya for a month?** Will this then help you to conceive? How qualified are the nutritional experts behind these products?

---

* This was written by a middle-class hippy.
** I made this up! It's not a suggestion! I then Googled "papaya infertility" and found one claim that it causes infertility and two claims that it cures it.

A proportion of people taking supplements will get pregnant anyway. This is part of the problem with assessing the effectiveness of interventions to support natural conception – are we looking at causation or correlation? Specialist prenatal nutrition programmes are probably going to help you make good dietary choices, but do they justify the cost? I suppose that depends on how rich you are.

When you start to consider environmental toxins, there is just *so much* to worry about. We live in a vast chemical soup. Air fresheners, optical brighteners, flame retardants, fuel additives, pesticides, insecticides, preservatives, antibiotic residues. It's one big uncontrolled experiment, and you can't remove yourself from it. Hanging crystals in your window won't protect you. There will be cases of human infertility, cancers or birth defects that are linked to chemicals in our environment – that's a good reason to stop putting them out there – but there's nothing we can do about the ones that are already there.

Living in the West, in the 21st century, we enjoy abundant food, heating, lighting, free medical care, and we don't die of common bacterial infections or the plague. That's a good trade-off against environmental pollutants. I'd still choose to live now.

Herbs to aid fertility

There are some interesting claims made for herbs to support fertility, but very few scientific trials that directly support them.

Take maca, for example (Latin name *Lepidium meyenii*). It's a Peruvian turnip-like plant which is said to improve mood and increase energy levels, mental clarity, sexual stamina and fertility. People in the Andes eat it to counteract the adverse effects of living at high altitude. Apparently, when the Spanish invaded, they were so impressed by it that there are records of *conquistadores* demanding to be paid in maca instead of gold.

Here's what I could find on scientific investigations into maca and human fertility. When nine healthy men were given black maca root tablets for four months, the quality and quantity of their sperm improved.[30] A separate, placebo-controlled, double-blind trial found that maca increased male sexual desire, but it did this without altering men's hormone levels.[31] A controlled study of maca in cattle found that it increased the sperm count of breeding bulls.[32] And when female mice were given black maca in combination with another herb *Turraeanthus africanus*, their oestrogen and progesterone levels increased compared to the control group, and they had larger litters of baby mice.[33] (Or would have done, if they hadn't been slaughtered while still pregnant in the name of scientific research.)

That's it. Nine men, 30 female mice and 78 breeding bulls. This plant could potentially replace IVF, Viagra, Prozac and coffee! Surely it's worthy of some large-scale trials?

If you ask your GP whether taking black maca root will increase your fertility, they will probably answer that there is little evidence that it works. (Because nobody has looked.) They might also say that the safety profile of the herb for the developing foetus has not been established. And it hasn't. The practicalities of testing herbs on pregnant women are daunting. The only indication that we have as to its safety in pregnancy is the fact that Andean Highlanders have been consuming maca bread, pancakes, jam, porridge, soup and beer for thousands of years, and they're still here.

Another herb with interesting possibilities is the Mediterranean flower Vitex agnus castus. Its traditional use is as a 'hormone normaliser'. It is said to act upon the pituitary gland, to improve the function of the entire endocrine system – whatever your hormones are meant to be doing, agnus castus should help them do it more effectively.

That's the theory. What's the evidence?

There are certainly indications that agnus castus works on the pituitary gland. One teenage girl with a benign tumour on her pituitary gland was referred to an endocrinologist: her periods had stopped, her hormone levels were strange and she was producing milk. By the time the appointment came up, she had started taking agnus castus supplements, and the doctor was surprised to note that the milk had disappeared, her menstrual cycles had restarted and her hormone levels were normal. He told her to stop taking the agnus castus, gave her a prescription drug that did the same thing but with strong side-effects, and wrote to a medical journal describing how agnus castus 'masked' her symptoms of pituitary dysfunction.[34] It's just as accurate to say that it 'cured' them.[35]

We know that agnus castus can cure pre-menstrual disorders.[36] It has been rated as effective as Prozac for premenstrual mood swings.[37] A review of available studies also recommends it for menopausal symptoms.[38] This suggests that it can 'tone up' your menstrual cycle, and help your fertility, but there are no studies that prove this.

Researchers have isolated compounds in agnus castus that are 'endocrinely active'.[39] It improves pituitary function in rats,[40] reduces their prolactin levels, and increases oestrogen and progesterone levels.[41] Given that agnus castus reduces prolactin levels,[42] it could help women with a short luteal phase. If it helps maintain progesterone levels, it could help women who miscarry because their corpus luteum doesn't produce enough hormone to sustain the pregnancy.

I found one double-blind, controlled study of agnus castus for corpus luteum insufficiency, and reference to another 12 non-controlled studies.[43] All the results were positive, but they need to be repeated on a much larger scale for this to amount to conclusive proof.

Researchers have been confused by agnus castus's apparently contradictory effects. The fact that it suppresses prolactin (the breastmilk-production hormone) in non-pregnant women has led to the advice that breastfeeding women shouldn't take it. But it has traditionally been used, very successfully, to increase breastmilk production in new mothers. It restores menstrual function to women who aren't ovulating, and so, because it gives women periods, it's not classed as safe to take during pregnancy, yet it has also been used to prevent miscarriage.[44]

Consult a medical herbalist if you want to take herbs to help you conceive. They will prescribe according to traditional usage – that is, based on what has helped people in the past. This is a valid way of ordering a system of knowledge: our legal system is organised by tradition, rather than by empirical testing. But in the absence of scientific trials doctors will continue to dismiss herbal medicines as 'untested', and therefore ineffective, when they could be very effective indeed. Since agnus castus works on the dopamine system in the brain, it could interfere with 'dopamine antagonist' medication. (This class of drugs are most commonly prescribed for nausea, depression, schizophrenia and bipolar disorder.) That's just

one reason why, if we're going to take herbal medicines, doctors should be knowledgeable about their effects.

Medicine Man vs Witch Doctor

This section touches on a theme that we'll return to later in the book: that of the limitations of Western medicine. Don't get me wrong, our system of medicine literally performs miracles – anaesthesia, antibiotics, insulin, cancer cures, organ transplants, assisted conception and more – but it is still open to critique. It is reductive, compartmentalising the body into separate fields of specialist medicine rather than viewing it as an interconnected whole. It focuses strongly on technological intervention. Research into new treatments is predominantly funded by the pharmaceutical industry, with all the attendant distortions of market forces. None of this adds up to best clinical practice.

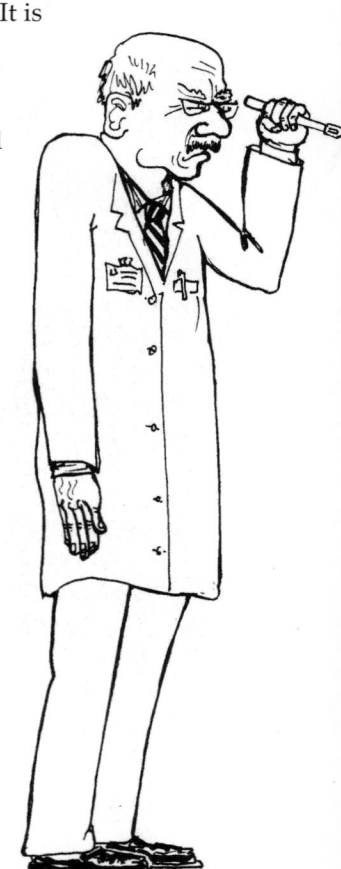

But then, the spectrum of alternative therapies does include some completely bonkers ideas being peddled by the mildly deranged. Statements like 'microwave cooking destroys all the nutrients in foods' abound on natural fertility forums. (It doesn't.[45]) We could do with sorting out the genuine wheaty wisdom in alternative therapies from the chaff. At the moment we have to choose between two parallel systems of health care that can conflict with each other. If conventional medicine were more receptive to the best that alternative therapies have to offer, then we would arrive at a more integrated, holistic model. We don't need either 'conventional' or 'alternative'. We need both. For example, if your oviducts are scarred from chlamydia, then a hysterosalpingogram is a very useful procedure. All the reiki in the world won't unblock your tubes. Try IVF.

On the other hand, a holistic model of health care, which encourages women to understand and monitor their bodies and which puts an emphasis on preventative medicine, would mean that you'd be monitoring your cervical secretions from a young age, and you'd have spotted that chlamydia infection before it had a chance to mess up your tubes.

Western medicine brings us clomiphene citrate, a drug that has an 80% success rate in prompting anovulatory women to bring forth eggs. But its side-effects include drying up cervical juices, and thinning the lush lining of the womb, so it does not necessarily help you to conceive. More understanding about the importance of cervical juice for natural conception would ensure that doctors work to overcome these side-effects.

Does it make sense for IVF clinics to drug women into temporary menopause, then hyperstimulate their ovaries in order to farm multiple eggs? The process has been likened to slamming the brakes on in a car, then throwing it into fourth gear. It can cause ovarian hyperstimulation syndrome, which, very very rarely, can be fatal.

There are no recommended maximum doses for drugs in IVF clinics. Doctors have been accused of a macho adherence to an unproven belief that maximal drugs and multiple embryo transfers result in more live births.

An alternative is 'mild IVF', where women are given lower doses of fertility drugs, and a single egg is removed, fertilised and reimplanted. This procedure seeks to work with a woman's menstrual cycle, rather than override it. It is cheaper than conventional IVF, cycles are shorter so may be repeated more often, and the side-effects of the drugs are far less severe.

The medical profession is male-dominated, within a culture that unconsciously posits 'male' as 'normal' and 'female' as 'aberrant'.* And it has historically viewed the female body as a dark, mysterious, dangerous place, to be dissected, 'assisted' and controlled.

I refuse to believe that the best we can offer infertile couples in the 21st century is to take the egg and sperm out of them and combine them in the lab. There must be ways to support our bodies to do this better. We need to find them.

* If you don't believe me, try dressing a small boy in a pink dress and see how people react.

Positive thinking

Conventional medicine separates 'mind' from 'body', and pays little attention to the way one can affect the other. Some alternative therapists attempt to redress this imbalance by encouraging 'positive thinking'. They tell you to think about babies, to visualise babies, to immerse yourself in babies, as though a fertile imagination will bring forth a fertile womb.

This may not be very helpful for your mental health.

Every month that you're trying to conceive, it can feel as though babies are being wrenched from your grasp. If you undergo IVF, then babies truly are created – just the first few cells of them. If you suffer miscarriages you can have weeks or months of growing a baby, but still end up bereft.

It's very difficult to be continually mourning unborn babies. There can come a point on the gynaecological rollercoaster where hope becomes more toxic than despair.

Do you know what? No one 'has' a baby. A baby is not a possession. It's not a thing, like a house or a car or an exam result. Becoming a mother is not about having a baby – it's about opening yourself up to unpredictability and to possibilities outside your control. It's about learning the power of unconditional love. You can be part of mothering whether or not you ever give birth.

Whatever happens on your fertility journey, be proud of yourself.

Appreciate your strength, and your beauty.

Give yourself love.

You deserve it.

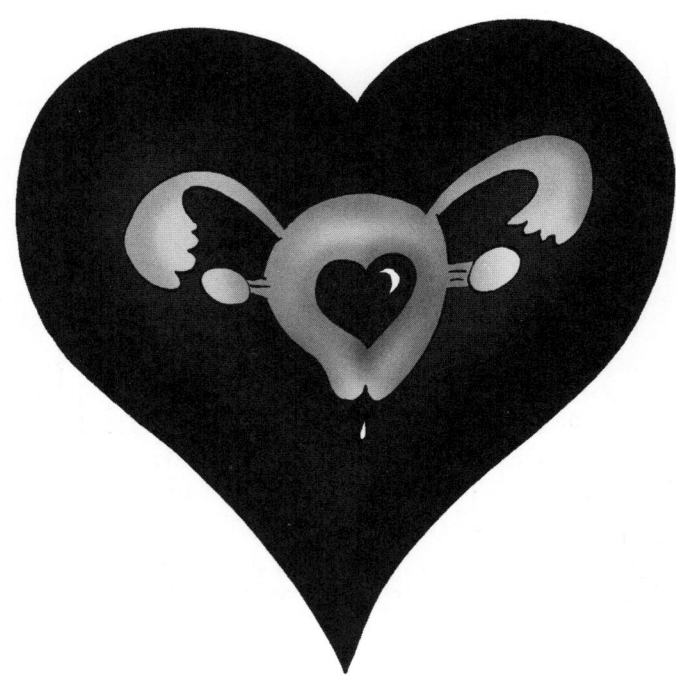

Book the Second

How to grow a baby

5 *Up the duff*

Your pregnancy is dated from the first day of your last period, on the assumption that you ovulated precisely two weeks later. Thus, for a textbook 28-day-cycle woman, on the day she conceived she was two weeks pregnant, when the mulberry-baby implanted she was three weeks pregnant (even though it was only six days old), and when she missed her period she was four weeks pregnant with an embryo that was two weeks old.

Confused? I am.

Anyway, between Week 2 and Week 12 of pregnancy your body does something absolutely amazing. You grow an entire person. It starts from a single cell, and ten short weeks later it has eyes and ears and the ability to suck its thumb. Not only that, you also grow some customised packaging – a balloon of amniotic fluid – and a specialised life-support system for the baby – the placenta and umbilical cord. This is an incredible transformation in a very short amount of time. Don't be surprised if it makes you want to go to sleep a lot.

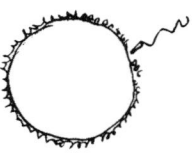

Week 2

Sperm meets your egg.
Actual size = smaller than this ⟶ .

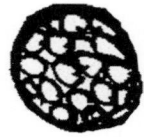

Week 3

Mulberry-baby floats down your oviduct.
Actual size = still smaller than this ⟶ .

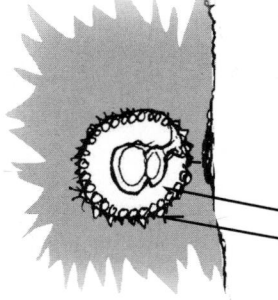

Week 4

Your womb lining engulfs it and nurtures it.
Still only about this big ⟶ .

These cells become the baby.
These cells become the placenta.

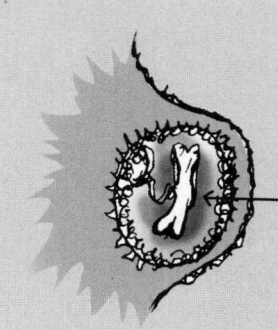

Week 5

Inner cells form into a primitive streak.
Actual size = grain of rice.

Amniotic fluid starts to fill this space.

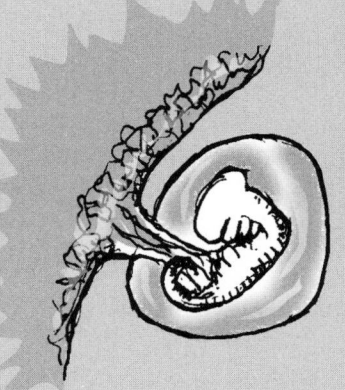

Week 6

A ball of amniotic fluid is now
floating in the womb, with something
that looks more like a baby in.
    Actually, who am I kidding? It
looks more like a sea horse. What's
with the tail?

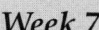

Week 7

Arms! Legs! The beginnings of lungs and
a beating heart!
    Let's hope it outgrows the tail, though.
Actual size = kidney bean.

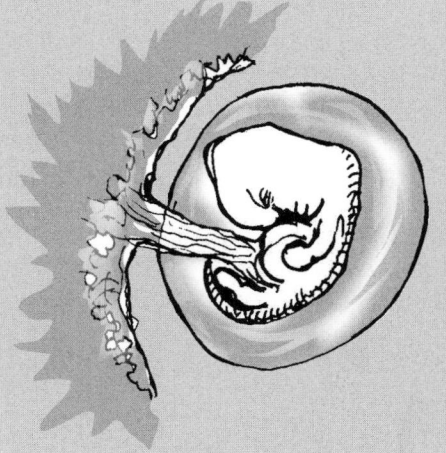

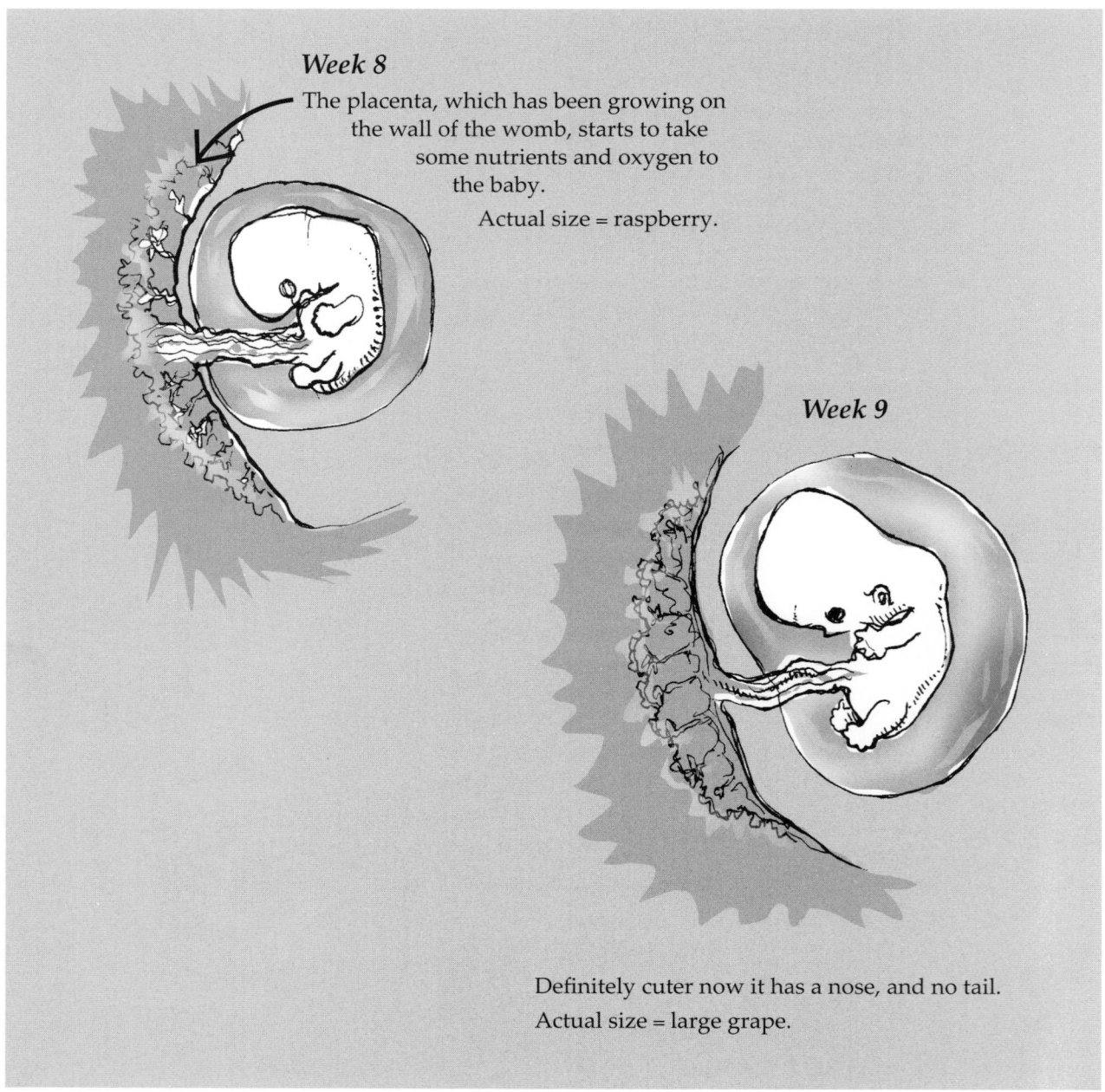

Week 8

The placenta, which has been growing on the wall of the womb, starts to take some nutrients and oxygen to the baby.

Actual size = raspberry.

Week 9

Definitely cuter now it has a nose, and no tail.

Actual size = large grape.

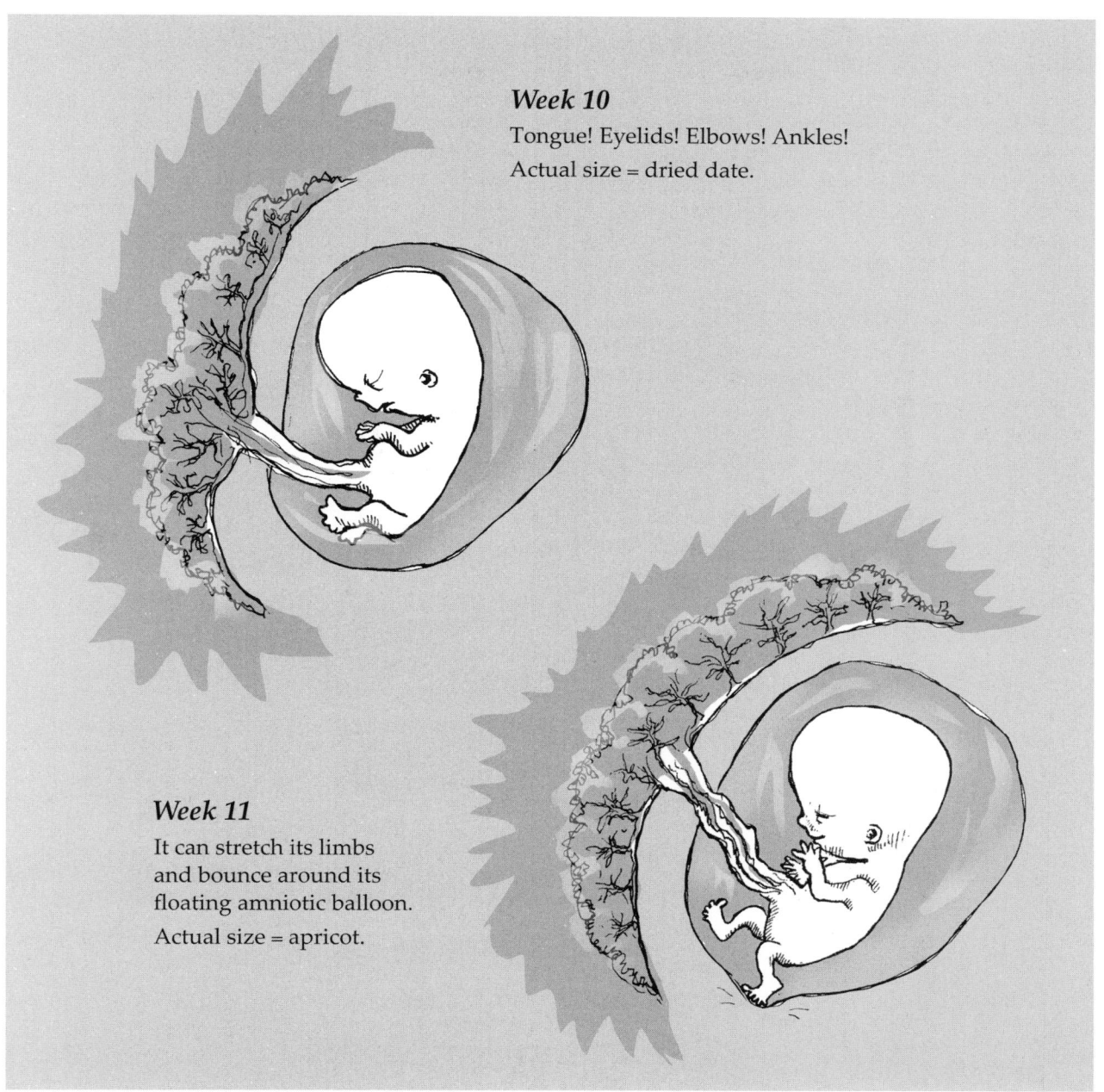

Week 10

Tongue! Eyelids! Elbows! Ankles!

Actual size = dried date.

Week 11

It can stretch its limbs and bounce around its floating amniotic balloon.

Actual size = apricot.

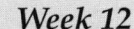

Week 12

It can swallow, and pee, and grab things.

Actual size = kiwi fruit.

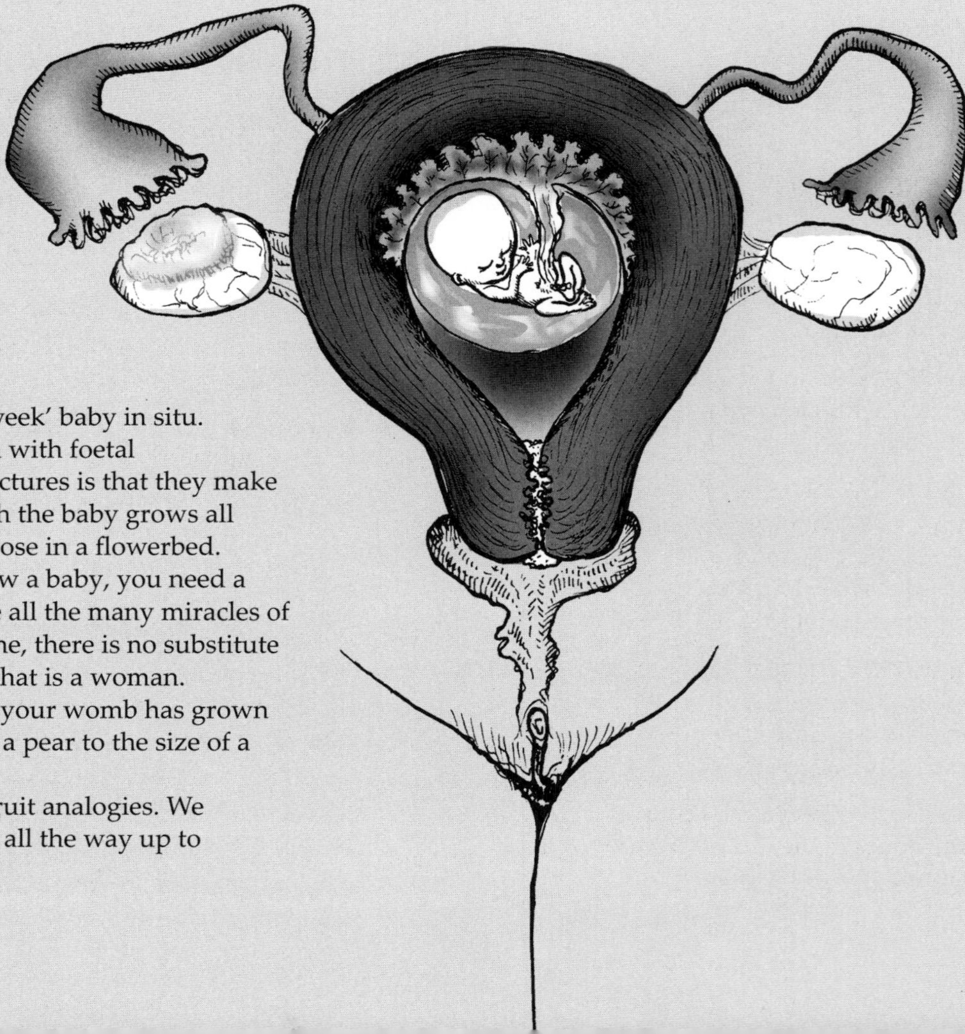

Here's the '12-week' baby in situ.

The problem with foetal development pictures is that they make it look as though the baby grows all by itself, like a rose in a flowerbed. Actually, to grow a baby, you need a mother. Despite all the many miracles of modern medicine, there is no substitute for the miracle that is a woman.

By Week 12, your womb has grown from the size of a pear to the size of a grapefruit.

I like these fruit analogies. We can keep going, all the way up to watermelon.

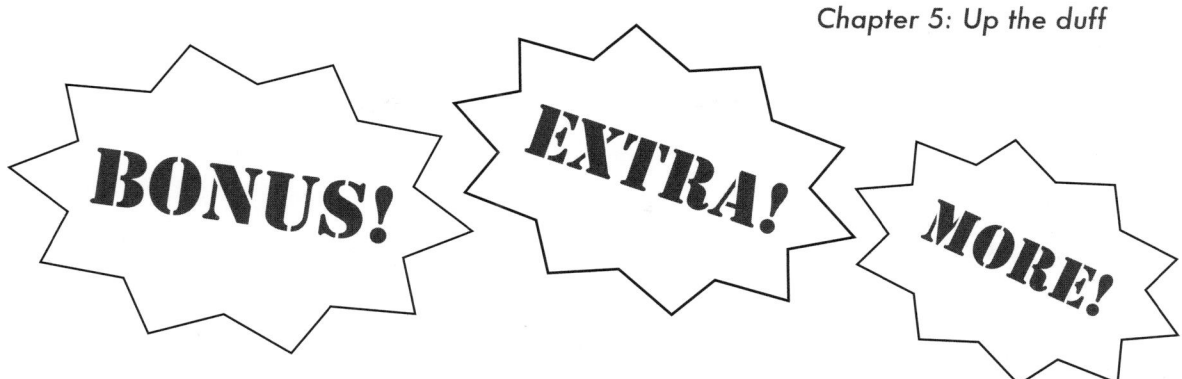

Not only do you grow a baby, a placenta, an umbilical cord and an amniotic sac, you also grow…

more blood! – 50% more by the end of the nine months…

a *larger heart!* to pump it, which beats faster – up to 30% faster by the time you're 30 weeks gone…

and *bigger blood vessels!* to rush nutrients to your baby…

wider ribs! and *fatter lungs!* which work more efficiently to get up to 50% more oxygen into the blood…

larger kidneys! that filter toxins faster, resulting in more urine. Unfortunately, your bladder doesn't increase in size; in fact, it gets quite squashed. To compensate, you will also grow more adept at spotting public toilets…

an *enormous womb!* (I guess you already knew that one.) It's 20 times it's previous size, with 10 times more blood flowing to it by the end of the pregnancy.

Some women get permanently *bigger feet!* as the bones in the arch of the foot change position…

and *fatter fun bits!* Your clitoris and vulva become a little larger, with a greatly increased blood supply, and thicker, more stretchy vaginal walls (which will be handy later on)…

and *fatter everywhere else bits!* You're meant to gain a little plumpness in early pregnancy. These are useful energy stores, in case of famine. Our evolutionary programming clearly doesn't know about 24-hour supermarkets.

You also get a *curvier back!* that sways backwards to counterbalance the great big weight out the front.

You have *bendier joints!* as your ligaments become stretchier…

and *larger breasts!* as with every pregnancy you grow more milk ducts and lobes…

you grow *thicker hair!*

You even get *stretchier eyeballs!* which change shape subtly, so contact lenses can become uncomfortable and you might be more short-sighted…

and up in the brain your *pituitary gland* increases in size by up to 50%. Together with the corpus luteum, the placenta and the baby itself, they pump out a bumper pack of hormones.

In Praise of the Placenta

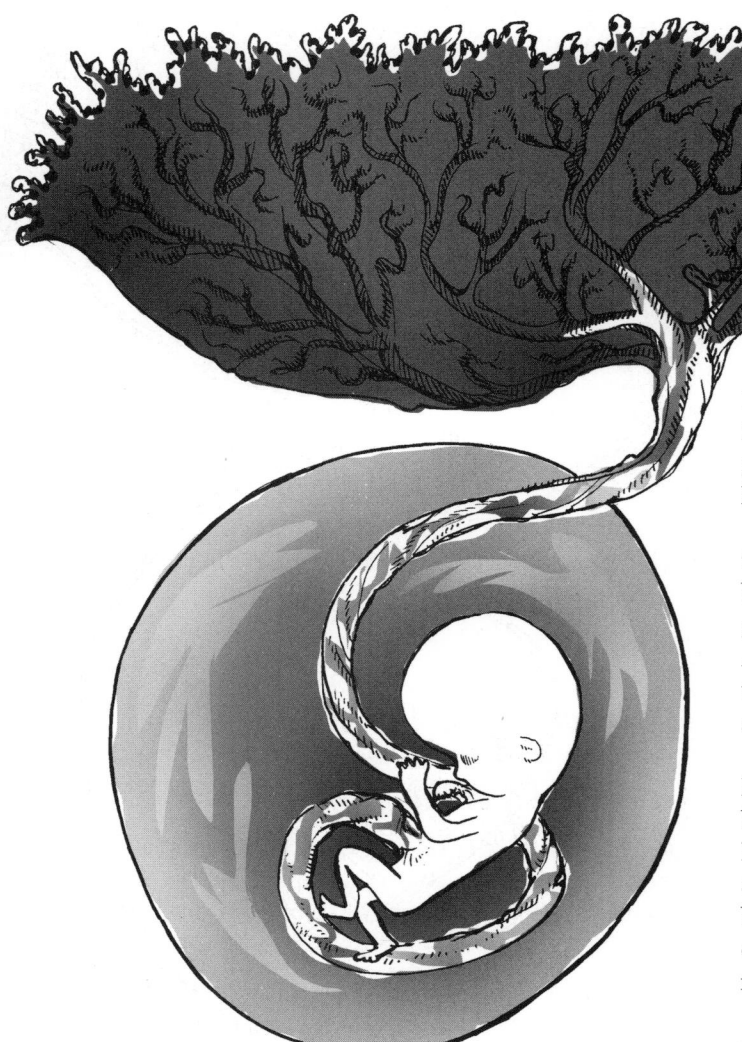

This little tiny potential baby is experiencing the trampoline-like properties of living in a bag of amniotic fluid, which cushions and protects it from bumps or falls. The baby drinks and breathes the fluid, like a funny little fish. Amniotic fluid is a complex mix of electrolytes, nutrients, growth factors and germ-killing agents. Scientists have never been able to recreate it in the lab.

As its heart beats, blood is pumped through the umbilical cord to the placenta. The cord, the baby's lifeline, is tough. It is covered in a layer of gloopy jelly to protect it from getting entangled. Around a third of babies are born with the cord wrapped round their necks, but this isn't usually a problem.

The placenta functions as the unborn baby's lungs, stomach, spleen and liver. It does this by burying little fine fingers into the womb lining, like a million tiny twigs. The mother's blood flows around these, transferring nutrients to the baby's bloodstream and picking up waste products to carry away. The placenta carefully regulates these nutrients, changing the menu as the baby matures.

But the placenta is more than a mere meal planner. It does clever things like carrying antibodies from the mother's bloodstream, yet at the same time creating an invisibility cloak of hormones phosphocholine and neurokinin B to hide the baby, so the mother's immune system doesn't spot, and reject, the foreign cells.

Basically, your placenta and womb lining (or 'decidua') are in charge of the show. All the main pregnancy hormones are produced in, around or with the help of the placenta and decidua. There are a lot of them. I'll explain some of main ones, but we're not going to cover them all.

We have already met **human chorionic gonadotropin**. This hormone suppresses your immune system to stop your body rejecting the baby. It's a growth hormone, helping build your womb. Its presence in your urine is what turns a pregnancy test positive. And it's probably the hormone that gives you morning sickness. It peaks in concentration at about the eighth week and starts going down after that, which hopefully means that your food will stay down too.

Then there's **human placental lactogen**. This stops contractions in smooth muscle – the muscle your womb is made of. It also helps your baby and your womb to grow. And it regulates your blood sugar, or rather, it quickly shunts sugars from your blood and feeds them direct to the baby. Hence the hunger pangs.

Relaxin. This does what it says on the tin – relaxes things. Your muscles, your ligaments, your blood vessels and all the soft tissues in your body become softer and spongier under its influence.

Prostaglandins help with wound healing. They're a good thing to help grow a baby.

Remember oestrogen and progesterone? The corpus luteum doesn't keep producing them indefinitely. From about Week 8, the placenta steps in and, in collaboration with some

hormone-producing glands in the foetus, it ramps up production.

Progesterone helps your body lay down fat stores, enlarges your blood vessels and kidneys and relaxes all your smooth muscles, including your guts and your womb. It increases your sensitivity to carbon dioxide, so you breathe out your baby's waste blood gases faster. It makes you hotter, and your womb needs to be a little warmer than usual for optimum baby growth. Progesterone triggers the creation of milk-making cells in your breasts, but it also stops you from making any milk just yet.

Progesterone also works on your nervous system to make you tired. You may have noticed this effect (as you prop your eyelids open with matchsticks and attempt to keep reading about complex hormone interactions).

Your progesterone levels are already running at twice the level you experienced when you were not pregnant, and they build from there. They'll be *ten times higher* by the end of the pregnancy.

You need all these 'smooth-muscle-relaxing' hormones for one reason. The placenta is pumping out **oestrogen**, and that's the hormone which makes the womb pulse, in nice co-ordinated contractions. (Remember? They helped the sperm up through the womb?) Under the influence of the huge amounts of oestrogen in your system, your womb is laying down masses of new muscle cells, and packing them all with oxytocin receptors. At the moment, the progesterone deactivates those receptors, but it's clear that some mighty big smooth-muscle movements are in store at the end of the nine months.

I wasn't lying about the 'huge amounts of oestrogen'. By the time you're 40 weeks gone, your oestrogen levels will be *one thousand times higher* than they were before you were pregnant. Blimey.

Oestrogen builds things. It builds nerves and lymphatic drainage for the womb. It builds your blood vessels, and milk ducts, and kidney cells, and hair follicles. It builds your fat stores. It helps build your baby. You name it, it builds it.

Oestrogen also increases the white blood cells in your blood, to protect you from the suppression of your immune system that accompanies pregnancy. It makes proteins in your blood more available to your baby. It ups the production of blood-clotting factors, so the soft, fat blood vessels that carry goodness to your baby don't haemorrhage.

Together with progesterone, oestrogen seals your womb tight shut with a solid plug of cervical juice. And it increases the acidity of your vagina, to protect the baby from germs.

There are three more hormones to mention, and they're rather pleasant. The placenta and the pituitary both give out **prolactin**, which co-ordinates the production of breastmilk, and it's present in pregnancy at 20 times anything you've experienced before. Prolactin makes you feel nurturing. You will previously have (hopefully) experienced a prolactin surge immediately after orgasm. That's what it feels like. Yum!

Your **oxytocin** levels increase. This hormone increases your gut's ability to extract nutrients from your food. It makes you feel sleepy (again, think 'post-orgasm') and less stressed. It helps you to feel connected to other people, loving and empathetic. The extra dose that you get of this hormone in pregnancy is nothing compared to the massive oxytocin rush that's in store when you give birth.

And you can look forward to a free hit of **beta-endorphin**, in the last few months of pregnancy, which is the same 'feel-good' chemical that runners get from a long-distance race. You'll not be looking much like a marathon runner, but you will be feeling like one. In a good way.

Basically, there's a lot going on behind the scenes.

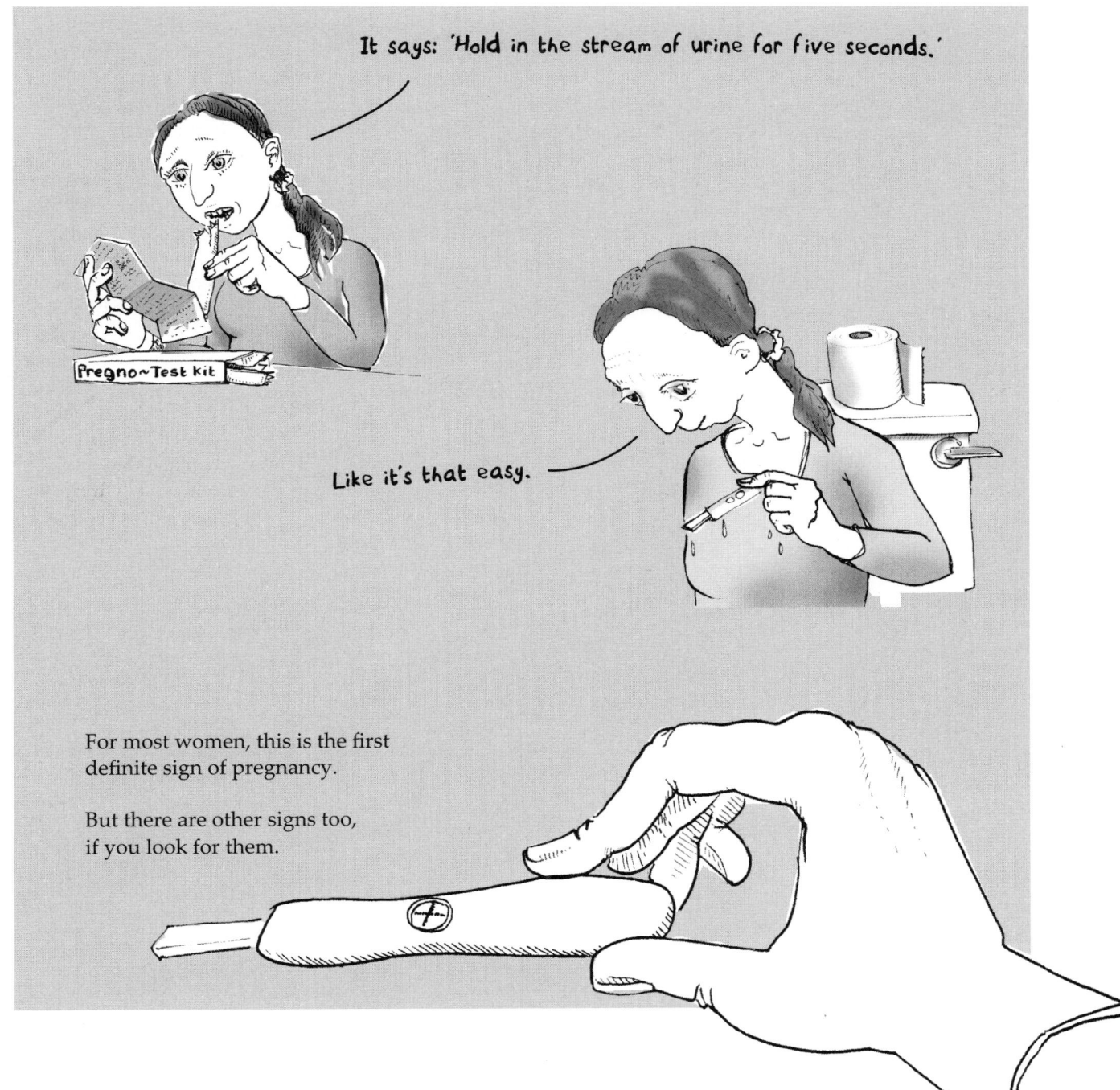

It says: 'Hold in the stream of urine for five seconds.'

Pregno~Test kit

Like it's that easy.

For most women, this is the first definite sign of pregnancy.

But there are other signs too, if you look for them.

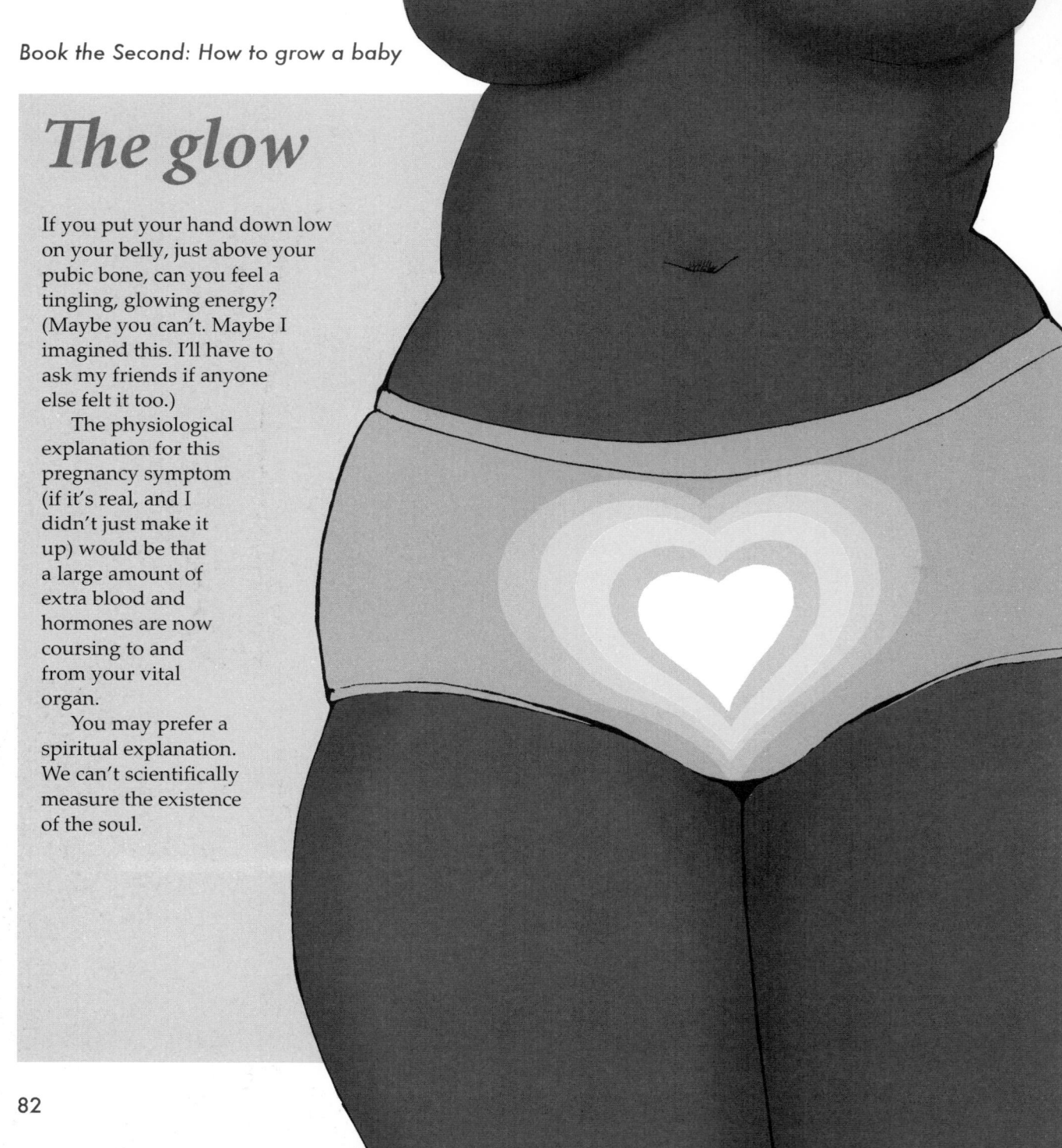

The glow

If you put your hand down low on your belly, just above your pubic bone, can you feel a tingling, glowing energy? (Maybe you can't. Maybe I imagined this. I'll have to ask my friends if anyone else felt it too.)

The physiological explanation for this pregnancy symptom (if it's real, and I didn't just make it up) would be that a large amount of extra blood and hormones are now coursing to and from your vital organ.

You may prefer a spiritual explanation. We can't scientifically measure the existence of the soul.

The 'contented cow' feeling

Oestrogen is powerful stuff. Remember, just the mini-dose that ovulating women get is enough to make them go dancing in low-cut dresses. Now you're high as a kite on the stuff, plus, your pituitary adds surges of prolactin and oxytocin, hormones that you will previously have only experienced immediately after orgasm. In the last months of pregnancy, you get some free endorphins in the mix as well.

Lots (not all!) pregnant women therefore feel mildly stoned much of the time, with a sense of contented rightness about the world. You can feel like this even if you know you're not going to keep the baby. It's bizarre.

It's a cunning stunt on the part of evolution to drug pregnant women up with feel-good hormones. And, given that birthing and raising a child involves a lot of effort, we deserve this. It's our bonus. Enjoy!

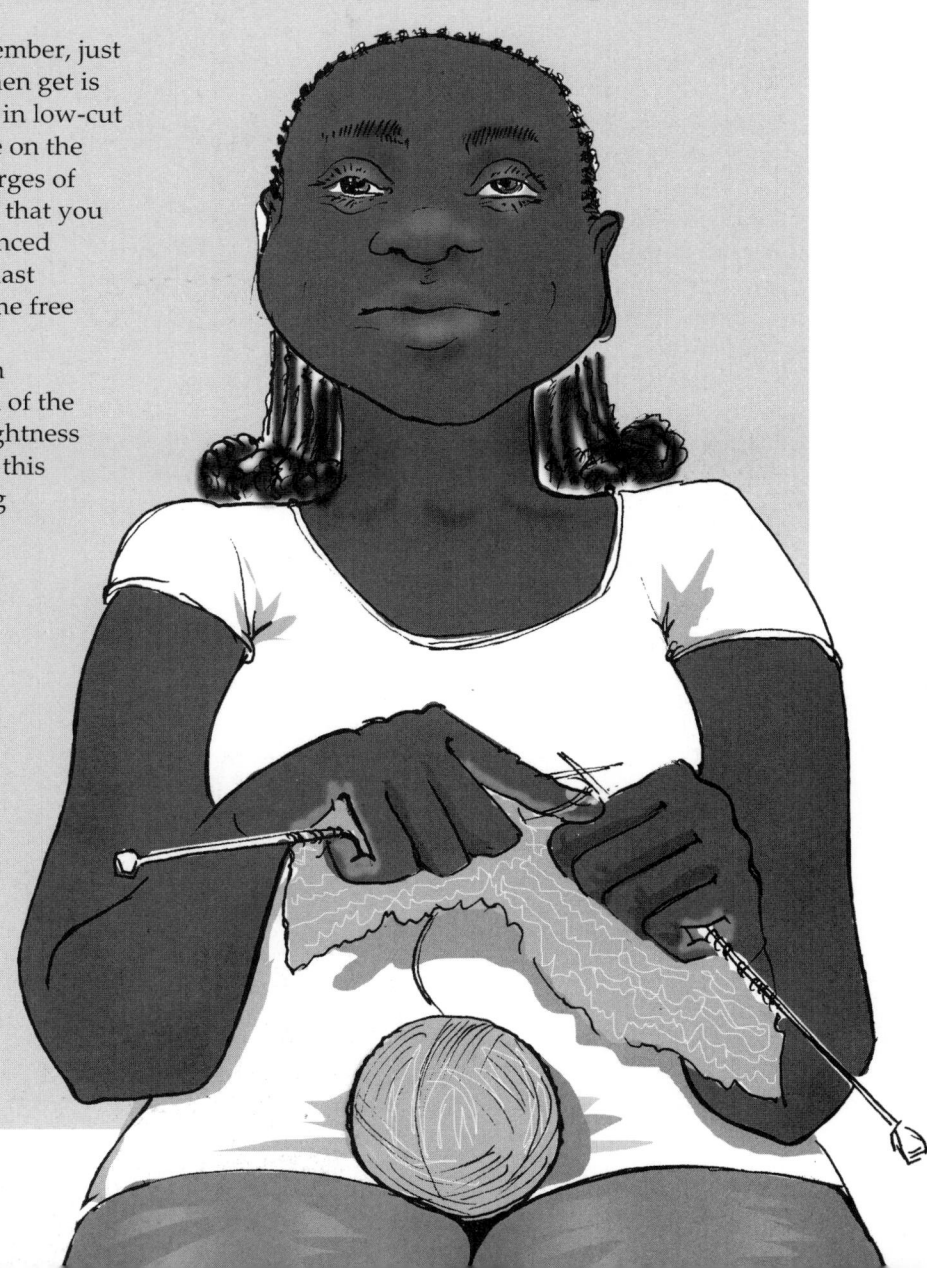

The 'psycho-bitch-from-hell' feeling

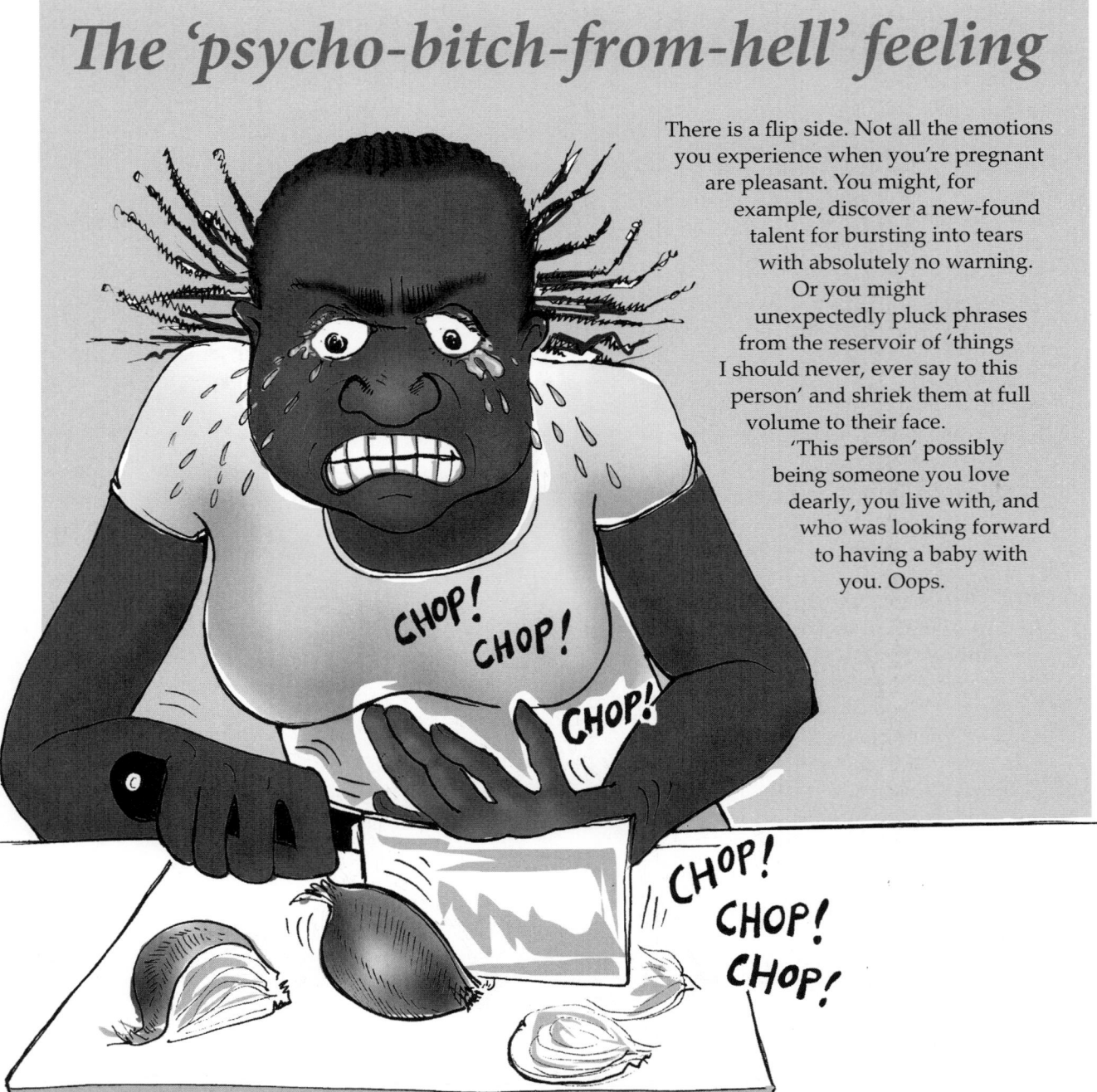

There is a flip side. Not all the emotions you experience when you're pregnant are pleasant. You might, for example, discover a new-found talent for bursting into tears with absolutely no warning. Or you might unexpectedly pluck phrases from the reservoir of 'things I should never, ever say to this person' and shriek them at full volume to their face.

'This person' possibly being someone you love dearly, you live with, and who was looking forward to having a baby with you. Oops.

As a feminist, I wasn't sure if the Sisterhood would approve of me letting everyone know that women can be biologically primed for extreme emotions. Then I had a think about patriarchal society in more detail.

There is an assumption that, when people (women in particular) show extreme emotion, they are being irrational. They are not. This opposition between 'rational' and 'emotional' is a false one – every truly intelligent decision is underpinned by emotional and intuitive understanding. We're suffering a hangover from Victorian values, where what masqueraded as a model of masculine 'rationality' was a psychopathic level of emotional repression, which was used to justify some extraordinarily widescale socially abusive behaviour. We still feel the need to apologise for having emotions that are 'too strong' (at least, here in England we do). Whatever you feel, it isn't wrong to feel it, in all its intensity.

Let's have a look at the personality changes some (not all!) pregnant women are prey to. There are rational evolutionary reasons for them all:

1. **Getting violently angry or upset when you are hungry.** This makes sense. It is extremely important for the unborn baby to be adequately nourished. Rage is a valuable resource to make darn sure that you, and consequently your baby, get some dinner.
2. **Getting incredibly upset or angry when you are tired.** Your energy is being diverted to the creation of another human being, so you will probably become more tired, more quickly than ever before in your life. Becoming tearful when you're overdoing it is a good warning strategy for you, and people around you. Ideally, rather than being embarrassed or discomfited by this, they would do something useful for you, to make your life easier. That would be in the best interests of the survival of the species.
3. **A newfound interest in babies**, or a willingness to tend plants or animals. So, pregnancy hormones might make you more nurturing. That's a good design feature. Well done, God (or whatever deity you prefer).
4. **An inability to watch horror films.** Your sensitivity to the stress hormone cortisol is very different in pregnancy, because it has a direct effect on the developing foetus. Watch a gardening programme instead.
5. **A heightened interest in hygiene.** Presumably, there has been evolutionary selection in favour of the offspring of pregnant women who washed their hands properly.
6. **A nesting instinct.** (This tends to kick in in the later months of pregnancy.) Like every mammal, we are biologically driven to prepare a safe place to give birth. Because we are humans, this gets subsumed into deliberations over wallpaper samples.

We are gradually emerging from several hundred years of oppression when women were *only allowed to be* mothers, nurses, nannies, cleaners and homemakers. We were regarded as crazy, oversensitive delicate creatures, unsuited for battle. That's sexist bullshit. Women are capable of everything men are, plus some, namely, the ability to bear children.

However, we have a way to go with sexual equality. Only women get pregnant. And all pregnant people are deserving of extra physical and emotional support. They are having babies for all of us. Think about it. If none of them does, we all die out.

It's OK to have mood swings when you're pregnant. It's society that's crazy, not you.

The smells

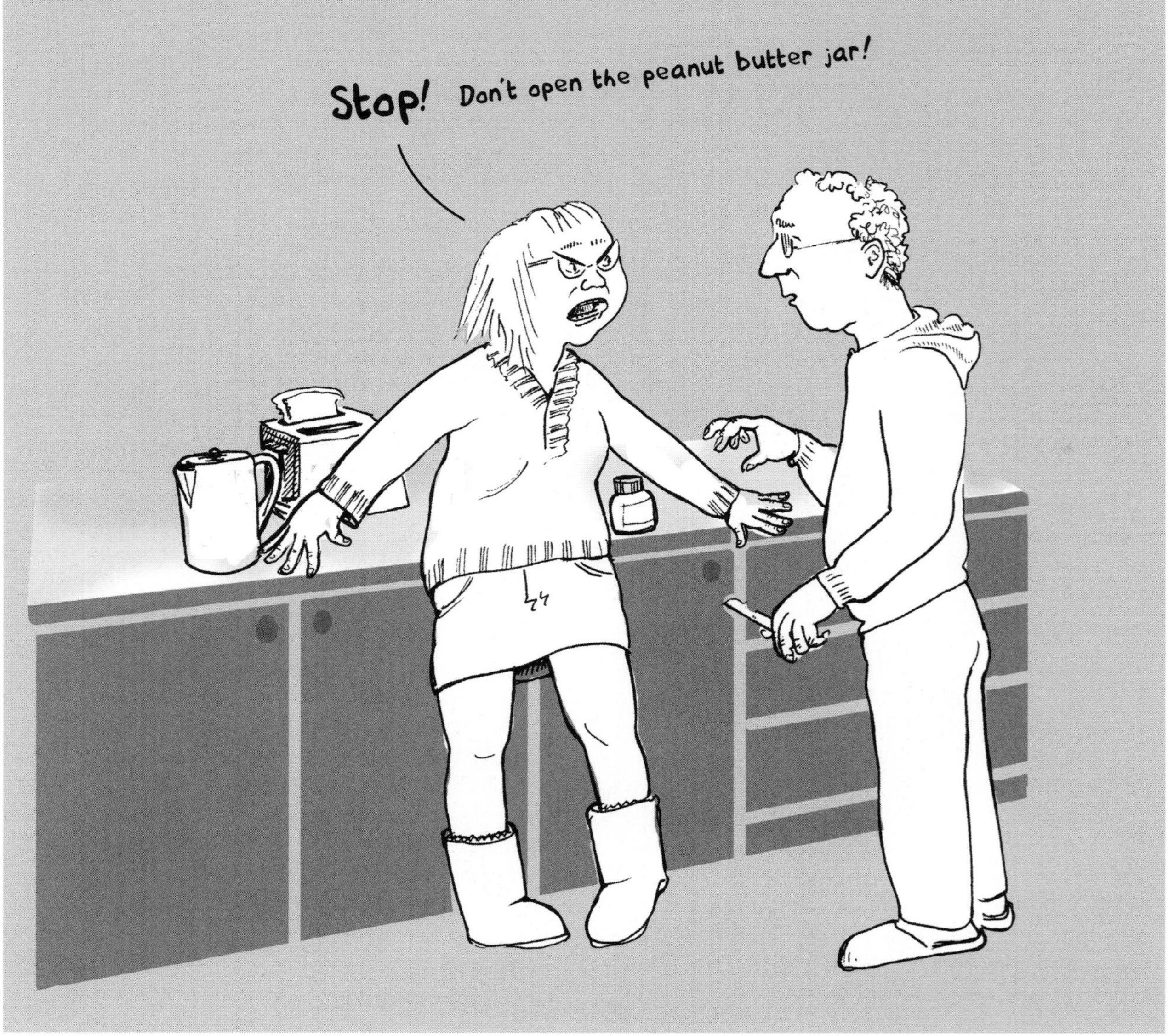
Stop! Don't open the peanut butter jar!

You don't understand: when you open the jar,

this is how peanut buttery it smells.

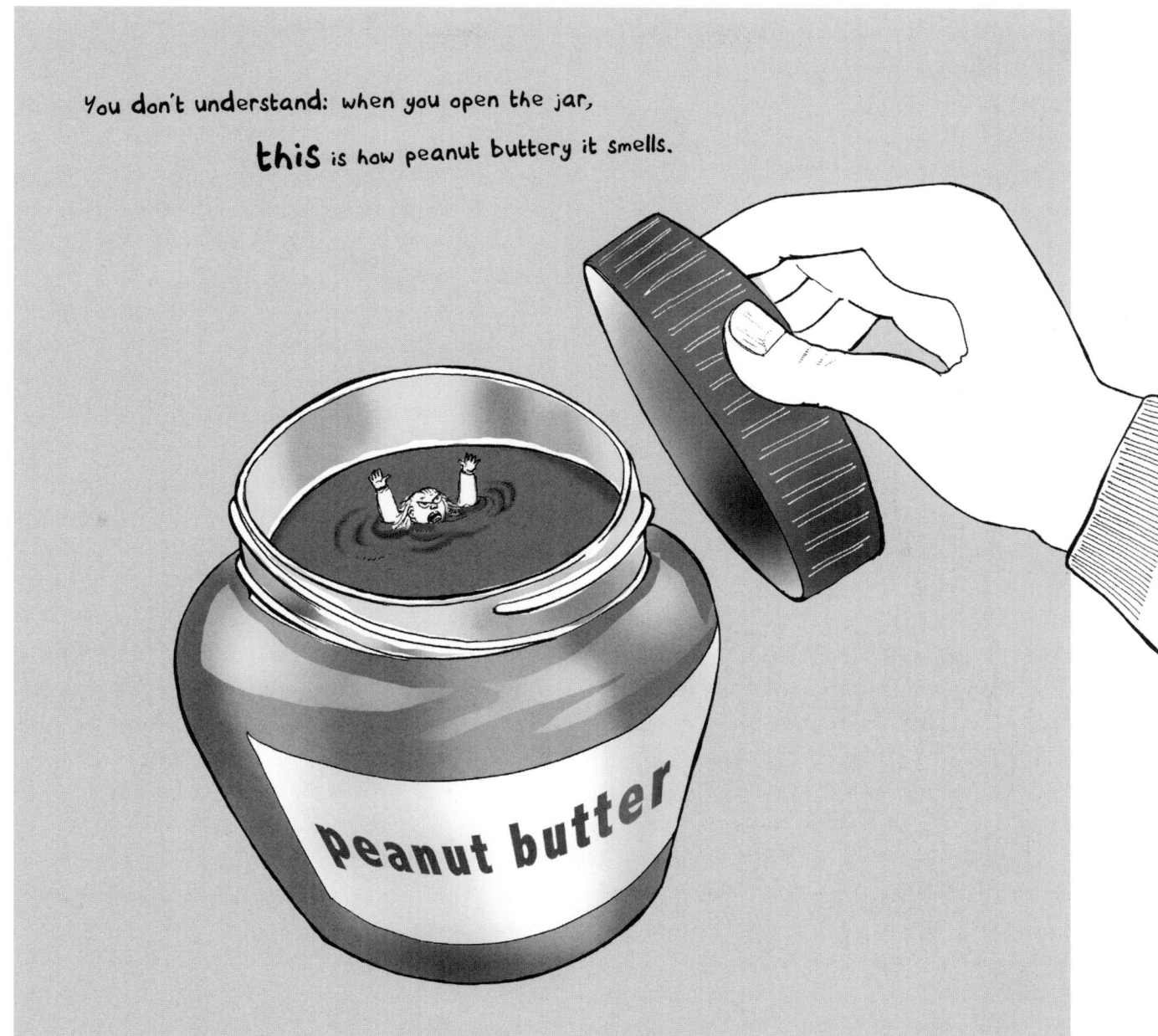

The sickness

'Morning' sickness is the clichéd sign of early pregnancy. It doesn't just happen in the morning. Eighty per cent of pregnant women experience some nausea, and it's most likely to be severe in the early months of pregnancy.

Opinion is divided about morning sickness. Some scientists believe is has evolved to protect the developing foetus from possible harm from dangerous toxins in food. Other scientists, the pregnant ones, who are currently throwing up, believe what the rest of us also think – that there can't possibly be an evolutionary advantage in making a pregnant woman eat everything twice, and that God is probably a man.

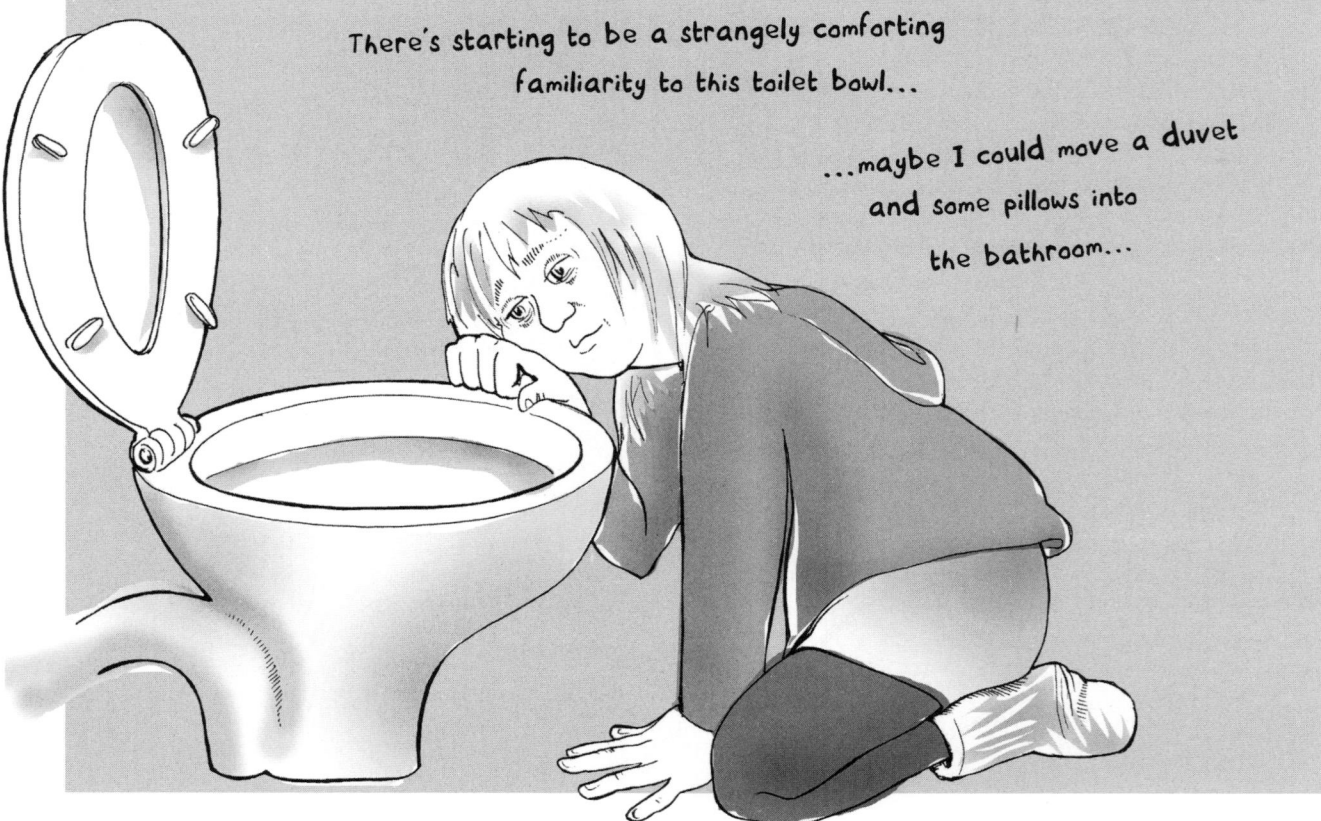

Blech! Peanut butter!

There's starting to be a strangely comforting familiarity to this toilet bowl...

...maybe I could move a duvet and some pillows into the bathroom...

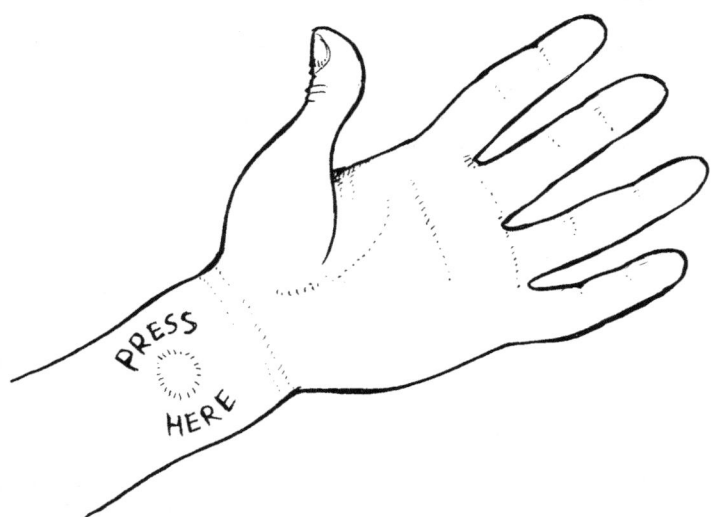

PRESS HERE

Things that help

- Try this acupressure point. It's on the inside of your wrist, underneath where your watch strap would go. Press firmly for a few minutes, breathe in through your nose and out through your mouth, and see if the feeling subsides. You can buy 'seasickness' bands which are an elastic bracelet with a plastic knobble which puts pressure on this point. Or you can wedge a pebble under your watch strap. Take them off if they give you pins and needles.
- Eat little and often. Cold food might be easier than hot, because it smells less.
- Try eating a dry biscuit when you first wake up, before you get out of bed.
- Ginger. Crystallised ginger, tea made from chopped fresh root ginger in boiling water, real brewed ginger ale such as Fentiman's (not the sugary ginger ale from the supermarket) or good quality ginger biscuits.
- Peppermint tea or fennel herbal tea.
- Ice lollies freeze the vagus nerve that controls the vomiting reflex. You can make your own out of any liquid that appeals, such as soup.
- Certain foods may trigger vomiting, even if they're ones you normally enjoy eating and have no problem with. This may persist throughout the pregnancy.
- Acupuncture can help.
- Hypnotherapy can help.
- Partner, friends and family of pregnant one – you can help. Prepare bland, non-greasy meals for her. Hold her hair when she's being sick. Clean the toilet daily, with a cleaner she likes the smell of.

Seek medical help if you can't keep any food and fluid down for 24 hours, if you vomit blood, have abdominal pain or a high fever. Vomiting during pregnancy can be severe enough to require hospital treatment.

Things that don't help

- People telling you 'it's a good sign, because it means you won't lose the baby'. This is not necessarily true, or appropriate. They should be careful saying annoying things to you at the moment, because you might be sick on them.
- Any mention or sight of food. Skip to page 100 now, because you won't want to read the next 11 pages.

The hunger

Pregnancy induces, in me, a very peculiar attitude to food. I know I need to eat, *right now*, but it's a particular, specific food that I need, and I'm not sure what that is.

At this point, a kind of mental fruit machine starts whirring in my head, and a series of foods pass through my mind in succession. It goes like this: 'Apple? No. Banana? No. Orange? No. Cherries? No. Radishes? YES! Definitely. Lots of radishes.'

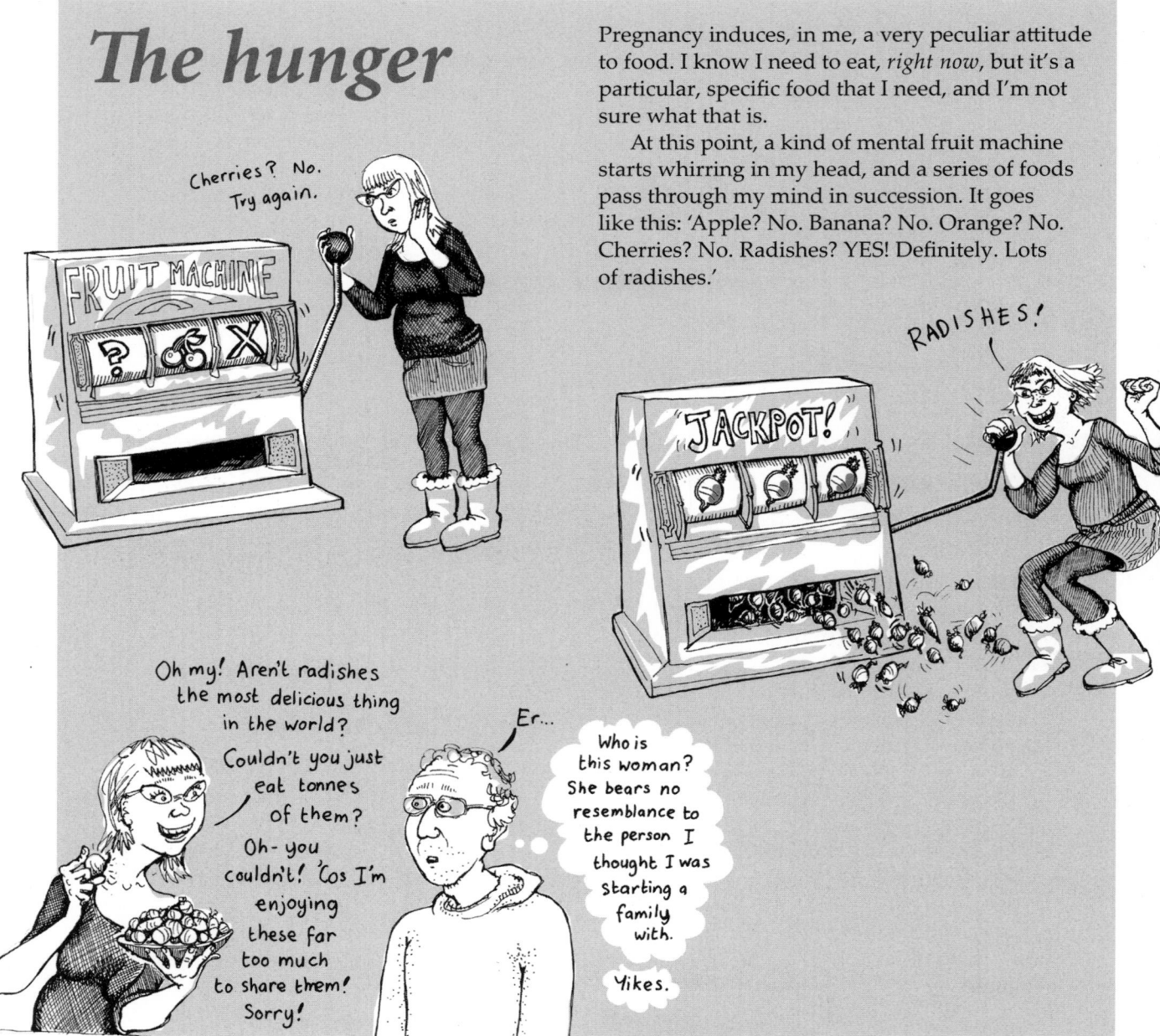

90

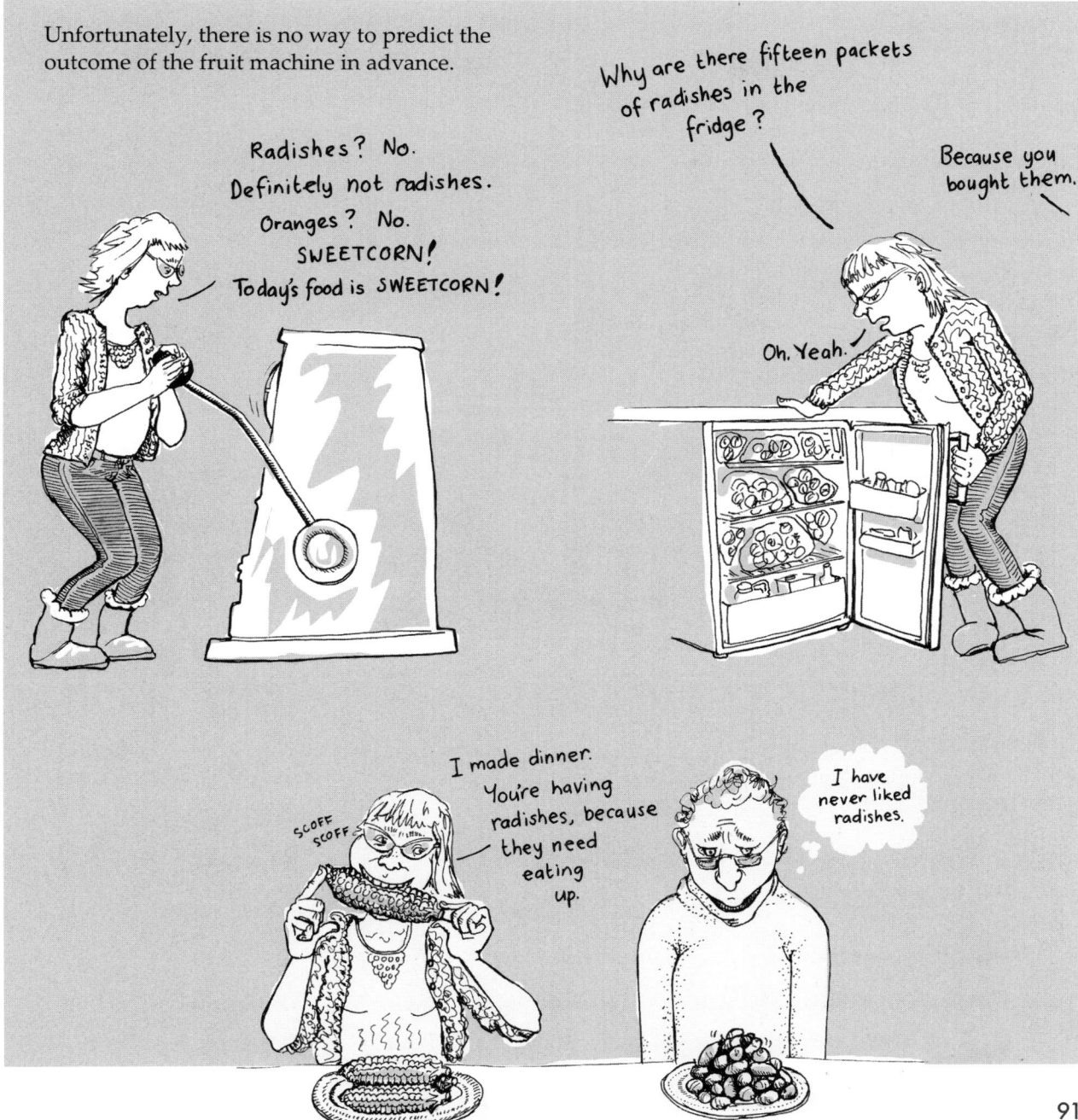

Unfortunately, there is no way to predict the outcome of the fruit machine in advance.

Radishes? No. Definitely not radishes. Oranges? No. SWEETCORN! Today's food is SWEETCORN!

Why are there fifteen packets of radishes in the fridge?

Because you bought them.

Oh. Yeah.

SCOFF SCOFF

I made dinner. You're having radishes, because they need eating up.

I have never liked radishes.

91

What to eat

As any farmer or dog-breeder will tell you, if you want to produce good quality offspring, it's best to eat a good-quality diet. This means eating regular meals of good, fresh food. This is harder than you might think.

Our economy is predicated on making ever-increasing amounts of money out of people. But there's not much profit to be made from good, fresh food: you grow it, transport it short distances to people, and they only eat as much of it as they need. The picture changes if you refine and process the food, add preservatives so that it keeps indefinitely, and lace it with an addictive combination of salt, fats, sugar, flavourings and flavour-enhancers. Dress it up in some fancy packaging and brainwash the population with a clever advertising campaign. Now you can get the population hooked on your 'food'. The additives in it will override their natural hunger limits so they'll overindulge, get withdrawal symptoms, and keep coming back for more.

It's a safe bet to say that if you have seen an advert for any given foodstuff, it's probably not good, fresh food.

To redress the balance, I have drawn some adverts for foods that are good for you to eat. (Take a pregnancy multivitamin too. Check that it contains iodine, as this is important for your baby's development.)

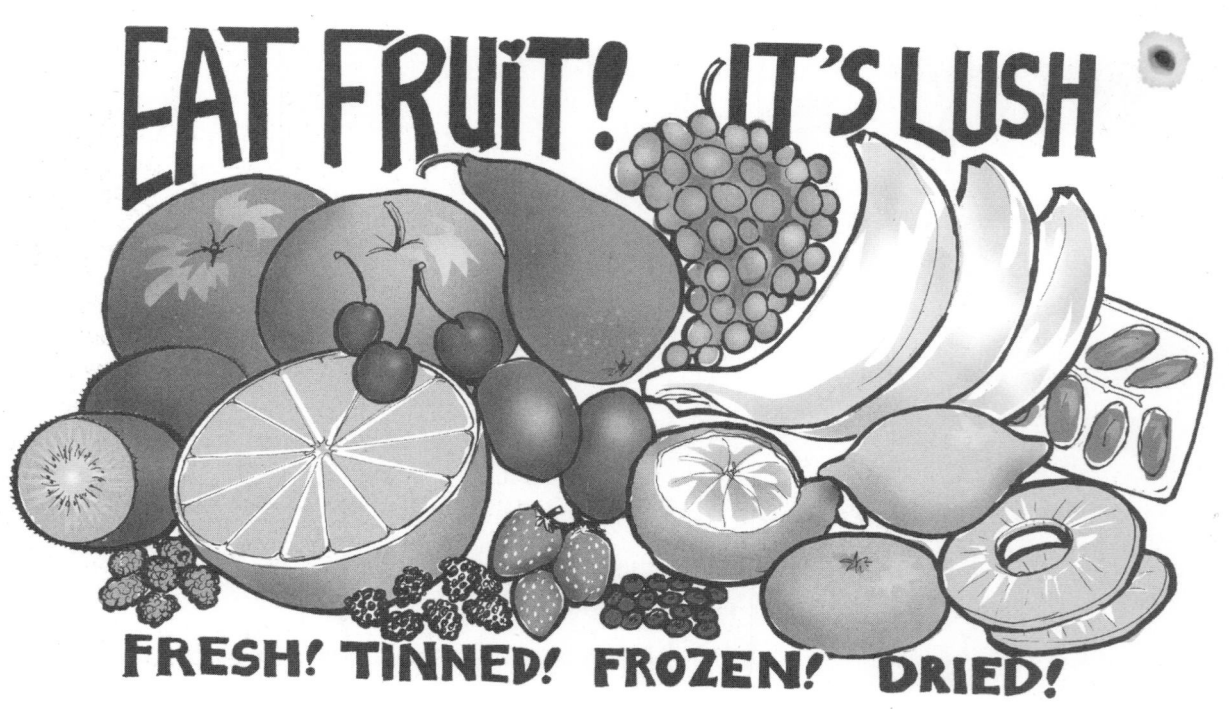

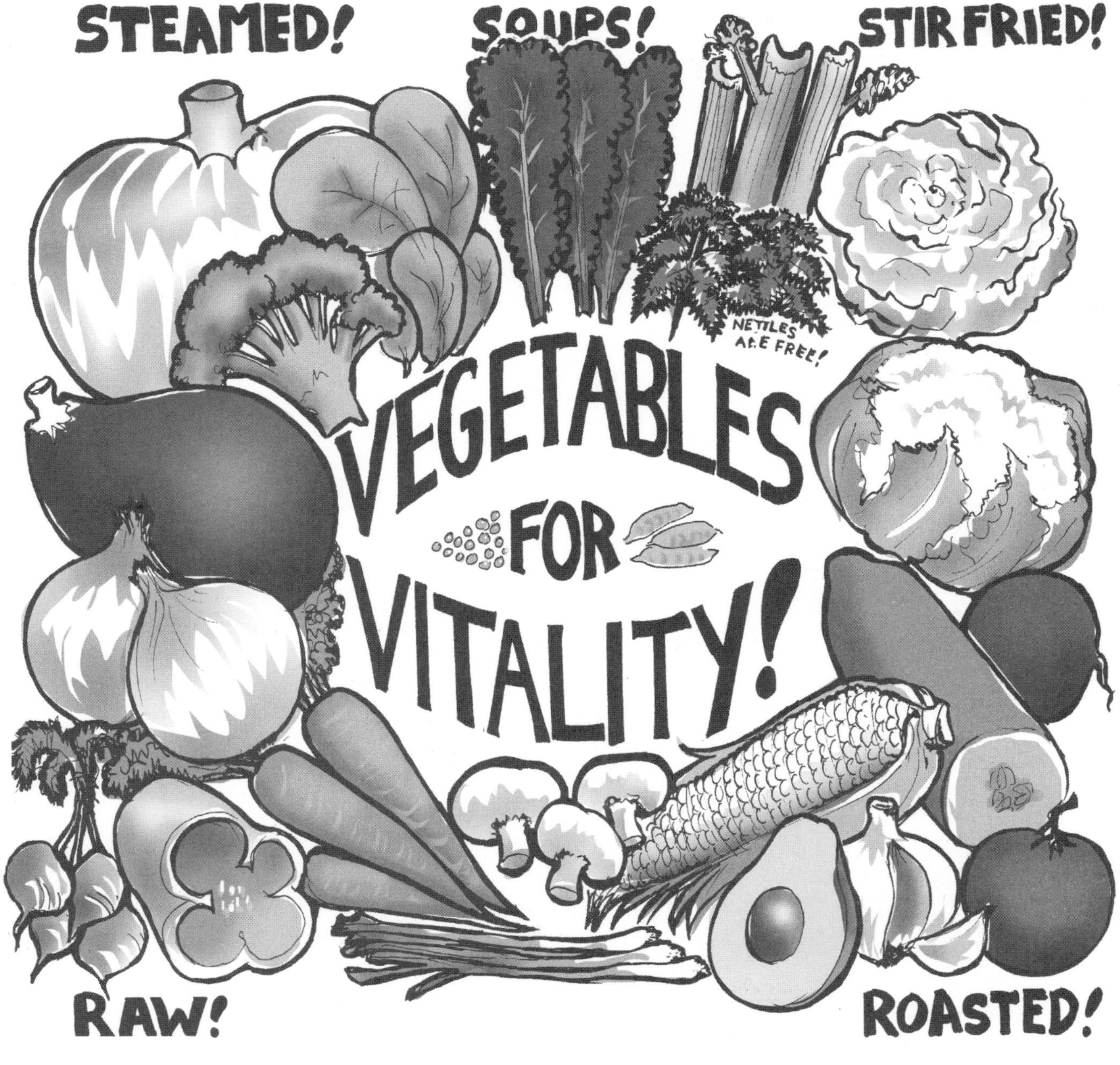
STEAMED!
SOUPS!
STIR FRIED!
NETTLES ARE FREE!
VEGETABLES FOR VITALITY!
RAW!
ROASTED!

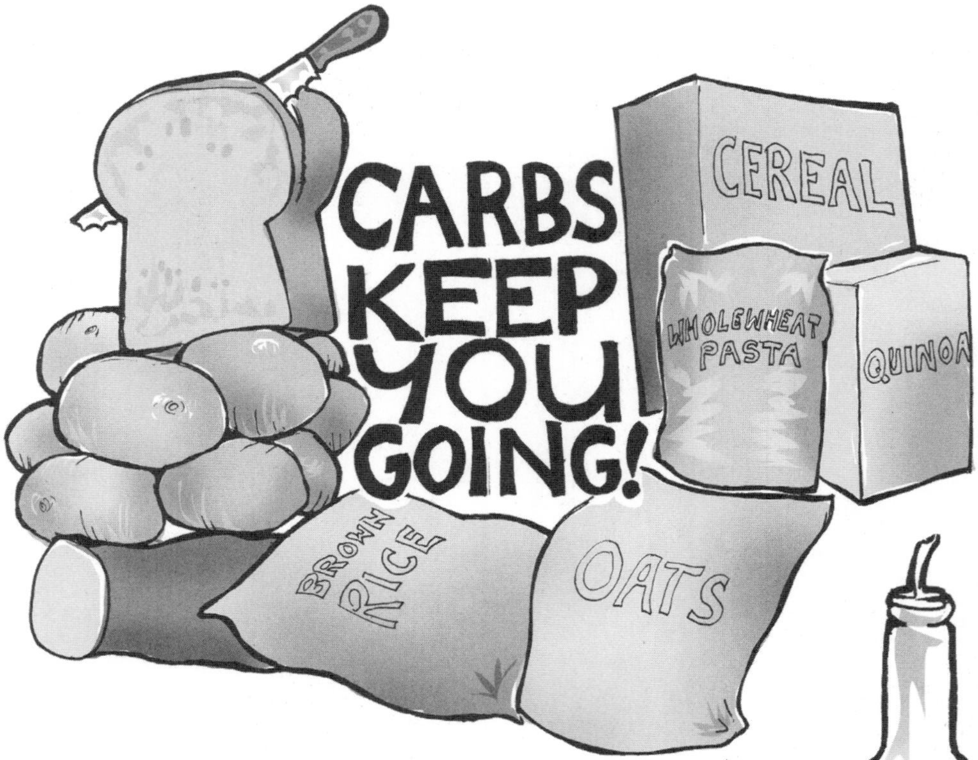
CARBS KEEP YOU GOING!
CEREAL
WHOLEWHEAT PASTA
QUINOA
BROWN RICE
OATS

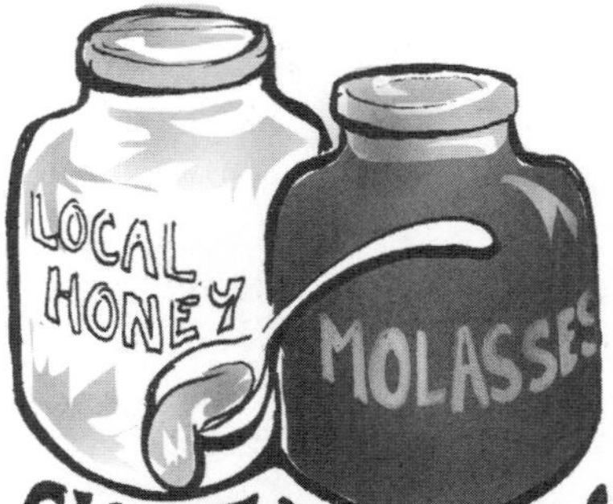
LOCAL HONEY
MOLASSES
SWEET TREATS!

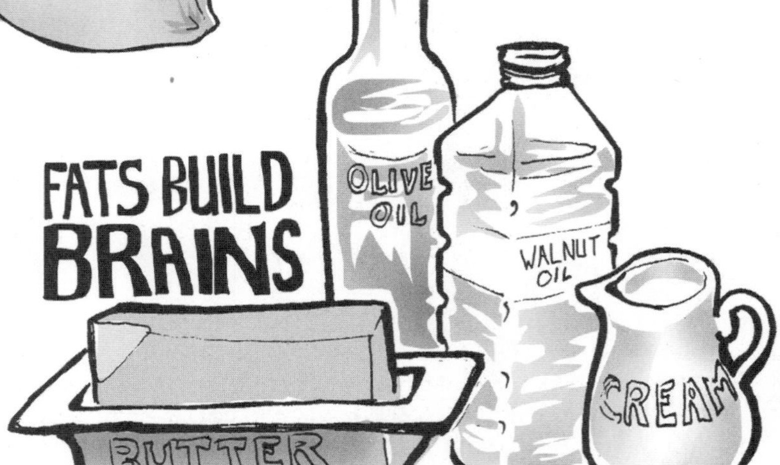
FATS BUILD BRAINS
OLIVE OIL
WALNUT OIL
CREAM
BUTTER
CHOOSE UNPROCESSED OILS!

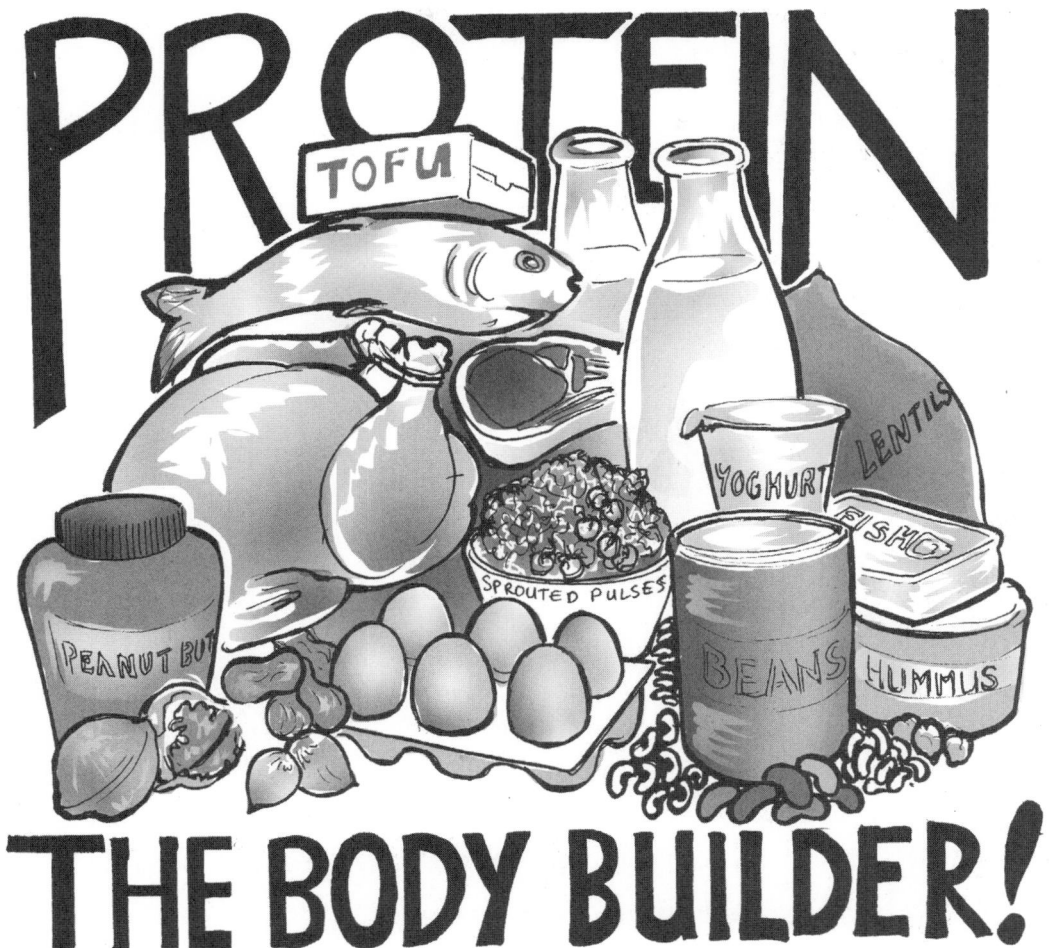

Read about best practice for fish, meat, cheese and milk consumption and preparation on pages 98–100.

Yes, vegetarians and vegans can get enough protein from plant-based foods. No, they don't need you to lecture them about nutrition.

I understand that you might not be feeling on top form for imaginative meal planning. Even glimpsing a photo of food could turn my stomach in early pregnancy. You'll have less energy for preparing meals (Partners! Friends! Family! Do some cooking and help out!) so make this as easy for yourself as you can.

It is not *bad* to eat chocolate biscuits. It won't *poison* the baby if you eat cake. If you're hungry, and you really want to eat chips, then do it. Just be aware that when you choose nutritious food you are doing your baby good.

Top breeders recommend it.

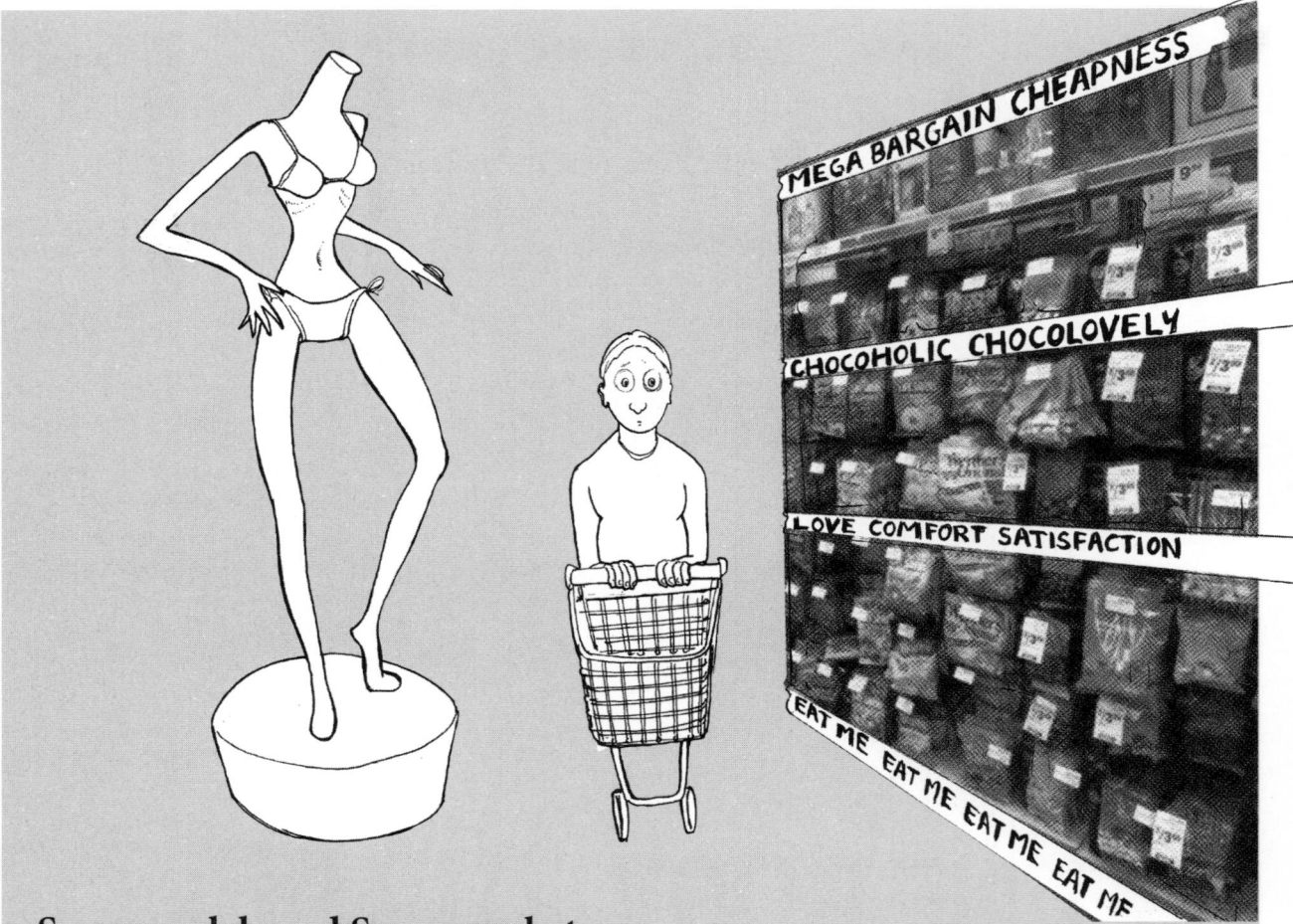

Supermodels and Supermarkets

When considering nutrition, accept that most food retailers set out to sabotage your good intentions. Takeaway menus are loaded with unhealthy options. Walk around a supermarket and take an objective look at its contents and you'll see that an astonishing percentage of the shelf space is dedicated to high-salt, high-sugar items. Economies of scale mean that frozen chips and chicken nuggets are the cheapest options, while fresh and whole foods have become expensive luxuries.

Back in 1950, British people were rationed to 16oz of sweets *a month*. Nowadays you can buy that amount of sugar in two cinema servings of soda. And they'll try to upsell you a family bag of chocolates along with it.

At the same time as society has become increasingly sugar-coated, our attitudes to body fat and female flesh have become skewed in the opposite direction. Since the 1960s, ideals of female beauty have become associated with semi-starvation, and the media has primed us with images of women whose body mass indices are dangerously low. So-called 'super'models suffer from life-threatening genetic conditions and eating disorders. You probably don't look like one, not least because most of them can't get pregnant – they don't have enough body fat to ovulate.

Pregnant women feel pressure from society to conform to this ideal of thinness, even though it puts their babies at risk.[1] When a woman's calorific intake is severly restricted in pregnancy, her baby is starved of nutrients. The baby is more likely to need special care after birth, and will have a lifetime's increased risk of serious illnesses such as diabetes and heart disease. That's how important it is for the unborn baby to be adequately nourished. And that's how irresponsible magazine articles are that praise celebrities for not 'piling on the baby pounds', dissect their diets, and fetishise pregnant women who are so thin that they look like a snake that has swallowed an orange.

You are going to become big and round and soft and curvy. Does this thought terrify you? Is becoming thinner associated in your mind with triumph, success and control? You may have an eating disorder. Be honest about this with yourself and other people who need to know. Many women find that focusing on the needs of their unborn child is the stimulus they need to overcome years of disordered eating.

- Tell your midwife or doctor.
- Ask for a referral to a nutritionist who has experience of eating disorders. If you have been regularly denying yourself food or binge-eating, you may have lost touch with your natural hunger cues, and could need a structured approach to your diet.
- Your midwife will ask to weigh you at some antenatal appointments. If you prefer, you can be weighed with your back to the scale.
- This isn't about your weight, it's about your self-image. Counselling can help you come to terms with your underlying motivation for wanting to be less.
- Attend a support group for people with eating disorders. Support groups rock!

If you have always been round and soft and curvy, pregnancy can be a liberation from self-loathing at your body shape. Skin-tight lycra becomes an option once you have a legitimate excuse for having fat ankles and a big belly.

Unfortunately, obese women are at risk of pre-eclampsia and diabetes in pregnancy, labour can be difficult, and their babies often need special care.[2] If you're overweight, you don't need any more fat-hate, shaming and blaming. That doesn't help you feel good about yourself, and, when you feel bad, food addiction is an easy comfort. But this isn't about how you look, it's about your baby and that's a good incentive. Either a 'low GI (glycaemic index) pregnancy diet', or a 'paleo pregnancy diet' may help to level out blood-sugar swings and ease refined carbohydrate cravings. See a nutritionist. You'll find exercise ideas on page 149.

Pregnant women who have had gastric bypass surgery can still grow healthy babies.[3] Make sure you eat protein at every meal. Tell your midwife, so she can monitor you. Take any prescribed vitamin supplements *as well as* your pregnancy vitamins, not instead of them.

What not to eat

What? Eight whole pages on food and pregnancy, and there hasn't yet been a mention of All the Things You're Not Allowed to Eat! Well, rather than treat you like a four-year-old and present you with a long list of Forbidden Foods, let's have a look at some of the actual risks presented by various foods and substances.[4] Then you can make up your own mind whether or not to eat them. If you are strongly craving a particular foodstuff, who am I to tell you you're Not Allowed?

Food poisoning

Being pregnant lowers your immune system – you're growing something foreign inside you, and you don't want your body's defences to attack it. This puts you at greater risk of food poisoning, and some kinds of food poisoning can harm your baby. Don't panic! The risks are slight, but they are avoidable. Vegans will be feeling slightly smug by the end of this list as the most hazardous foods tend to be meat, milk, eggs and fish.

Basic food safety:

- Wash your hands before you cook.
- Check that your fridge is colder than 5°C and put leftovers in there once they are cool.
- Don't leave your shopping in a hot car boot for hours.
- Don't eat old food. Trust your nose (there's a reason why it's supersensitive) and throw food away if you think it has gone off.

Salmonella

This is a bacterial infection that causes vomiting and diarrhoea. It can be passed to your unborn baby, and very rarely, can cause stillbirth. You can get it from eating meat, especially poultry, unpasteurised milk products and eggs. To put this in perspective, it has been estimated that one egg in 20,000 is infected with salmonella. Best practice for avoiding salmonella poisoning is to:

- Always wash your hands, kitchen surfaces, chopping boards and utensils immediately after preparing raw meat.
- Cook all meat thoroughly, so that no trace of pink remains. Barbecues are particularly dodgy for undercooked meat.
- Reheat food that contains meat until it's piping, steaming hot and bubbling. Stir food that is re-heated in a microwave, and then heat a bit more.
- Cook eggs until the yolks are firm.
- Don't eat or make home-made mayonnaise, ice-cream, drinks or sauces with raw egg in. Shop-bought mayonnaise, commercially prepared sandwiches and salads with mayonnaise in and other commercial raw egg products are fine because the egg will have been pasteurised.
- Don't lick the raw cake batter off the spoon (this is so hard to not do!)

Listeriosis

The bacterium *Listeria monocytogenes* likes to multiply in milk, some soft cheeses and meat products. It's a nasty one: 22% of cases of listeria poisoning in pregnancy result in the death of the foetus (78% don't, though. Statistics can be scary).

- Avoid unpasteurised milk and dairy products. If unpasteurised milk is the only milk available, you can make it safe by boiling it.
- Avoid pâté, including vegetable pâté (sorry, vegans!)
- Avoid soft camembert/brie type cheese, the ones which are squidgy with a white rind, and

soft blue cheeses such as Dolcelatte, Roquefort or Danish blue. These are OK to eat cooked in a pie or melted onto toast as long as they are completely melted and bubbling hot all the way through.

- Hard cheeses like cheddar, stilton, Red Leicester and edam are fine.
- Other soft cheeses and cheese spreads are safe, as long as they are made from pasteurised milk. So you can eat mozzarella, feta, cottage cheese, ricotta, halloumi and goat's cheese, as long as it's the standard stuff from the supermarket, not made by an artisan in a Greek village and left to swelter on a warm restaurant plate for hours.
- Keep all ready-to-eat meat and fish products in the fridge, and throw them away when they're past their sell-by date.

Campylobacter

The risks and the causes are as for salmonella, but campylobacter bacteria can also be carried in untreated water. So don't drink water from rivers, lakes or streams. Like you were going to.

Toxoplasmosis

This is caused by the common parasite *Toxoplasma gondii* that can be carried in meat, unpasteurised goat's milk, and sheep and cat poo. About a third of people in the UK will get toxoplasmosis at some point, and if you know you already had it before you were pregnant, you will be immune and you don't need to worry about it. About five women in a thousand contract it for the first time when they are pregnant, and about three babies in 100,000 have the illness at birth. If those statistics scare you, they shouldn't, because you have a 99.5% chance of not getting toxoplasmosis, and

your baby is 99.997% likely to not be born with it, particularly if you:

- Follow all previous recommendations for preparing and cooking meat safely, and avoid unpasteurised milk products.
- Don't change the cat litter yourself. If you have to, use disposable rubber gloves and wash your hands extremely well. It's best practice to get the litter tray changed daily and fill it with boiling water for five minutes to neutralise bugs.
- Cats could, theoretically, poo anywhere. If you think this is a risk, wear gloves when gardening and wash soil from fruit and vegetables.
- Avoid lambing ewes and newborn lambs.

If these restrictions aren't practical – say, you're a hill farmer or work in a cat sanctuary – it is possible to be tested to see if you have already had toxoplasmosis and are immune to it.

Shellfish and sushi

- Raw shellfish carry a whole host of food poisoning bugs, so don't slurp raw oysters or similar. Freshly and thoroughly cooked shellfish is OK.
- Raw, unsmoked fish in sushi might possibly have anisakids (parasitic worms) in. If that knowledge hasn't just put you off ever eating sushi again, you should know that freezing the fish at –20°C for 24 hours makes it safe. Ready-prepared sushi in the supermarket will have been frozen, so that's fine. Sushi that is freshly prepared in a fancy Japanese restaurant – well, you don't know. You can ask if it has been made from frozen fish, or you can stick to the cooked fish, smoked fish and vegetarian varieties.

Mercury poisoning

Unfortunately, our oceans are polluted with mercury, so although fish are tasty and nutritious we now have to be careful how much we eat.

- Fish that eat other fish contain appreciably higher levels of mercury, so avoid shark, marlin and swordfish.
- The recommended limit is two portions a week of oily fish such as tuna, salmon, mackerel, sardines or trout.

Vitamin A overdose

Too much vitamin A could be harmful to the developing foetus.

- This explains why you take pregnancy multivitamins, not ordinary multivitamins, even though they're twice the price.
- Liver and liver pâté contain vitamin A. Avoid, unless you're majorly craving it.

Hydrogenated fats

These pass through the placenta, and do no one any good at all. Check the label.

Caffeine

Very high caffeine consumption has been linked to miscarriage and low-birthweight babies. You don't have to cut it out altogether, but, if you're worried:

- Cut down to about five cups of tea or three cups of instant coffee or two filter coffees a day. It's OK if you occasionally exceed this limit.
- Remember, there is also caffeine in cola, chocolate and lucozade.
- Avoid high-caffeine 'energy' drinks.

Peanuts

They're fine. Eating peanuts in pregnancy won't give your child a peanut allergy.

What not to do

There are other things to fret about, besides the sell-by date on a ready meal.

Don't smoke

You probably already know that smoking in pregnancy is not a good idea, but did you know why?

Tobacco smoke contains 4,000 toxic chemicals, including at least 60 that cause cancer. With every puff of a cigarette, these toxins enter your bloodstream and many pass through the placenta to your baby. The most dangerous one is the one you're addicted to: nicotine. This narrows the blood vessels in your body, including ones in the umbilical cord. It's like forcing your baby to breathe through a narrow straw.[5]

Not only that, but the carbon monoxide in the smoke replaces oxygen in your blood, so even less oxygen is available to your baby.

The result? Your baby's growth is stunted, it is more likely to be born premature, and is at twice the risk of stillbirth. The placentas of smokers are 'aged' and inefficient, and are more likely to peel away inside the womb.[6]

If just part of your brain is thinking 'Oh, great – a smaller baby will be easier to give birth to', then have a rethink. You really don't want your baby to be smaller than it's meant to be. The growing your baby does in the womb sets it up for life. And so the babies of smokers are more likely to have breathing problems at birth, to develop asthma in later life, and are at more than double the risk of sudden infant death syndrome (cot death). They tend to have lower intelligence, more behavioural problems and learning disabilities. They have a higher incidence of congenital heart defects, and, bizarrely, are more likely to be obese as teenagers.[7]

And the really, really bad thing about smoking is, if you're a smoker, reading all that probably made you want a cigarette.

Every cigarette you don't smoke helps your baby grow the best it can. You'll never find a better reason to quit.

Stopping smoking is easier with help from family, friends and specialist support services.

Don't drink

This is another biggie. The children of women who drink regularly or heavily are at risk of foetal alcohol syndrome. They have slightly deformed facial features, small heads, lowered intelligence and lifelong problems with rage, impulsiveness, disorganisation and trouble learning how to love. It is the only entirely preventable intellectual disability.[8]

Having said that, it's not necessarily the mothers who are to blame. We live in a strongly pro-alcohol culture, where powerful corporations are making vast amounts of money from trying to sell us fun in a cocktail glass. It can be very difficult to not drink. Flip back to page 63, read the definition of 'alcohol abuse' and 'alcoholic', and think hard about whether it applies to you. If it does (be honest, now!) then follow the Government's recommendations. Do not drink anything at all for the duration of your pregnancy. If you can't stop once you start, then don't start.

But if you don't have a problematic relationship with alcohol, is it OK to have a drink or two? There have been conflicting results from scientific research into this issue. Some pregnant women feel patronised and infantilised by a blanket ban on alcohol when there's not much research to support it. Others feel outraged that people risk ingesting toxins in pregnancy in any case.

One major longitudinal study[9] has helped untangle the contradictions. It turns out that there are four different variations in your genes that determine how your body processes alcohol. The genes of women who drank just a few units a week in pregnancy were compared against the IQ of their children at eight years of age. For every one of these unlucky gene variations, the child's intelligence dropped by two IQ points. So, if you have a few drinks a week in pregnancy, depending on your genes, it might not affect your child at all, or it might knock up to eight points off their IQ. You don't know your genetic type, so you can't tell whether it will affect them or not.

If you are considering drinking, the timing is important, as well as the amount. The first 12 weeks are a bad time to ingest alcohol. There's a lot of organogenesis going on down there. Vodka is not going to help.

That's the science. Now you can choose whether to drink some champagne at your sister's wedding. It's not going to do your baby any good, but the amount of harm it will do is not easy to quantify.

*Whoa there. That was a lot of information; a mass of rules and restrictions (and we're not done yet). You've only just found out you're pregnant, and now you've been told to buy gardening gloves, and you're wondering how to measure the temperature of your fridge. This is itself a sign of pregnancy: **feeling confused and guilty**.*

Welcome to motherhood.

Don't feel guilty

Our society is bad at meeting the needs of pregnant women and mothers. One of the ways this manifests is that there is strong pressure on women to make the Right Choices absolutely every step of the way through motherhood.

Feeling confused? Guilty? We've hardly started yet. There are a whole heap of choices in store: where to give birth, where the baby should sleep, what the baby should eat, when your infant should start childcare, what school your child should go to… These are couched in very individualistic terms, as if you, the mother, are solely responsible for your child's welfare and as though you alone have the power to shape their character, their happiness and their future prospects.

In fact, society is collectively responsible for all our children. Why should it matter what school you choose? All schools should be good schools. Why should the place of birth be so significant? All births should be empowered births.

With this in mind, I'm going to give you the only piece of advice I want you to take away from this book and internalise.

Do not feel guilty.

Guilt is a pointless emotion. Guilt is all about blaming yourself, and blame is destructive. When you blame someone else, you stop seeing the wider picture – you're no longer honestly evaluating all the multiple factors that influence events. When you blame yourself, you do the same, and you suffer.

This book is dedicated to giving you accurate and accessible information about your body. This is to help you make your own decisions. Accept that whatever you choose in motherhood, you do it with the best intentions, considering the information, and the support that is available to you at the time. And then get on with it.

Smoking and drinking do pose real risks to foetal development, and there are genuine reasons to abstain. But what if you didn't realise you were pregnant until some weeks or months had passed? What if you unknowingly exposed your baby to toxins? Should you feel guilty about that?

No. You can't rewind time and undo it. Just trust that your baby will be OK. Perfection is not attainable in motherhood. Love is.

Foetal alcohol syndrome is a terrible blight on our society, but the way to tackle it is to dedicate money and resources to top-quality social care, and offer vulnerable people an alternative to self-destructive spirals of addiction. It's not just alcohol that's the issue, it's the pressure that people feel to drink, which is compounded by advertising and alcohol-based social rituals and places of entertainment. Likewise, tobacco was once just a wild Mexican weed. It was only once it was processed and packaged and pushed on people that it became a problem.

As a pregnant woman you occupy a unique niche in society. Complete strangers can assume a right over your unborn baby, as though you, the mother, cannot be trusted. There have been incidents where a pregnant woman has raised a glass of wine to her lips in a restaurant only to be accosted by an outraged member of the public. Why should our peers intervene to tell us we're doing things wrong, rather than congratulate us for doing things right? Those strangers, with their opinions, are not going to offer to carry your shopping for you, or buy you a nutritious snack, so how much do they really care about your baby? They don't even necessarily know what they're talking about.

Here's another top tip.

Any time a stranger feels motivated to tell you, as a pregnant woman or as a mother that you're doing something wrong for your child, ask them one question in return: 'Are you a parent?'

They probably aren't. That's why they still think they've got all the answers.

I digress. Let's get back on with listing some more things to stress about.

Don't take drugs

Let's start with the prescription varieties.

In 1957, German drug company Chemie Grumenthal released a new wonder drug for insomnia, thalidomide. It was meant to be safer than any other drug on the market, because it was impossible to overdose on it. In many countries it was available without prescription. When women took thalidomide between days 35 and 49 of their pregnancies it resulted in catastrophic birth defects. And many women did, because it was also marketed as a cure for morning sickness. Ten thousand children were affected before the drug was withdrawn from sale.

Before the thalidomide scandal, there was very little awareness of the potential for drugs to harm the unborn baby. It was thought that such substances couldn't cross the placenta to the baby. Now the thinking has reversed completely, and the assumption is that any medication could be unsafe, until it is proven otherwise. It's not very ethical to conduct pharmaceutical trials on pregnant humans, so there are many drugs where we simply don't yet know whether they are safe or not.

So, as with many other aspects of life as a pregnant woman, the advice is to employ the precautionary principle – if in doubt, don't.

- If you take regular medications, discuss them with your doctor, ideally before you get pregnant, or as soon as you realise you are.
- Remind your doctor that you're pregnant before they prescribe you any medication.
- Tell the pharmacist that you're pregnant when you buy anything from the chemist.
- Don't take remedies that you have stored at home unless you have checked with your midwife or pharmacist that they are appropriate for use in pregnancy.
- For pain relief, choose paracetamol, or very occasionally paracetamol with codeine if the pain is severe. Try not to take paracetamol every day unless you have good reason. Don't take ibruprofen or asprin as these have both been associated with possible birth defects, miscarriage and bleeding in pregnancy. Don't take codeine in the last few weeks of pregnancy.

Not all drugs are taken by mouth. The active ingredients in hair dyes, self-tanning creams and sprays and hair removal creams are all absorbed into your body through your skin, and their safety is unproven. If using these products is essential for your self-image, consider waiting a while until you're more than 12 weeks pregnant.

Vaginal deodorants should definitely not be used in pregnancy. They are also unneccessary. If you're concerned about your natural odour, mention this to your midwife or doctor, because you could have an infection.

There are active ingredients in herbal remedies. Consult a herbalist or, at the very least, do some internet research into whether your chosen herbal supplements or teas are recommended for use in pregnancy.

Don't take illegal drugs, either

Heroin, cocaine, ecstasy, ketamine and speed are all bad for babies.[10] Women who use them risk stillbirth, and give birth to low-birthweight, developmentally delayed babies. However, because they are illegal, it can be hard to know what adverse effects are due to the drugs themselves, as opposed to being attributable to stress, poor nutrition, attendant addictions to tobacco and alcohol, or the horrendous array of dodgy chemicals that they are cut with.

Once again, I am going to argue this from both sides. When you're pregnant, don't do drugs, because they definitely harm your unborn child. If you're addicted to drugs, get referred to a programme to help you gradually quit, because going cold turkey without medical supervision might also harm your baby.

On the other hand, if you have taken drugs in pregnancy, the outlook for your baby is not all bad. The moral panic about severly disabled 'crack babies' turned out to be unfounded, and, although children exposed to drugs are disadvantaged, they do grow, and many do very well.[11] It may not be the best start in life, but it could still be the start of something good. It's up to you to sort your life out, but one study has found that drug-users who have children are 60% to 80% more likely to stop using drugs than people who don't.[12] You'll never find a better reason to get clean.

Cannabis isn't good for babies either, although its effects are less severe.[13] Studies have shown a link with slightly lower birth weight,[14] with behaviour problems in toddlers (though, strangely, only for girls)[15] and with poorer educational outcomes for teenagers who were exposed to cannabis in the womb.[16] There has also been research which shows no ill effects.[17] Cannabis use in pregnancy has been linked to severe morning sickness.[18]

However bad street drugs are, the effect of tobacco and alcohol addiction on unborn babies is far worse.[19] That's a sobering thought.

Avoid germs

If you have a choice, stay away from people with 'slapped cheek' disease, chickenpox, rubella, measles, mumps, or cytomegalovirus. (If you've already had these infections, you're immune and not at risk.) Malaria, yellow fever, West Nile virus and polio are also to be avoided. If you're having sex with a new partner, use a condom to protect your baby from sexually transmitted infections. *Wash, wash, wash your hands* (particularly after changing nappies), don't share cups and cutlery, and kiss little children on the cheek or forehead, not on the lips.

Don't lift heavy things

You are just all-round stretchier when you're pregnant, so repeatedly lifting heavy objects is not recommended. Or avoidable, if you already have a young child.

If your job involves heavy lifting, your employer should move you to lighter duties.

Not more than ten minutes in a sauna

But hot baths are not a problem.

What about exercise?

It's fine! Do as much as you want to. But, since getting out of bed can be a marathon effort in the first 12 weeks, you're currently excused from PE. See page 148.

The bosoms

Bonus bosoms are another early pregnancy sign. They get bigger, tingly, and can be incredibly sensitive.

I have no way to know for sure, but I think that pregnant breasts are as vulnerable to pain from crushing or hitting as a man's testicles are. And breasts are much larger. And many pregnant women have toddlers to look after, who have hard little knees and elbows, and like to use their mothers as climbing frames. Ouch.

This is not the only way your pregnancy starts to show. Nipples become darker, larger and more clearly defined. A dark stripe of skin, the '*lina nigra*', may show down the middle of your belly. Some women also get darker skin on their face.

The skin on your vulva also changes from pink to dark purple. The medical profession knew this back in Victorian times, but this simple pregnancy test was never widely used, because… you'd have to look! Instead, doctors spent much of the early 20th century injecting animals with pregnant women's urine and slaughtering them to study their internal organs, which was more morally acceptable.

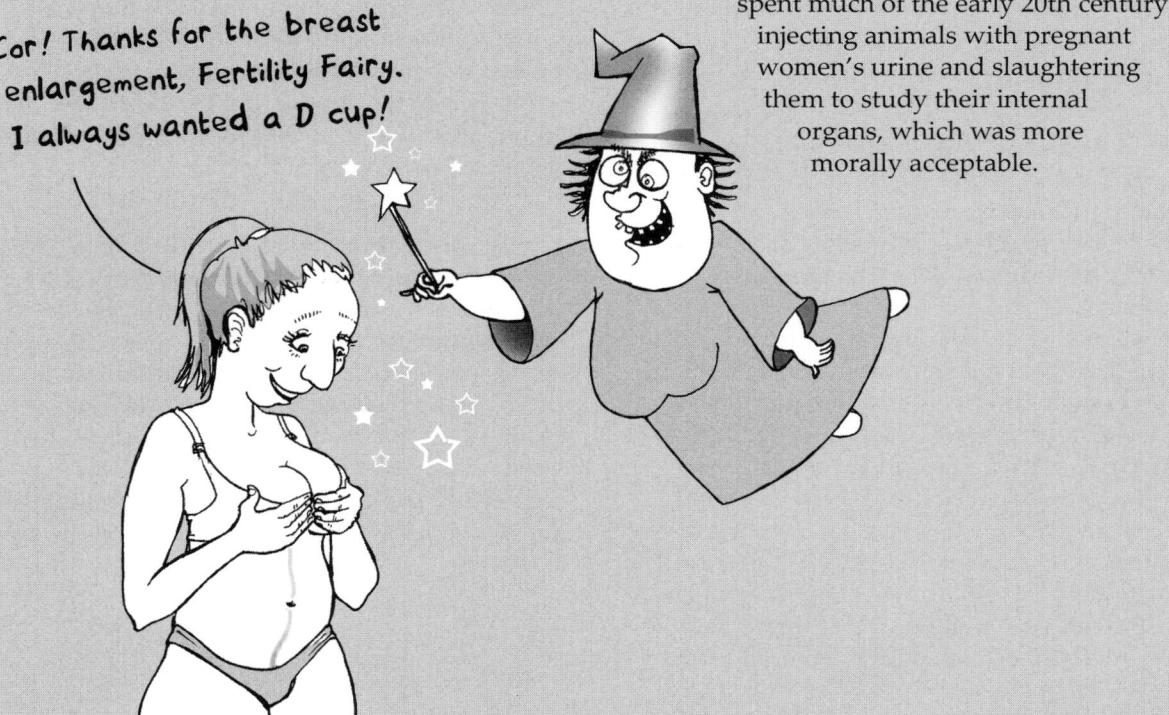

Cor! Thanks for the breast enlargement, Fertility Fairy. I always wanted a D cup!

The juices

Too Much Information warning: read on at your own risk…

Unsurprisingly, with all that oestrogen and progesterone rushing around your system, your cervical juices go into overdrive. A thick plug forms across your cervix, which nothing, I mean nothing, is going to swim past. And you also get a steady dampness of whitish, unslippery juice. If you're paranoid about getting your period, or desperately wishing you would, early pregnancy involves a lot of rushing to the bathroom to check that you haven't come on.

While we're on the subject of intimate details, can you have a shag? Is it safe? Yes! It is! If you're having sex with a man, his semen contains hormones that actually help maintain the pregnancy. And, whoever you're having sex with (including yourself!), orgasm increases blood flow to the womb, which is good for the baby. Post-orgasmic endorphins cross the placenta and make your baby feel nice too.

Lovemaking is not going to harm a healthy foetus. The only time your midwife might advise you to abstain from sex is if your waters have broken, if your cervix is dilated (opened up) or if you have had premature labour pains.

Some women really enjoy sex in pregnancy. They no longer have to worry about trying to get pregnant, or trying to avoid getting pregnant. The extra blood flow to their vital organs, and a good mix of pregnancy hormones, give their sex drive a zing. Others feel fat and sore, too tired at night, and too sick in the morning (top tip – try in the afternoon). Although it's very juicy down there,

it's infertile juice, which is not as slippery and fun as fertile juice. Pregnant women are also prone to thrush – suspect this if your vagina feels itchy or sore.

- Using a sexual lubricant which contains grapefruit seed extract could counteract mild thrush, and might revitalise your love life. Try ordering 'Probe Light' lube from Sh! women's sex shop online.
- Eating unsweetened live yoghurt, raw garlic or a probiotic health food supplement could help with thrush.
- Try cutting out sugar and fruit juice from your diet.
- Don't wear nylon tights, and choose loose-fitting cotton underwear.
- You can buy creams and pessaries to treat thrush from your chemist, but don't take oral tablets of fluconazole to treat it, as these are not safe to use in pregnancy.
- Your partner may need to be treated too.

If your partner is acting as if you're under an obligation to provide him* with sex, and you can't or don't want to, then he needs to rethink his priorities. He can take care of his own sexual needs, can't he? He has hands! You can still be close, and not have sex. A relationship is about intimacy, not just bonking. The important thing is that you communicate about how you are feeling, and spend time together having fun. You're going to be parents, so you'll need to work as a team.

---

* I think it's fair to assume that this is a particularly masculine model of entitlement to, and expectation of, female sexual availability.

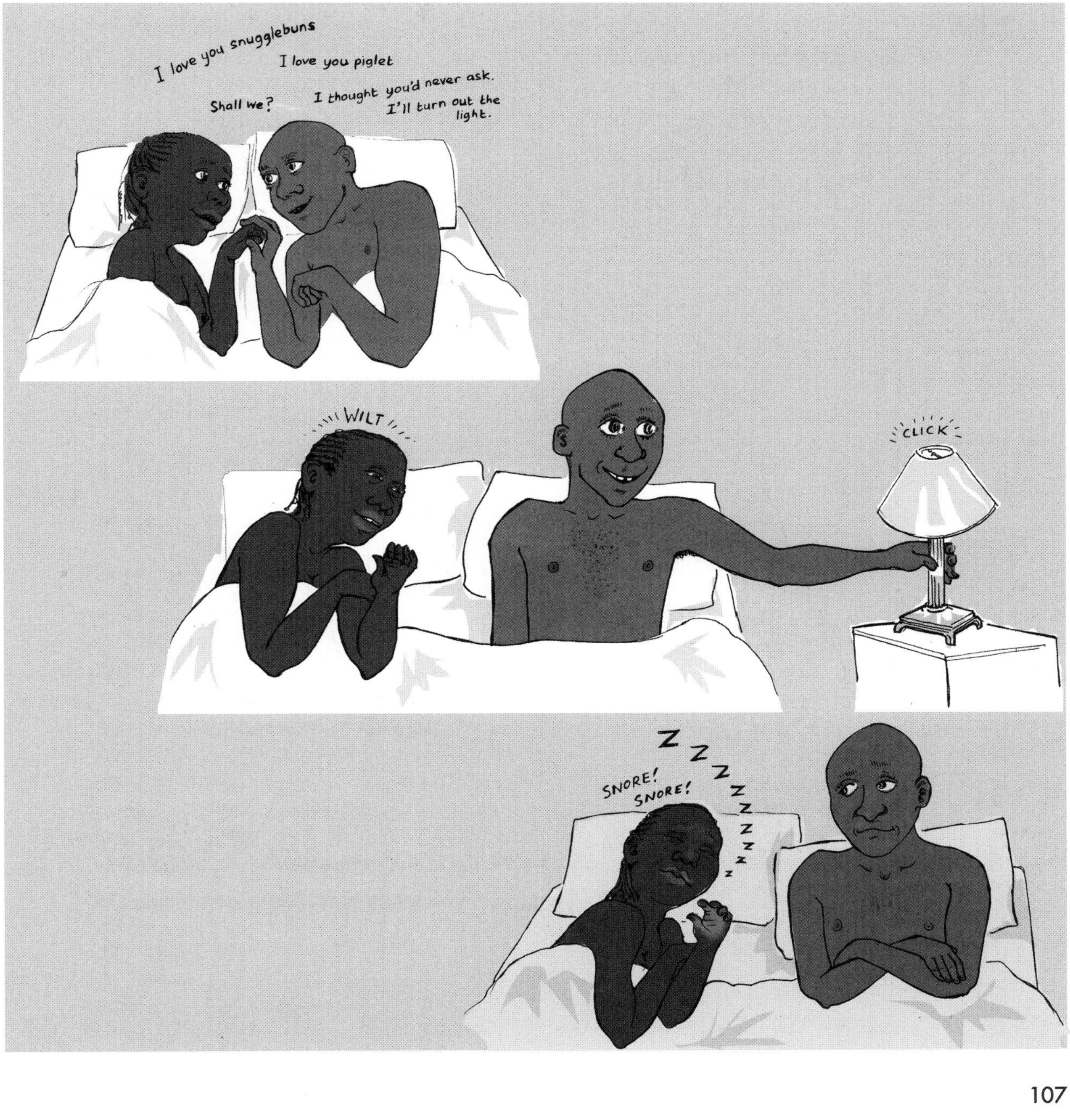
I love you snugglebuns
I love you piglet
Shall we?
I thought you'd never ask.
I'll turn out the light.
WILT
CLICK
SNORE!
SNORE!
Z Z Z Z Z Z Z Z

The sleeping

Apparently, some women sail through pregnancy without any appreciable drop in their energy levels, gaily getting things done. And there are women who find in pregnancy a source of untapped creative inspiration that they channel into writing novels, or other mammoth projects.

I was not one of those women.

Quite possibly, you're not either.

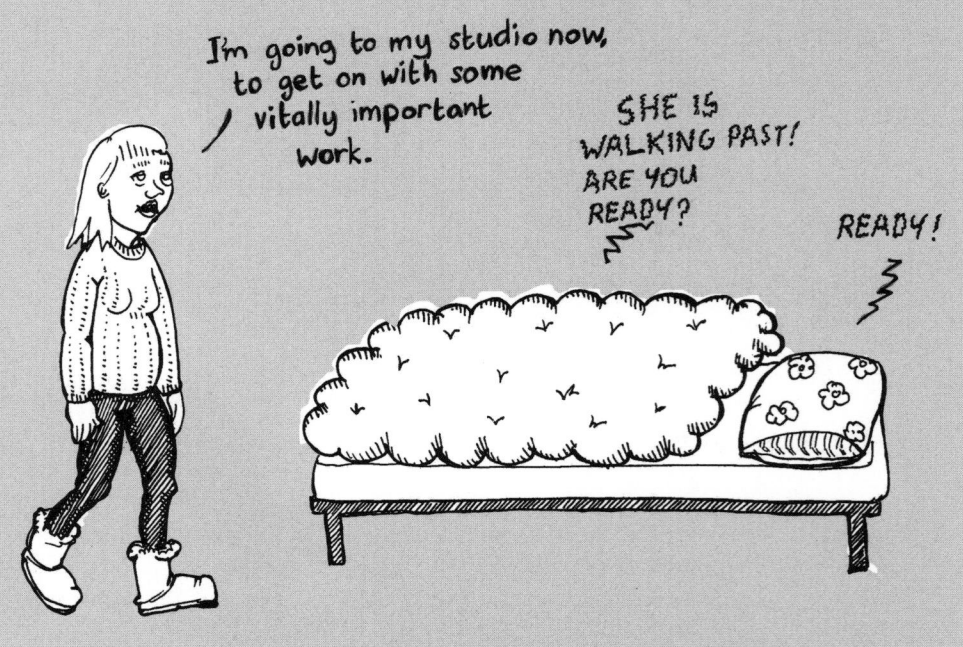

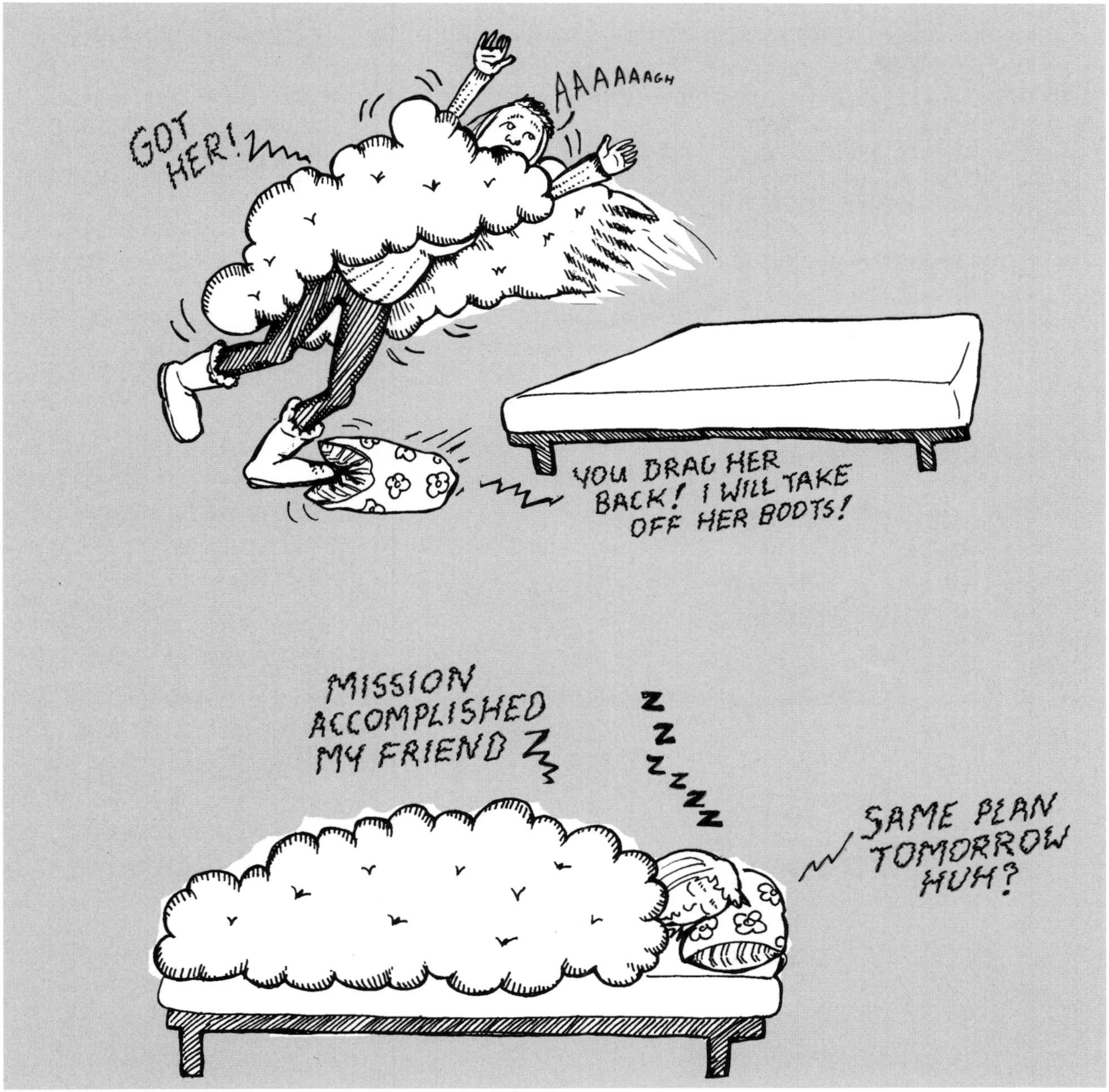
AAAAAAGH
GOT HER!
YOU DRAG HER BACK! I WILL TAKE OFF HER BOOTS!
MISSION ACCOMPLISHED MY FRIEND
ZZZZZZ
SAME PLAN TOMORROW HUH?

I'm not denigrating women's abilities if I say that pregnant women can find it difficult to get stuff done. In fact, the opposite is true. In the ten weeks following conception a woman takes a single cell and transforms it into an entire, miniature human being. In the following 30 weeks (or so), she incubates it to sleek, fully functioning perfection. This is a job in itself. No one else can do it. Men can't do it; it can't be done in test-tubes, in labs. So, any time you feel like you're not getting stuff done when you're pregnant, remind yourself that you are. You're creating a person. Technically, anything else is multitasking.

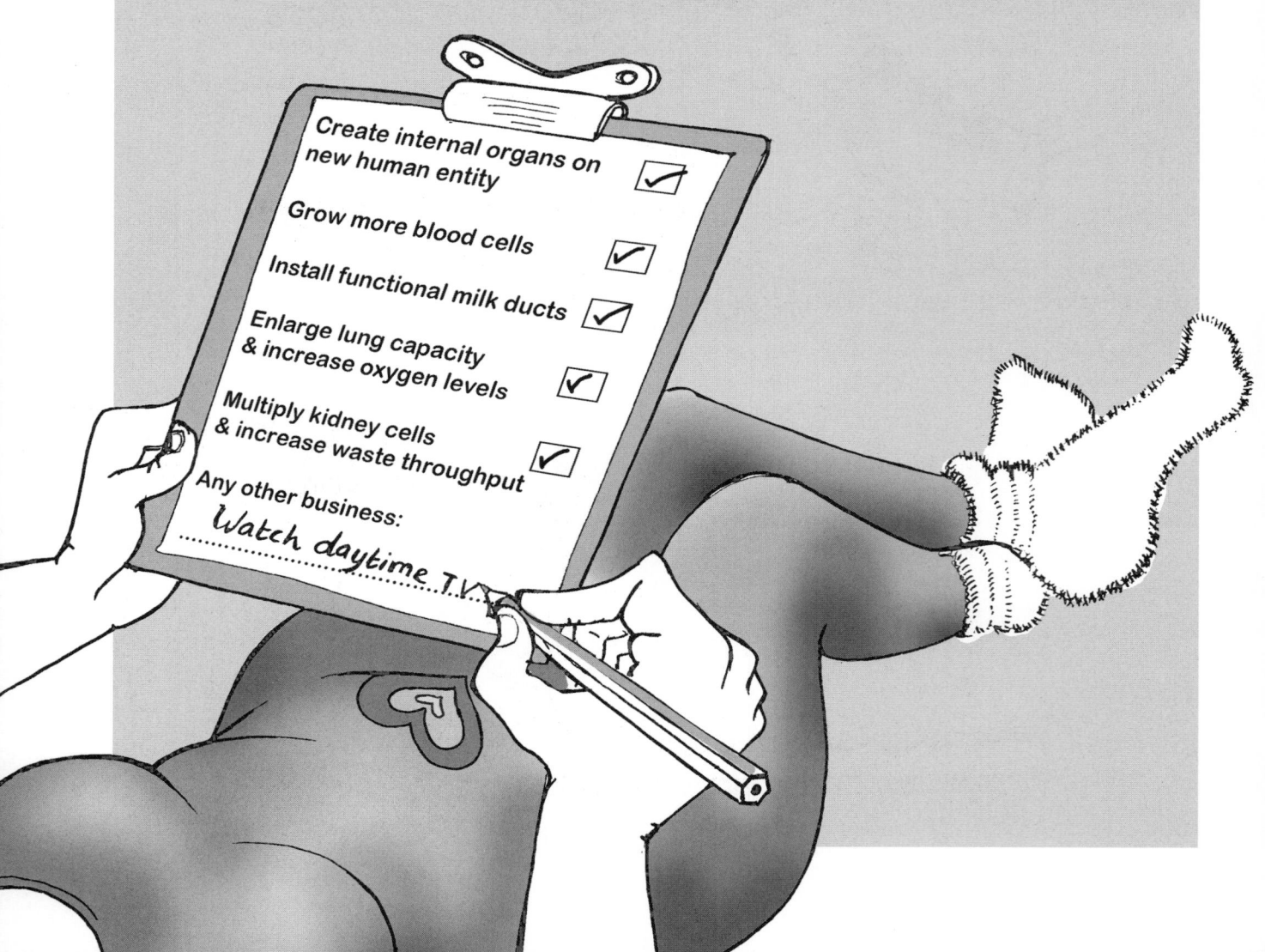

Create internal organs on new human entity ✓

Grow more blood cells ✓

Install functional milk ducts ✓

Enlarge lung capacity & increase oxygen levels ✓

Multiply kidney cells & increase waste throughput ✓

Any other business:
Watch daytime T.V.

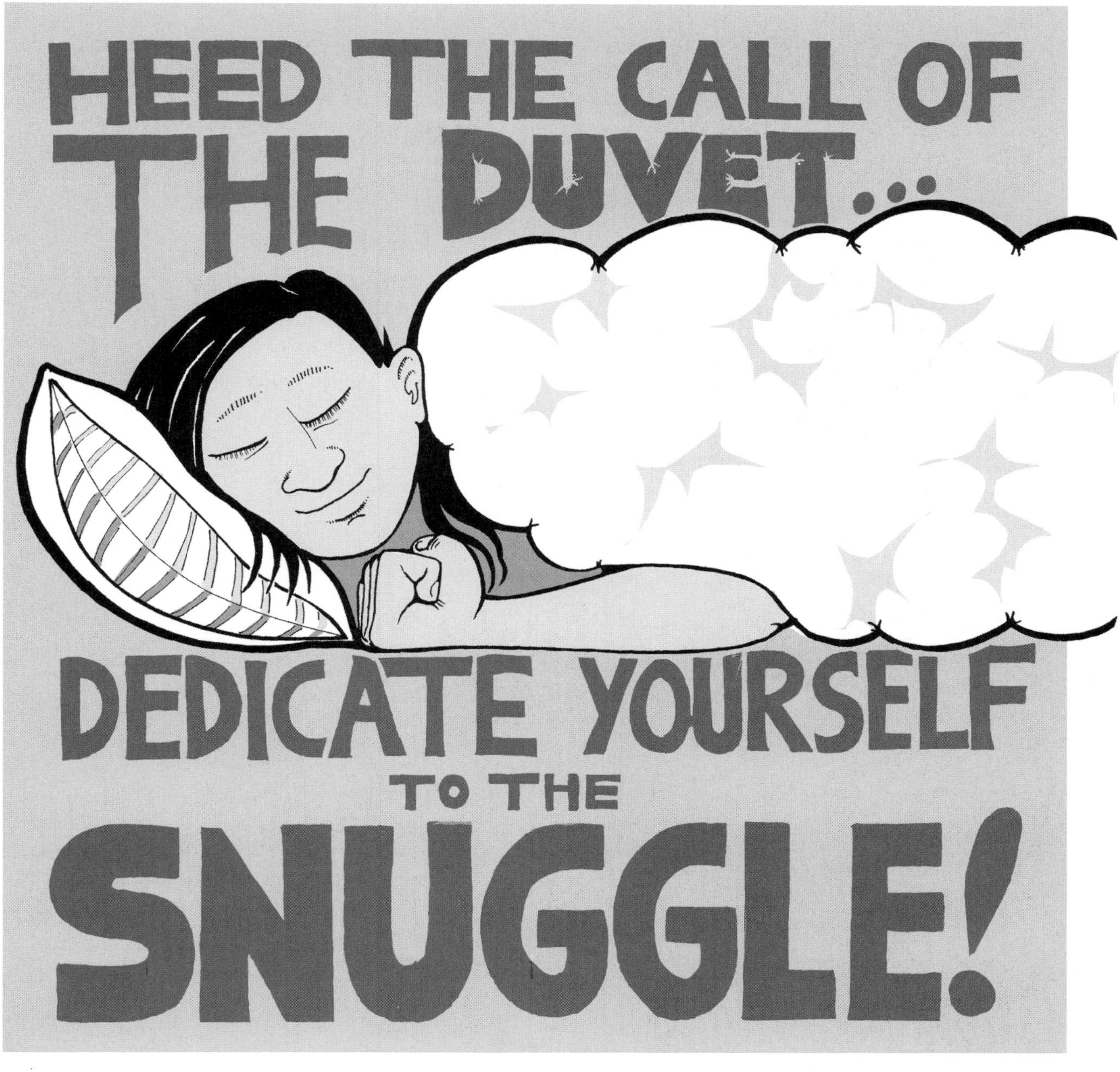
HEED THE CALL OF
THE DUVET...
DEDICATE YOURSELF
TO THE
SNUGGLE!

The waking

You're only a few weeks pregnant, but already your body forces you to get up in the middle of the night, to go for a wee.

It's as if you're in training for something…

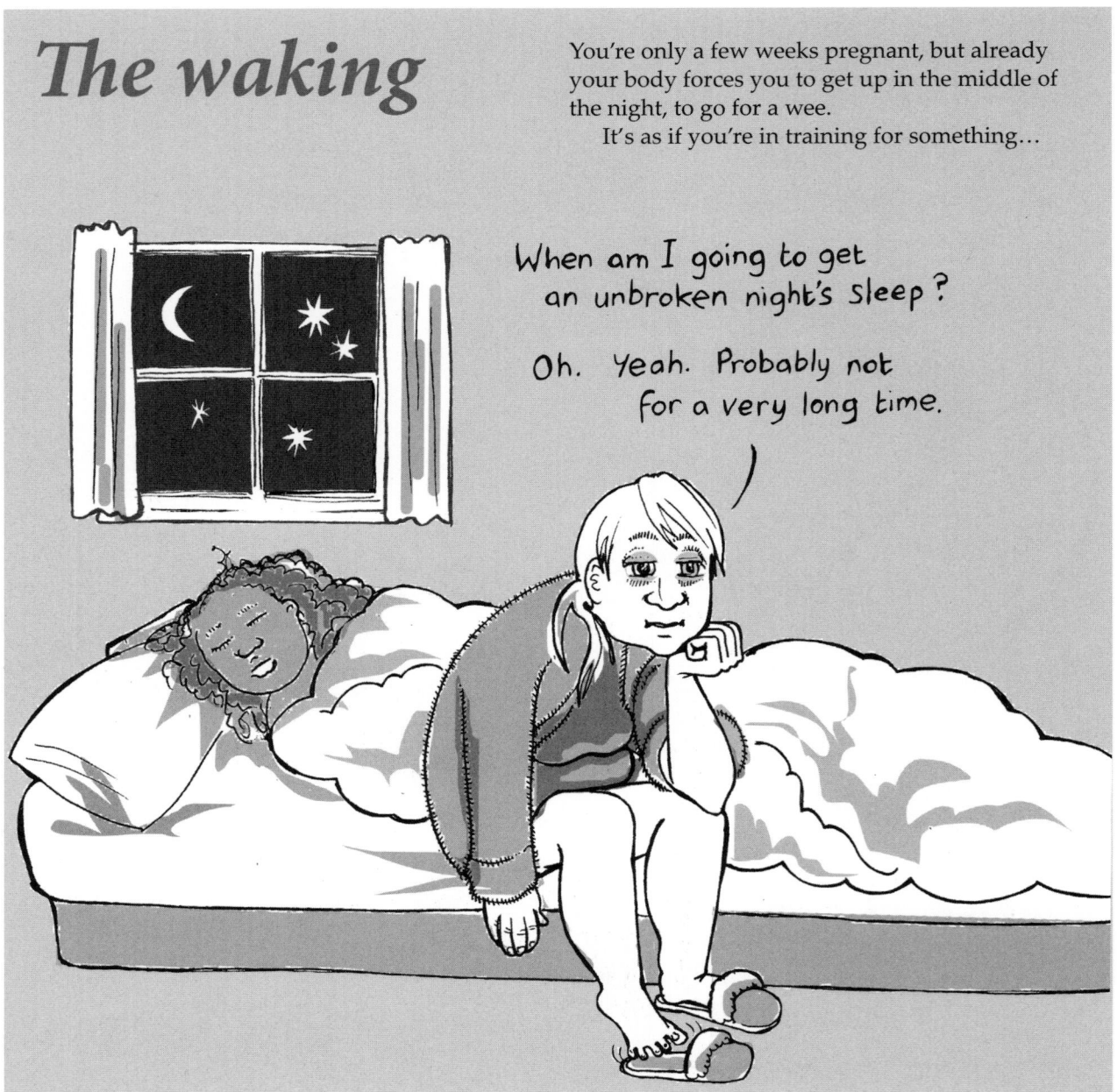

When am I going to get an unbroken night's sleep?

Oh. Yeah. Probably not for a very long time.

The fog

It's not just that you're tired. Your brain does actually work differently when you're pregnant.

Your brain is the one thing that doesn't get larger in pregnancy. It actually gets very slightly smaller, but don't worry, it all grows back by the time the baby's six months old.[20]

You might forget what you're saying midway through a sentence, fluff text messages or spell things wrong. Pregnant women tend to score less well on tests of verbal recall. They can also suffer from short-term memory deficits.[21] It can feel as if a kind of fog has descended on your mind:

'What did you do last Thursday?' You have absolutely no idea. What's a Thursday?

This doesn't mean that you become more stupid. Being responsible for the survival of a small baby is the most enduring mentally taxing activity that any human being undertakes: once the baby gets here, you don't get any time off from being a mother. The multiple tasks of baby-monitoring that new mums do involve a kind of extra-sensory hypervigilance, and pregnancy gears your brain up for that.

So your working memory, the part of your intelligence that processes multiple pieces of information, remains just as good. As does your spatial memory. Your ability to read emotions actually improves,[22] and you may become more unflappable in potentially stressful situations.[23]

When you concentrate on the task in hand, your performance is undiminished. Right now, there are pregnant brain surgeons doing neuro-surgery and pregnant pilots landing planes. But you might be wise to invest in a diary or a calendar on your phone to help you remember what's happening next week.

Once again, I wasn't sure if the cause of feminism was best served by discussing the biological changes that occur in pregnant women's brains. The history of feminism has centred around proving that women are as good as men in the workplace, and, to do this, we have minimised biological differences between the sexes. Many women in employment are scared – with reason – that their pregnancy and impending motherhood will be viewed as an inconvenience by their employer and their career prospects will be harmed.* Maybe it's best if their boss doesn't know that their brain has just shrunk!

You dedicate your time and energy to your employer, and they make money from your efforts. They should be grateful that you work for them, not the other way around. Best managerial practice is for employers to treat employees like human beings, not robots: staff loyalty and performance improve if they do. That's why we need more women in managerial positions. You, with your enhanced emotional recognition skills and unflappable attitude – you'd be a good person to promote.

I find another useful tool for feminist analysis is to ask the question 'What would it be like if men could…?' about any given area of sexual difference. Like, if men menstruated, the working month would include a five-day 'period leave' where they would retire to menstrual massage clinics for pampering. If men could lactate, breastfeeding would be an Olympic sport. And if men could get pregnant? Just imagine! Men regularly elevate the humble cold to flu status. They wouldn't be trying to pretend that pregnancy doesn't affect them and that they don't need special treatment.

The job of feminism isn't to prove that women are 'as good as' men; it's to enable men to see the worth of women.

---

* Maternity Action are very helpful for negotiating your employment rights in pregnancy and beyond.

The first appointment

Positive pregnancy test? Better get some antenatal medical care. You don't have to visit your doctor (unless you want to). You can refer yourself straight to the midwives, the experts in pregnancy and birth.

Ideally, you will see the same midwife all the way through your pregnancy, you build a personal relationship with her, and she'll be the person who will help you give birth. This is the best way to ensure that your medical needs are monitored and your emotional requirements met.

The NHS isn't currently organised like this, although it could be! This is called caseload midwifery, you can request it, and there's more information about it on page 263. If you don't get it, you will see quite a few different midwives at your antenatal appointments. And so you can discover that there are a lot of exceptionally cool people doing midwifery. Antenatal appointments are a very good thing to go to. You have a legal right to time off work to attend them.

To start off your maternity notes, your midwife or doctor will ask you the date of your last menstrual period, take out a little round cardboard wheel and do some calculations. They will then announce how many weeks pregnant you are, and give you your due date – the day you can expect your baby to be born.

Except it won't, and you can't.

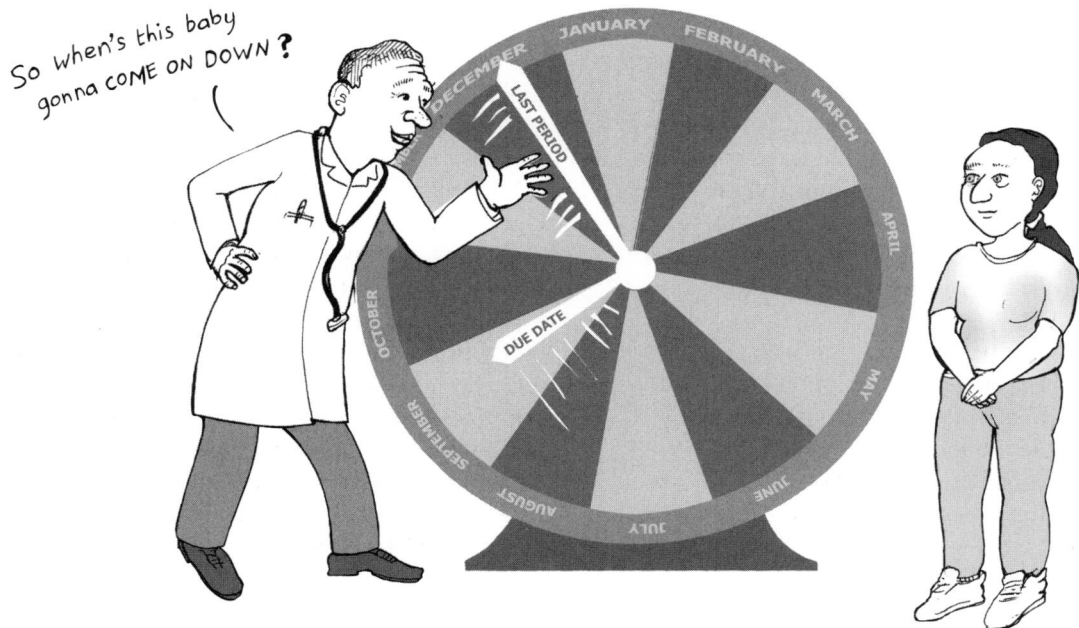

They might as well pull out a crystal ball and gaze into it. Nobody, not even respected members of the medical profession, can predict the future.

Your 'due date' is based on two assumptions. The first is that babies take exactly 38 weeks to grow from conception to fully cooked. In reality, growing a baby, like everything else in nature, is subject to natural variation. Some come out earlier. Many are happy to stay in a little longer. You're not in control of this, and neither is your doctor.

Do not go home and put a big red X through 'September 20th' (or whatever day they said). Instead, draw a red line all the way from two weeks before that date to three weeks after. And when people ask you your due date, tell them 'September, or maybe October' and leave it at that. If your pregnancy lasts longer than your 'due date', the last thing you want is people phoning you every day from September 21st saying 'Haven't you had it yet?'

There is another assumption at work here – that you conceived the baby two weeks after your last period started. As you'll know, if you've read page 39 of this book, that's simply not true for many women. If your menstrual cycles were irregular, or very long, you could have ovulated several weeks or even months later. When doctors used to insist on artificial induction of every labour at 40 weeks past the last menstrual period, a significant number of babies were born premature.

And what if what you thought was your last period wasn't true menstruation? If it was implantation bleeding, or bleeding in early pregnancy, your 'due date' will be wrong as well, although too late rather than too early.

If you know the date you conceived your baby, and it wasn't two weeks after your last menstrual period, you have two choices. You can tell the doctor or midwife the date of conception, and ask them to adjust their figures. This will work best if you can show them a fertility chart with ovulation and intercourse marked on it, preferably with some temperatures on too. Doctors like charts. You are taking a risk, though, that they will believe you over the 'Pregnancy-lasts-for-40-weeks-dated-from-the-last-menstrual-period' mantra that they learned at medical school.

So your other option is to work out when you conceived, count backwards 14 days, and tell them that's when your last period was. They're never going to know any different.

Can't remember when your last period was? You're not alone. The other method that the medical profession use to calculate your 'due date' is a 12-week dating scan. The theory is that all 12- week embryos are developmentally identical, and an ultrasound scan at that point can precisely date your pregnancy. Of course, in reality, not every embryo does grow at the same rate, and not every ultrasound machine is high-quality, and not every sonographer is experienced. Still, that's the due date that gets entered on your records.

Your midwife will then ask to check your height and weight and blood pressure. If having your blood pressure taken makes you feel stressed, tell her this – it's a phenomenon known as 'white coat hypertension'. She will sensitively ask about previous pregnancies, medical history and lifestyle. She will offer to test a sample of your blood for some infections that could affect your baby. If you have had mental health issues or are in an abusive relationship, your midwife can get you extra help. If you have been circumcised and infibulated, you can be referred to a specialist midwife to help with your options in childbirth.

And you'll be offered screening tests to see if your baby has thalassaemia, sickle-cell disease if your ethnicity makes it likely, or Down's Syndrome.

The field of prenatal screening has seen some recent major advances, so there is now a more accurate blood test for Down's Syndrome, which doesn't carry a risk of miscarriage. The potential is there for a whole range of genetic conditions to be detected in early pregnancy. This will increase the dilemmas faced by parents-to-be.

Because what do you do if you get a positive result? Once you know your baby has something that is genetically or chromosomally undesirable, do you necessarily terminate the pregnancy? The language of testing suggests that it's possible to 'screen' out undesirable conditions from the general population. But many of these are wanted, longed-for and loved potential babies. The assumption that you test and then you terminate underestimates how psychologically devastating it can be to lose a child that you desperately want.

Some genetic conditions are inherited, so any subsequent children you have could also be affected. It's possible to have IVF treatment and screen embyros before implantation to find ones that are defect-free, but this has a poor success rate and is incredibly expensive. So do you keep trying? And keep testing? And, potentially, keep terminating? It's a really tough situation for the parents. Once we can easily analyse unborn babies' DNA, where are the ethical limits? Say they develop a test for deafness. Would parents terminate for that? But deaf people aren't disabled if everyone learns sign language.

I'll declare my hand here. My nephew has Down's Syndrome. Maybe that makes me an expert, or maybe it makes me biased. But I'm not alone in finding Down's can be an unexpected blessing rather than a curse. One study[24] of people with Down's found that 99% of their parents loved them and 79% of parents felt their outlook on life was more positive because of their child; 94% of siblings were proud of them and 88% felt they were better people because of their relative; 99% of people with Down's were happy; and 96% liked the way they look. Check out that last statistic! Ninety-six per cent of us people with 'Normal Syndrome' don't enjoy that level of self-confidence.

Having said that, it's good that pre-natal diagnoses exist, because some parents do want to know and, however difficult it is for them, they make the best decision for their circumstances. I just want you to remember that the choices are for you to make, not the medical profession.

Ultrasound scans are also not compulsory, although many women like having them. Surprisingly, their safety in pregnancy has never been conclusively established.

Antenatal care is truly a pick-your-own-adventure scenario. You are being offered medical care and you can choose what to accept. You can ask for more information about the risks and benefits of any given procedure, and take your time to make up your mind. As we'll discover when we get to the birth chapter, hospitals develop protocols for treatment where they group people together according to 'risk factors'. But you are an individual, not a statistic, and you can ask to be treated as one.

You'll be given your notes to take home, read if you want to, and bring back at every appointment, which is great, because it puts you in control of your care.

And there's one more question you should be asked:

So, where do you want to have the baby? At home or in hospital?

What?!! I can't think about having a baby! I've only just got my head round the fact that I'm pregnant!

The reality

There's a baby in there. Even though it's only a little bean of a baby at the moment, it's still a freaky thought – you're carrying *someone else* inside your tummy. When other people get pregnant, it seems the most natural thing in the world. But when it's you? And there is actually *somebody inside you*? Weird.

Maybe that's why we get doped up on chill-out pregnancy hormones – so we don't think about it too hard.

What is your baby like? Do you have an idea? Do you get flashes of insight into its character? Boy or girl? Are you really hoping for one or the other? Don't worry though, you can't be disappointed, because parenthood's a profound lesson in loving what you get. What about names? Are you mulling over a shortlist?

Maybe you're not. Perhaps you're very pragmatic, or distracted, or determined not to think about all this just yet.

Do you suddenly see babies everywhere you go? Have you ever held a baby? Sniffed a baby – inhaled that sweet smell of new baby at the back of its fat neck? Are you scared of babies?

You don't discuss these kinds of things at antenatal appointments. In our culture, the social rituals that accompany pregnancy centre around medical care and, later on, shopping for the new arrival. It's all very practical – it's about blood tests and ultrasound scans, then different makes of car seats and pushchairs. We don't explore the philosophical, emotional or spiritual ramifications of pregnancy. That's not very British.

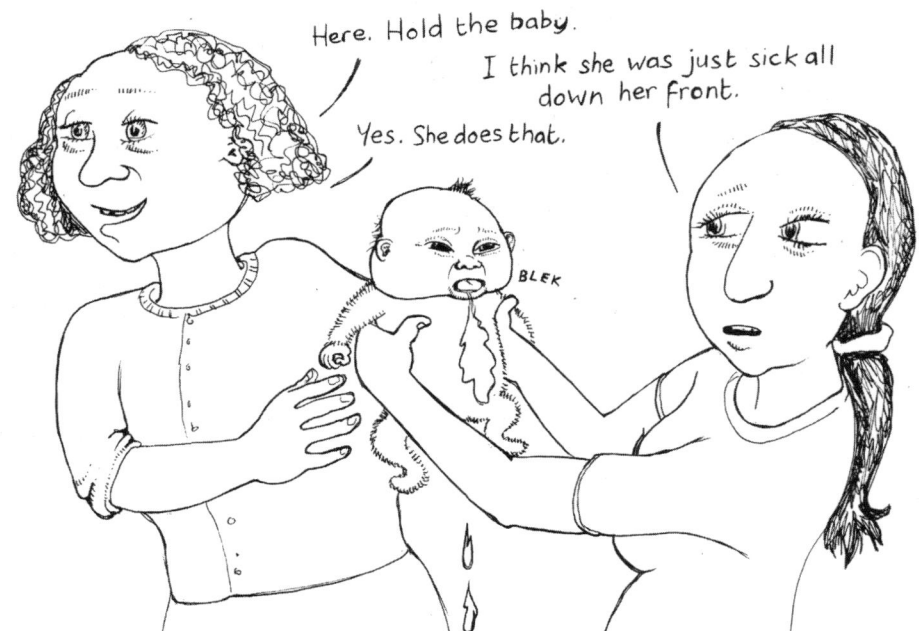

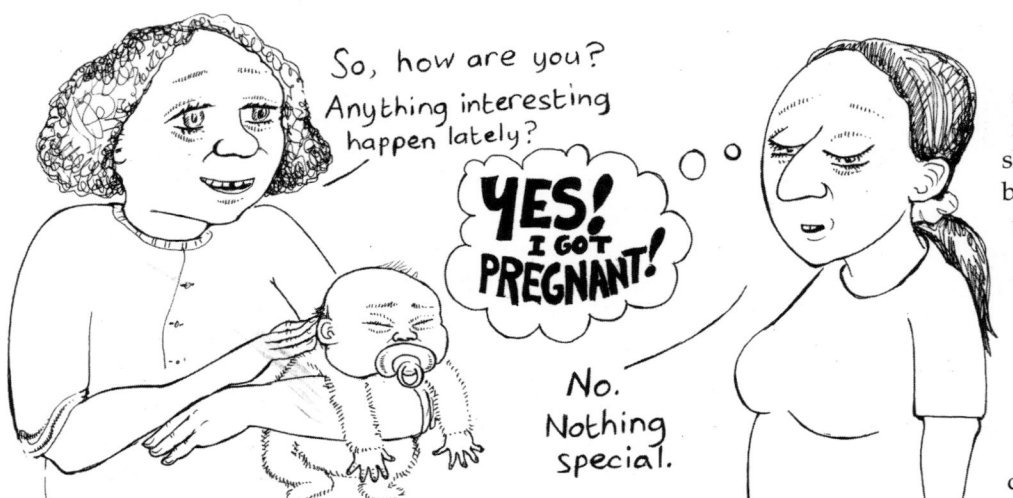

So, how are you? Anything interesting happen lately?

YES! I GOT PREGNANT!

No. Nothing special.

The secrecy

It's a big deal, finding out that you're pregnant. The prospect of parenthood can be wildly exciting, or terrifying, or both. And it's a big deal being pregnant. Your body changes dramatically well before your bump starts to show, and you may find that your mind does a bit too. The first 12 weeks of pregnancy is the part where you do the hard work of creating the baby – it's exhausting and all encompassing.

Yet there is a conspiracy of silence around early pregnancy. Shh! Don't tell! When you do tell people, they reply, 'Ooh. Early days!' As though you're *not really pregnant* until the magic 12-week mark has passed, and the risk of miscarriage has receded.

Why is this? Why the secrecy? Why the shame?

Of course some women may not want to share details of their personal life, and I'm not suggesting that women should be obliged broadcast the news that they're pregnant, particularly when, sadly, they may not get a supportive, positive reception. But neither should pregnant women be sworn to silence for the first three months. It doesn't serve their best interests, or their baby's.

On a practical level, the foetus is most sensitive to environmental toxins during the period when its internal organs are forming. Routine heavy lifting is to be avoided where possible. So employers should prioritise the safety of pregnant women from day one, and not wait for the visible later stages of pregnancy.

On an emotional level, women are encouraged not to announce they are pregnant in case they miscarry. This is superstitious nonsense. You're not going to jinx the pregnancy if you talk about it! For women who do miscarry, society's refusal to recognise the validity of early pregnancy compounds their loss and their grief. You and your partner will find it much harder to come to terms with losing a baby if no one else knew you were carrying it.

So tell your good friends and family that you're pregnant. Sure, before 12 weeks there is still a risk you could miscarry, but in that tragic event, you will need their help and their love.

Unfortunately, you will have to use your judgement as to when to tell your employer. If you work in a supportive environment, where staff are valued, then it's information that they need to know straight away. If only all workplaces were like that.

The support

There was an assumption made, on the previous page, that, when your family and friends find out that you are pregnant, they will be loving and supportive. Of course, that's not necessarily the case…

Your friends

You can divide your female friends into those who have already had babies, and those who haven't.

The first set are more useful. They offer you snacks and tell you to put your feet up, and cluck over you, and get excited on your behalf. They are a potentially useful source of free baby clothes and accessories, and a fount of unsolicited advice.

Your friends who haven't been pregnant yet might be a bit bewildered by you. Why are you crying? Fools! You need to eat something, and they haven't offered you any biscuits! Of course you're crying! They're lucky you haven't stabbed them.

It's hard being the first person in a circle of friends to get pregnant, traipsing soberly around nightclubs and trying to go to sleep on the tables. It's no fun at all. In time, your friends will catch you up. They'll get pregnant in turn, and then you can cluck over them, and offer them snacks, and get excited on their behalf, and jovially remind them how useless they were back when you were expecting.

A friend who is struggling to get pregnant, or who suffers a miscarriage or stillbirth, needs special treatment. Don't cut her out of your life. It is hard enough for her, being cruelly left out of the motherhood club, without her losing her old friends too. Stay in touch with her and *ask her how she is feeling* – that simple question, sincerely asked, can be enough to bridge the gulf between you. Don't automatically show her your scan pictures, or photos of the birth – first consider whether she wants to see them. Make your friendship about you, and her, and not just about your baby – in time, she can forge her own relationship with your child. Your friendship can survive this, if you show sensitivity and tact.

There is one sort of friend you should actively avoid when you're pregnant. It's the one who has had a child and is keen to tell you all about the most horrendous aspects of their birth. You don't need to hear this. You're not them. You're not having their baby. Every birth is different. This is a useful posture to adopt in this situation:

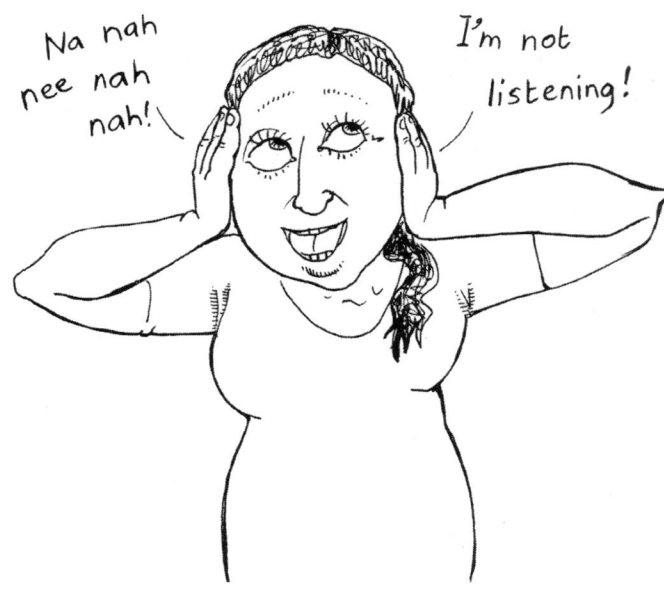

121

Your mother

Ideally, you would be able to turn to your mum for advice and practical help. She would share your joy and embrace the role of grandmother. It's a very special thing to raise a daughter, and for her to go on to raise a child herself.

However, this is a major readjustment in your respective roles, and it isn't always easy. You are vulnerable and supersensitive: if your mother is unsupportive, things can be very difficult.

Is this not what she wanted for you? Did she want you to further your education or career before getting pregnant? Maybe this is a reflection of her own sense of self-worth, and the career opportunities she had, or missed out on. You may need to gently explain that you're living your own life, not hers.

Does she think she's too young to be a grandma? Is she worried about getting old? Our society values older women less than younger ones, because it's all about beauty, not brains.

Perhaps, on some level, she's scared for you because she struggled with traumatic experiences or undiagnosed post-natal depression when she had children herself. Still, once again, this is your life, not hers.

Does she dislike your partner? Maybe she has reason to (see the next section). Or she could be reacting out of classist, homophobic or racist prejudice, in which case she can go and stuff herself. If she wants the privilege of being a grandmother, she had better sort out her attitude.

Some women internalise repressive cultural expectations of absolute female obedience, and then attempt to control their children's reproductive choices accordingly. If this is your mum, remember that women like you have successfully rebelled against this kind of parental pressure. Find them. They can help you come to terms with this.

Becoming a mother throws the issue of your own parenting into sharp focus. Counselling can help.

Your partner

Let's talk about what a healthy relationship is like.

A non-abusive partner:

* listens to you;
* encourages you;
* makes you feel good about yourself;
* calls you by your name;
* communicates honestly with you;
* likes your friends;
* is pleasant to your family;
* is faithful;
* aims to please you sexually;
* shares household chores.

It's not a lot to ask.

An abusive partner:

* threatens you;
* controls you;
* blames you;
* never admits that he's in the wrong;
* tells you you're stupid;
* tells you you're ugly;
* calls you a derogatory nickname or refers to you as 'babe' or 'darling' or 'the wife';
* stops you from seeing friends and family;
* aims to please himself sexually (abusers are overwhelmingly, but not exclusively, male);
* may be unfaithful;
* is certainly dishonest.

Do you feel anxious? Walking on eggshells? Worried you're about to do something wrong at any moment? Are you subjected to unpredictable outbursts of rage? And then tender, tearful reconciliations? You can be being abused even if your partner has never physically hurt you. And now you are pregnant, you are vulnerable, and you are more likely to be attacked.

It can be very hard to recognise abuse for what it is, because when the person you're in love with dedicates their energy to manipulating your thoughts, actions and emotions, they very often succeed. Abusive people can be charming, powerful and charismatic. They come in every colour, social class and sexuality.

We're not helped by books and movies that romanticise arrogant, emotionally unavailable men, which blame women for being victims ('It takes two to tango!' 'You must have done something to provoke this.') and which promise that dysfunctional behaviour can be 'cured' by the love of a good woman. If there is a positive future for your relationship, 'more love' from you will not bring it about.

It's not you – it's him.You're trying; he's abusing. (Substitute 'she' if appropriate. Lesbians can replicate dysfunctional gender roles.) You both need insight into your partner's destructive patterns of behaviour, and he (or she) will need to completely revise the way they interact with you. Properly. Not just enough to persuade you that it's all OK now and wheedle their way back into your life.

You're pregnant. This isn't a good time to have to contemplate ending your relationship, but, if your partner is incapable of treating you with love and respect, they will not be an equal, fair and appropriate parent. Maybe you can cope with your partner's abuse, but will you be able to protect your child? Single parenthood is daunting, but staying in a relationship that is corrosive can be worse. If your baby shares your partner's DNA, that fact alone doesn't give him parental rights. Parenting is about investing love and effort in a child, not genetics.

Having said that, this is a decision that only you can make, and not all women choose to leave. Services to help victims of domestic violence are there for you whatever you decide.

Whether you stay or leave, you need to take steps to increase your safety. This is serious. Two women a week in the UK are killed by their male partners or ex-partners.

Tell your midwife you are being abused. Read the books *Living with the Dominator* by Pat Craven, and *Why does he do that?* by Lundy Bancroft. Contact Women's Aid, which works with women of every age, class, ethnicity and sexual orientation. There is help available. Take it.

PICK YOUR OWN ADVENTURE MOMENT!

Are you happy?
Are you healthy?
Is everything going well?

NO →

↓ **YES**

DON'T READ THE NEXT CHAPTER!

It's about losing the baby,
by accident, or design.

Fear of your baby dying is primal and pervasive: pregnant women and new mothers are haunted by it. You really don't need to read about losing babies if it's not happening to you, and the next 14 pages are likely to make you upset. *So please skip them.*

Turn to page 140.

NOW!

Do you want to
have a baby?

NO

I don't know

If you don't want to give birth to or raise a child, you don't have to. The next section discusses the ethics, the practicalities and some feelings surrounding abortion and adoption.

YES

If you desperately don't want to lose your baby but might suffer miscarriage or stillbirth, turn to page 130.

This section is also for parents who terminate a pregnancy in difficult circumstances, because it's about grieving for someone you loved, who didn't get to live.

6 Lost (1): Abortion and Adoption

If you're pregnant, and you don't know whether you want to be, you're not alone. Nearly half of all pregnancies in the UK are unintended[1] – 'mistimed' or completely unplanned. Forget whatever ideas you might have about 'what sort' of girl gets herself knocked up accidentally. Women get pregnant when they are using contraception. Women get pregnant against their will. Single women get pregnant, married women get pregnant, older, younger, black, white, mainly straight, but some gay – they all face the same dilemma. And then there are planned pregnancies that go wrong, where a change of circumstances forces a woman to reconsider her future.

Your choices are: motherhood, abortion or adoption. Sometimes it's easy to decide – you know you just *can't* continue with the pregnancy, or on the other hand, there's *no way* you would give up your child. Sometimes it's very difficult.

Abortion

Abortion is readily available. Around a fifth of all pregnancies are terminated every year in the UK.[2] It is a straightforward procedure[3] which, although not entirely risk-free (no operation is), carries far fewer risks to your health than carrying a baby to term.[4]

Abortion does not cause cancer.[5] It will not make you infertile, and is extremely unlikely to cause complications in a subsequent pregnancy.[6]

In Britain, you shouldn't have to pay. Your GP should refer you for NHS services, and may also be able to arrange an NHS-funded abortion at a private clinic. Your doctor will keep your decision confidential. If you are under 16 and you don't want to tell your parents, they can't force you to.

If your GP is ethically opposed to abortion, they have to refer you to another doctor who will help.

It is possible to access an abortion up until you are 24 weeks pregnant, but the earlier in the pregnancy it is carried out, the lower the risk of complications.

There are two methods: medical (using drugs) or surgical (an operation).

Medical abortion

For this procedure, you are given two drugs. First, a tablet of mifepristone, 'the abortion pill', ends the pregnancy, by blocking the action of progesterone in your body. Some time later, possibly at home, a pessary of misoprostol is placed in the vagina, which causes heavy cramps and bleeding. Essentially, these drugs cause miscarriage, which is an experience that is not at all like a heavy period: the blood loss is more dramatic and the pain is more intense.

If your pregnancy is more advanced than eight weeks you will deliver a tiny but possibly recognisable baby, so be mentally prepared for this. Medical abortion doesn't carry the very small risk of uterine injury that a surgical abortion does. It is the preferred method for women who are less than seven weeks pregnant.

Surgical abortion

If you are less than 14 weeks pregnant, this can be done under 'local anaesthetic'. You are awake throughout the experience and it will probably hurt a lot. I'm just being honest! They kinda downplay the pain side of it in the literature. On the plus side, it is a hundred quid cheaper than an abortion under general anaesthetic, and you can drive yourself home afterwards.

Otherwise, your option is surgery under general anaesthetic, which is the one I would recommend. You can wake up afterwards, and this whole pregnancy thing can just have been like a bad dream.

You will probably bleed for a few days or weeks after an abortion. Use pads, not tampons. It shouldn't be heavier than a normal period, or smell strange.

Abortion issues

There are people who disagree with my opinion that abortion is a morally acceptable outcome for an unwanted pregnancy. This is a human life that is being terminated, and therefore abortion is murder. This might be your sincerely held belief.

It is interesting to compare this to the issue of vegetarianism. A comparable percentage of the British population are vegetarian as are pro-life. Eating animal products causes avoidable suffering. Meat is murder too.

Having an opinion about abortion if you have never faced the reality of an unwanted pregnancy is like taking a stance over meat-eating when you have never been hungry. There are women who are devoutly opposed to abortion until the choice becomes real for them, and who then make an incredibly painful decision to terminate. Because they go against deeply held moral beliefs, they carry a heavy burden of guilt and shame. And there are also women who have no ethical objection to abortion, but who choose not to terminate a pregnancy, because it doesn't feel right, even though they always assumed that they would.

I agree with right-to-life activists that this is a human life we're talking about – you, me, and everyone we know were once a little bundle of cells in someone's womb. But, there is another human life involved, a walking, breathing, thinking human – the potential mother.

The issue is not whether the foetus is a person or not. The issue is consent. Conceiving and bearing a baby, and raising a child, can be a wonderful, transformative experience, but *you have to want to do it*. If you don't, it's hell. If you don't understand how consent makes a difference, consider this. If you consent to give away a large amount of money, that's a soul-enriching act of philanthropy. If you don't, it's robbery. Consensual sex forms a loving, magical bond between two people. Without the consent, it's rape.

The pro-life movement underestimates what it is they expect of women when they call for abortion to be banned. You give your time, your energy, your blood, tears and a year of your life to make another person. Once you have given birth, you become a mother. This is not something that should happen to you against your will.

Access to abortion changes society for the better. Having a choice allows women to *choose to* have a baby, as well as to choose not to. Because motherhood is a huge undertaking, people need to enter into it willingly. Just knowing that an alternative exists stops unexpectedly pregnant women from feeling trapped and frees them to commit to being a parent. It's an amazing thing, to make every child a wanted child.

Since the central issue legitimising abortion is the consent of the woman involved, it is very important that people respect that it should be her choice to make alone.

Fathers and non-biological co-parents, I admit, this is hard for you. I know that it's your kid, but it's growing in her body. You have the option to walk away and not devote an ounce of effort to its creation and upbringing. She does not. And so you don't have the right to decide whether it is brought into this world. If she asks you, of course, you can explain the extent to which you're willing to support the child practically, and this may be a factor in her decision, but it's her decision to make.

It is as unacceptable for anyone to tell a pregnant woman that she should have an abortion as it is for them to tell her that she should not.

And the sole factor behind her decision should be whether or not she wants to have this child. Women should not be forced into this for lack of adequate welfare benefits, decent state-funded healthcare and childcare. If the anti-abortion lobby diverted their energies to fighting for redistribution of wealth and social justice, they could potentially cause a lot more children to be born.

Please, once you have made your decision, respect your own judgement enough to accept that it was the right choice. Part of my reasoning for exploring the issue of abortion in a book about pregnancy and birth is that there are women who suffer from enduring sorrow at a previous termination, and find that a subsequent, very different, wanted pregnancy rekindles the feelings of shame and self-blame.

It's OK to feel sad. It's OK to feel sorry. You have lost a baby, even though it was one you couldn't keep, so you may feel empty, and you might have some grieving to do. If the decision wasn't truly yours, if you were coerced into it, however subtly, you have the right to feel angry about that. Please, don't feel angry with yourself.

We are under intense pressure, as women, to be mothers – and not just that: to be good mothers, perfect mothers, not that ultimate evil, the Bad Mother. This is bullshit social conditioning. Because having an abortion, by definition, is an unmotherly thing to do, the act can cause you to run up hard against some unarticulated aspects of your own self-image. But you can't live a stereotype. Sometimes choosing not to be a mother can be the best decision. Allow yourself to accept that.

Anti-abortionists like to claim that abortion causes mental illness. It doesn't.[7] They then go around blaming women who do it, in very personal and emotive terms. So perhaps it would be more honest of them to say, 'Abortion doesn't cause mental illness but we will try our hardest to ensure that it will.'

Part of the reason why women blame themselves once they've had an abortion is that other people blame them. And this means that abortion is usually secret. And so it's hard to find the other women who have gone through it and to be able to honestly discuss the complexities of the feelings involved. You can't even go on an internet chatroom for support without religious fundamentalists popping up and telling you you'll burn in hell. Please don't internalise their vitriol: they have no right to stand in judgement on you. It's not their body and it wasn't their child.

On the subject of mental illness, be prepared to be *horrendously* pre-menstrual about a month after the abortion. Your hormones will be out of balance during this first cycle. A consultation with a herbalist or an acupuncturist could help.

Adoption

Giving the baby up for adoption is commonly perceived to be far less morally contentious than abortion. I was surprised to discover that it's not. It's an ethical minefield.

This is the nice story:

A woman chooses life for her baby, then nobly and selflessly gifts it to a new loving family who can give it a two-parent home. She gives her baby everything she can't afford to provide for herself. Everyone lives happily ever after.

The reality can be a little more complicated:

Once you create a child and offer it up for adoption, then that child has two mothers. There is the mother who does the work of parenting and who forges a bond of love with that child, and then there's you, the birth mother, who carries a genetic key to their looks, their medical history, and to some extent their personality.

You will have a degree of attachment to your baby, because you made them and birthed them with your body. You are likely to grieve when they go.

Some adopted children grow up feeling wounded by perceived rejection by their birth mother. Others feel blessed by having two sets of parents. A lot depends on the honesty and the love involved.

You are taking a gamble that the life the adoptive parents can give your child will be qualitatively better than the one you could. It is not necessarily the case that wealthier parents can give your child opportunities that you can't. Mothering is about emotional as well as financial riches.

The concept of 'open adoption' has been created, to help address these concerns. You choose the adoptive parents, and you then stay in touch with your adopted child through letters and visits. This can be a tricky relationship to negotiate. You will have relinquished all rights to your child irrevocably once the adoption papers have been signed. Some 'open' adoptions go on to become 'closed'.

As with abortion, this should be your free choice. You shouldn't be coerced into this, by emotional blackmail or by financial necessity. As with abortion, other people have no right to judge the morality of your choice.

The element of coercion is particularly acute once commercial adoption agencies are involved. If you arrange an adoption with an agency while you are still pregnant, you may find yourself financially or emotionally obliged to relinquish the child at birth.

The history of adoption has been tainted by some appalling episodes of what is essentially baby-snatching, leaving birth mothers mourning all their lives for children who are yet living.

Inter-country adoptions have been criticised as a form of colonialism. It would be better to close the huge disparities of wealth between poor and rich nations rather than ship babies from the former to the latter.

Despite everything I have just written, *it can work*. It can be a really positive experience for everyone involved. I didn't make you read that to put you off, but to help you think it through. There are all kinds of families in the world and there is a lot of love to go around.

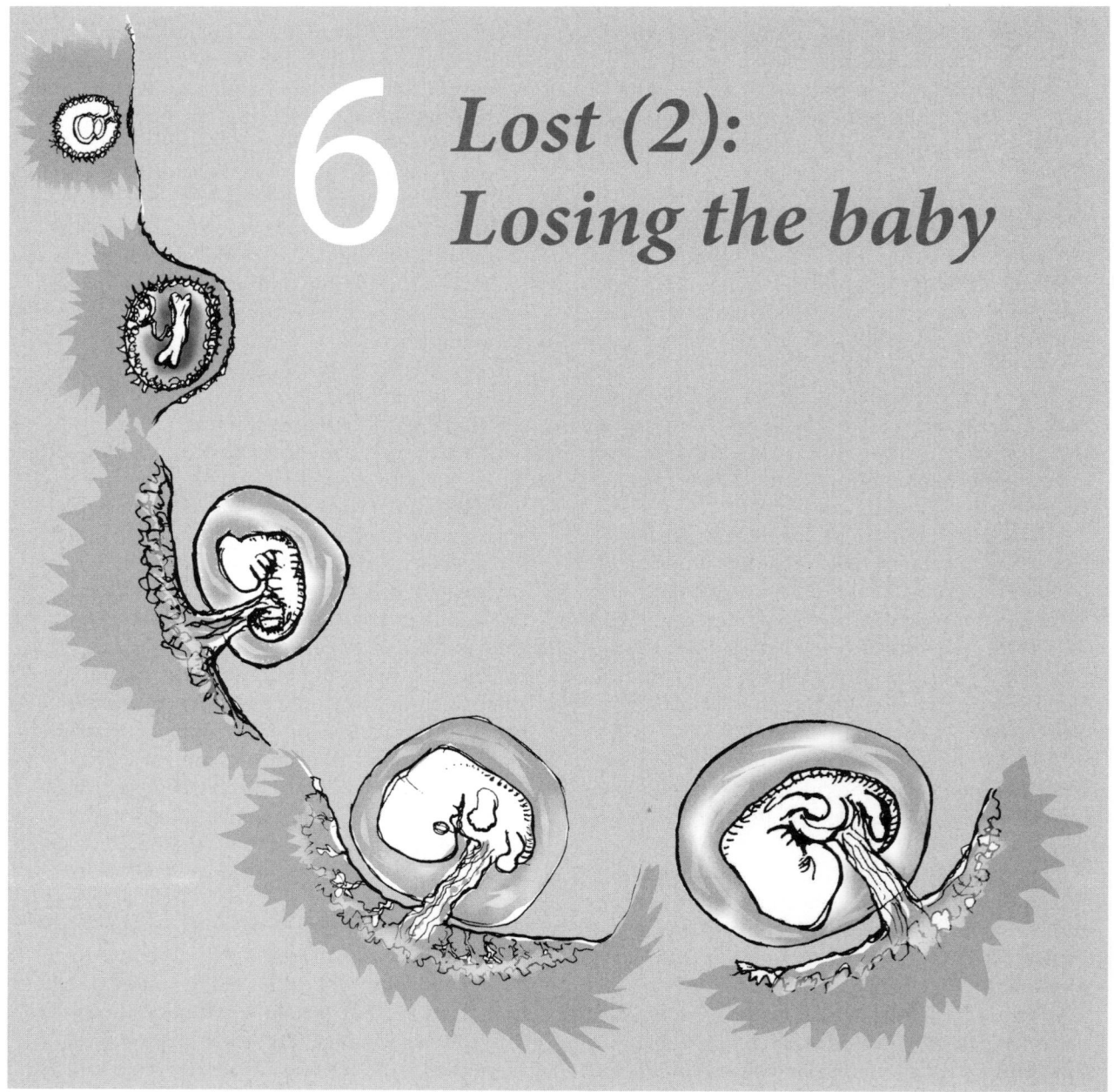

6 *Lost (2): Losing the baby*

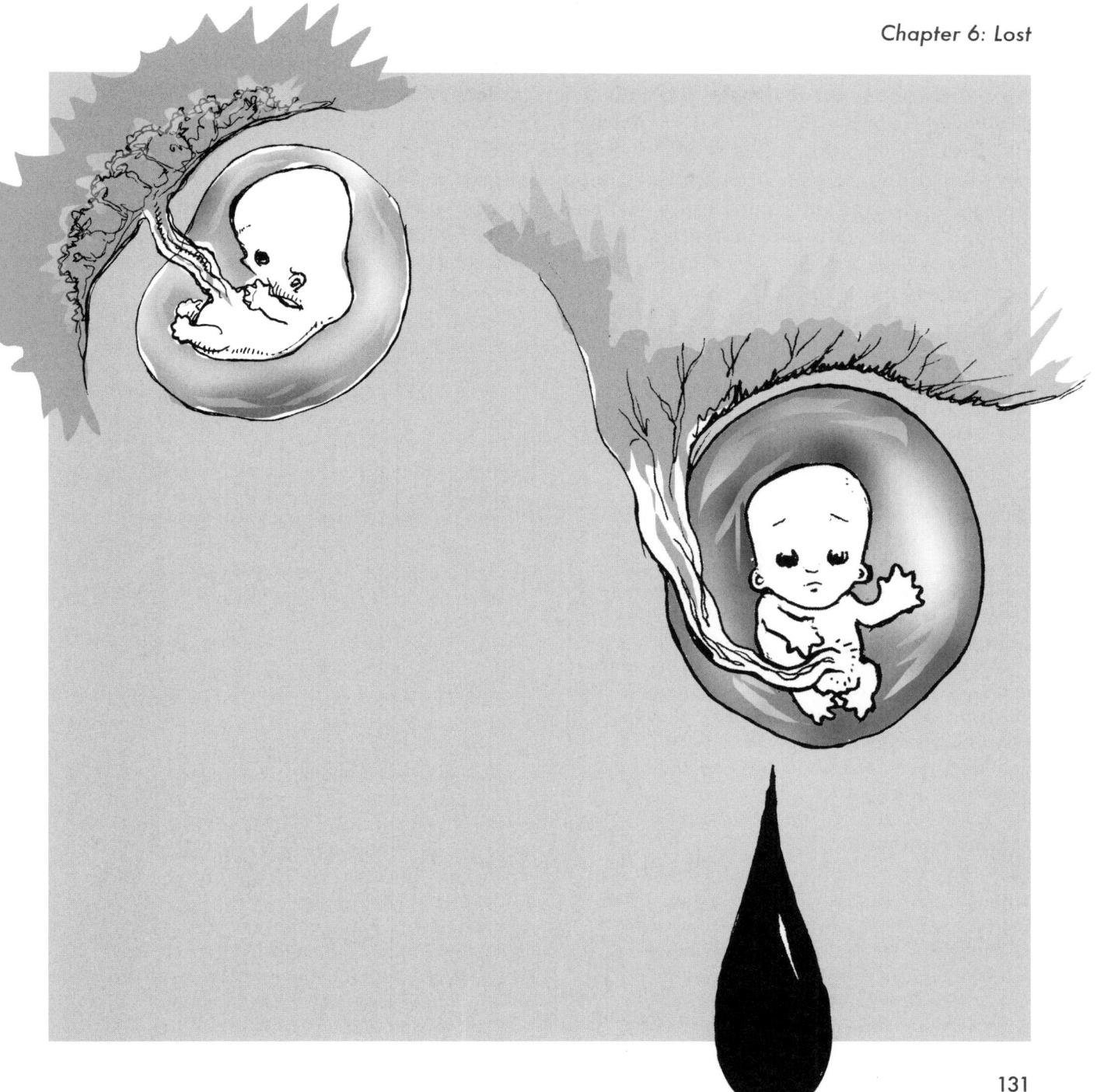

An estimated one pregnancy in four ends in miscarriage, 99% of which occur in the first twelve weeks of pregnancy. That's a quarter of a million miscarriages every year in the UK. It's a very big thing, that is talked about very little. I think I had an idea, from what representations there are of miscarriage in popular culture, that it would involve somebody waiting, swooning and dramatically heamorraghing, possibly while wearing a white satin gown. It's not usually like that in real life.

Initial signs

The first sign is usually a few steady streaks of blood loss. Some women don't get this, and only discover they are miscarrying at a routine scan. (But light bleeding in pregnancy can also be perfectly normal, so if it happens to you, it doesn't necessarily mean you're going to lose the baby.)

If you are bleeding

See your GP or midwife or phone an out-of-hours medical service. If you are more than six weeks pregnant, you can be referred to your local Early Pregnancy Advisory Clinic (EPAC) for an ultrasound scan to check everything's OK.

Bed rest won't prevent a miscarriage, if that's what's occurring, so you can carry on quietly with your normal routine. It is reasonable, though, to take time off work if you can, and if you want to go to bed, then do. Rest is always good in early pregnancy in any case.

If you are in pain

Pain could also be a worrying sign, with or without bleeding. If you have severe one-sided pain, or pain in the tip of your shoulder, seek urgent medical assistance as this could indicate an ectopic pregnancy. Otherwise, take paracetamol if you need to, and seek medical advice as to whether a referral is required.

At the EPAC

The EPAC waiting room is my personal idea of hell. The walls are lined with chairs filled with women who are so desperately worried that they can't even look each other in the eye. The telly is blaring, but no one can watch it. I could suggest that you take a good book with you, but you probably won't be able to read it. Time ticks by at a snail's pace.

The EPAC is invariably located right in the middle of a busy maternity unit, so the corridors around are filled with proud new parents clutching bouncing babies in car seats. Nice one, hospital architects. Thanks for that.

The only thing I can say that might help you while you wait is that half the women who attend an EPAC go on to have a fine, healthy baby. That might be you! You just don't know it yet. It's a real Schrödinger's cat moment.

Eventually you will be called in for a scan. If you are less than ten weeks pregnant, the scan will be done with a smooth white wand that is placed in your vagina. This is because the baby is low down and difficult to see. At later than ten weeks it will be a regular ultrasound, with gel on your tummy, though if the baby is not very obvious an internal ultrasound might still be necessary. The scan will hopefully reveal that everything is fine and there is nothing to worry about. Hooray!

Or it might not.

When the sonographer has finished handing you tissues, you will be given an appointment with a doctor where you can ask questions and discuss what happens next.

Why has this happened?

We don't know.

Some babies don't grow right. The sperm meets the egg and the chromosomes arrange themselves in the wrong way. Miscarriage is nature's way of letting these babies go.

Maybe the hormones of pregnancy weren't strong enough to sustain the baby. Nobody knows why this happens in some pregnancies but not in others. Sometimes the baby grows in the wrong place, the Fallopian tube, which is triply traumatic: you've lost the baby, your life is endangered, and your future fertility is compromised.

In some cases, a scan reveals that no baby is visible, either because its cells didn't form, because your womb has reabsorbed it, or it has slipped away unnoticed. This can make you think that you were never really pregnant, and you were fooling yourself all along. Nonsense. You *are* pregnant, and you were right to invest as much love and excitement in your future baby as any other, luckier mother.

I can tell you why it *hasn't* happened. This wasn't your fault and you haven't done something wrong.

It is good that scientists study whether common foods, drugs or activities might be harmful to the unborn baby, but the legacy of such studies is that, when babies die or suffer birth defects, mothers assume a huge burden of guilt, as if by their actions they are somehow responsible. This is almost always untrue and inappropriate.

What the scientists are describing are tiny increments of risk, spread out over the general population. The mothers are inferring a direct causal link, when it doesn't exist. For example, a bereaved woman reads a headline such as 'Coffee increases miscarriage risk' (which is itself a sensationalist misinterpretation of some scrap of scientific evidence). She then goes on a massive downer, obsessing over a cappuccino frappé that she drank a week before she miscarried *for an unknown reason*. But the coffee didn't kill the baby. Millions of women drank way more coffee than her, and all their babies were fine.

This has not happened because you are a bad person who deserved to be punished. It can feel like that, though. That's grief for you – being so sad makes your brain play tricks. If you are religious, please remember that your God is about love, not revenge. It just happened because it happened, and now you have to come to terms with it.

What now?

First there's a practical decision to be made, which you're probably in no fit state to make. Your options are for medical or surgical intervention to remove the baby, or to wait and let nature take its course. None of these options is inherently safer or more effective than any other, and none of them will harm your ability to get pregnant again and carry a subsequent baby to term.

Surgical management

This is sometimes referred to by the incredibly offensive and hurtful name of 'Evacuation of Retained Products of Conception'. We are not talking about 'Products'. This is your *baby*! How *dare* they? The correct terminology is Surgical

Management of Miscarriage (SMM). Words are important. There is no excuse for medical terminology that wounds.

SMM involves using gentle suction to remove the baby from your womb. It is usually done under general anaesthetic, although you may be offered a local anaesthetic. With the local option, although your cervix is numbed, you will still be able to feel the operation in your womb, and this can be quite painful.

Think about what you want to happen to your baby. You can ask for it to be returned to you to take home for a private ceremony, or the hospital can sensitively arrange for it to be cremated in accordance with their policies.

Medical management

You can be given drugs to speed up the process of miscarriage. First you will be given a tablet of mifepristone, then, the next day, admitted to hospital, where a pessary of misoprostol is placed in your vagina (you can insert this yourself – you don't have to let the midwife do it). This will bring on cramps, which can be severe, and blood loss, which can be heavy. You should be given strong pain relief if you need it.

Birthing a baby at this early stage involves passing large pieces of placenta and womb lining as well as the baby. Your baby may be recognisably formed, with limbs and a face, or it may be a tiny pale bean. (Too Much Information alert! It is common to pass the baby in the toilet by mistake, but you can take it out again if you want to see it.)

Natural management

You don't have to have any further medical intervention if you don't want it. You can just go home and wait for the baby to come away in time.

There may be some weeks of waiting involved. Although most losses occur before nine weeks, some women's bodies wait until nearer the 12-week mark to miscarry. Don't worry, there isn't 'something dead' inside you. Your body created this baby, and now your body has a way to take care of it.

A miscarriage is not 'like a heavy period'; it is like a miscarriage. The blood loss can be heavy enough to turn the bath water red. The pains you experience are akin to labour pains, as your cervix has to open up to let the baby out. It would be nice if they gave you prescription-strength pain killers to take home with you, but they don't. I don't know why. I assume that doctors have tended to underestimate the pain involved.

But, in a strange way, suffering with a miscarriage can be helpful. I mean, you're hurting inside anyway, so there can be some meaning in giving it physical form. Opiate painkillers dull the pain but they also remove you from your thoughts and feelings, which then have a habit of catching up with you once the drugs wear off.

Probably the best reason to miscarry at home is that you can be entirely private with your grief. You can decide what to do with what there is of your baby, and you don't have to negotiate with medical staff about this.

There is also a very, very slim chance that you have been given an incorrect diagnosis, and the baby is still viable. Miscarrying without intervention eliminates this doubt.

With all forms of miscarriage management there is a small (1%) risk of infection and/or small pieces of tissue being left behind. Your blood loss shouldn't continue to be heavy or smell strange. Use pads, not tampons for any bleeding and don't have penetrative sex until it has stopped.

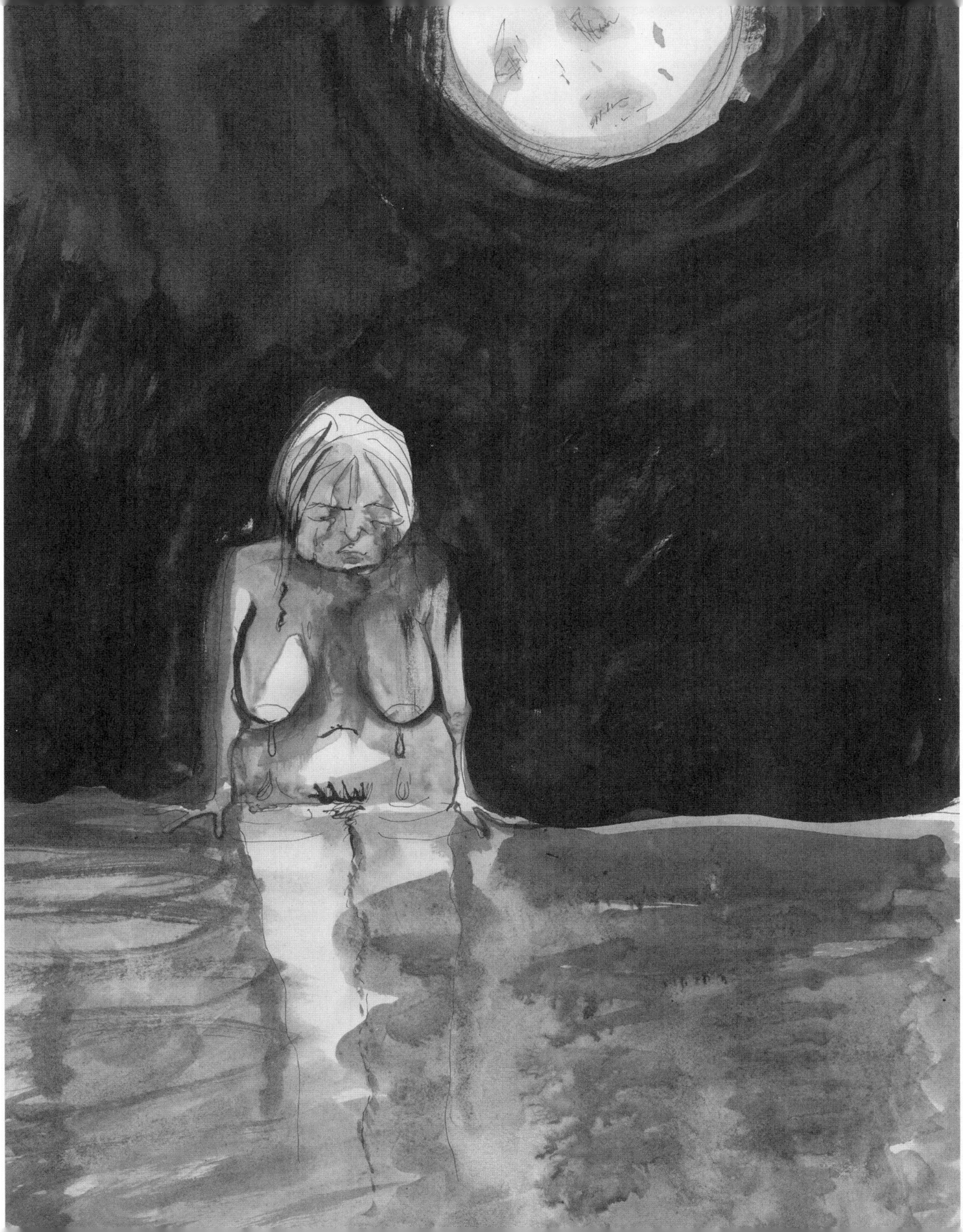

Hang on, what just happened?

This may be different for you, but I found that none of the staff at the EPAC ever used the word 'baby' when talking about miscarriage, and this made it much harder to come to terms with what had just happened. First-trimester pregnancy loss puts bereaved parents-to-be in the unique position of grieving for a child who never lived, and whose physical form, if they see it at all, is so frail and slight as to be inconsequential. That tiny smudge of tissue is far too small for all the hopes and dreams with which it was invested.

Grieving is made more difficult when staff persist in referring to your (potential) child as 'the pregnancy' or as 'the products of conception'. If you think about it, even the word 'miscarriage' is a euphemism. Nobody speaks the truth – that you were meant to have a baby, but it died.

I wonder why this is?

Perhaps the staff who have to announce this tragedy daily, or hourly, become desensitised to it, and prefer to use medicalese to distance themselves from the rawness of people's grief. Maybe it's because if they use the word 'baby' you'll cry and they think that's unkind, that it's making you more upset. Of course, it wouldn't make you more upset – it would allow you to be as upset as you actually are. It does people no good to hold back the tears when they have a reason to cry.

But maybe it has something to do with abortion. Our medical system respects a woman's right to choose to terminate a pregnancy, but it does this by according the unborn child the status of a non-person. This is a philosophically unsustainable position (see page 127 for the correct ethical justification for abortion) and it's exceptionally unhelpful when women lose a wanted baby. Because they receive no official recognition of their loss, it gives them nowhere to go with their grief.

You are mourning someone who really existed, but who never properly became flesh. That is hard. You can name this baby if you want to, or use an affectionate nickname like Baby Bean. Have a ceremony for your child. You could plant a tree or a rose bush, go to a beautiful place and talk to them, or write them a letter from the heart.

You may find life particularly hard just before your next period, because your hormones are out of balance when you suddenly stop being pregnant. See a herbalist or acupuncturist for help with this.

The Miscarriage Association is a wonderful organisation. Their support groups really help.

Termination for foetal abnormality

It is usually inappropriate to state that one form of tragedy is 'worse' or 'more traumatic' than another. Having said that, I can't think of a harder decision for a mother to be faced with than to have to choose whether to terminate for foetal abnormality. Some problems with the baby may not be picked up until the 20-week scan, which, considering the time needed for further investigations and diagnoses, can leave parents with an agonisingly short amount of time to decide what is best for their child, their future and their family.

It can be cripplingly difficult to grieve for a baby when you feel responsible for their death. It may help you to be reminded that *all* mothers feel responsible for the death of their child, whenever or however it occurs. As a parent, your role is to protect and nurture your child. If you can't do that, for whatever reason, it feels as if you have failed.

It is very important that all medical staff are aware of the importance of consent around this procedure. It is possible for a doctor to blithely state 'we recommend termination' as though that is the only thing to do. It's not the only option, and the choice is the mother's to make, not the doctor's.

'Late miscarriage' and stillbirth

The medical profession perversely insists on categorising a baby that dies after 13 weeks up until 24 weeks as a 'late miscarriage'. 'Stillbirth' would be a more accurate and respectful classification.

There is a continuum of tragedy here, from the loss of a baby in the earlier months, all the way up to full-term stillbirth. Some babies die in the womb, some arrive too soon to live, some die during labour. It is rare – 99.5% of women who give birth in the UK do so to a live baby – here we are discussing the 0.5%. As with miscarriage, we don't always know why babies die. There are more medical investigations and diagnoses that are applicable to these later deaths, but, even today, over half of all stillbirths happen for no clear reason.

If you have discovered that your baby has died (or is likely to die) in the womb, you will have to go into labour and give birth. The prospect of enduring this pain can be frightening, but afterwards women are glad that they had the opportunity to birth and meet their baby. You could consider a water birth to help with the pain.

Hospital staff will help you to spend time with your baby, to take photos, and to assemble a memory box of special items. There may be the opportunity to take tiny handprints and footprints. You may be uncertain how you will cope with

seeing the body; you don't have to, and staff won't make you, but nobody who does this regrets it later. Even if they have a physical abnormality, your baby will still be unforgettably perfect in their own unique way.

If your baby dies before birth before 24 weeks gestation, you can take the body home with you for a private burial. Or the hospital can arrange a funeral. You will not be entitled to maternity leave or benefits, but you can claim sick pay (although that's not much) and may be granted compassionate leave from work.

If your baby is born alive, no matter how early, or dies and is delivered at 24 weeks or later, there is a legal requirement to register the death and conduct an official funeral. You are entitled to standard maternity leave and pay.

You will probably produce milk for your baby. You will also need postnatal care.

Contact SANDS, the Stillbirth and Neonatal Death Society, because you can get help there from people who have gone through this before.

Grief

After you have dealt with the practicalities, endured the medical procedures, completed the bureaucracy and held whatever funeral ceremony is appropriate, at the end of the day there is just you, your partner if you have one, and your grief.

And it's a very dark place.

Generally, when someone dies, you have a store of reminiscences to sustain you, and a community of bereaved people, your mutual friends and family, with whom to share them. This doesn't apply when a woman loses her child at or before birth. A common reaction to death is to feel a sense of disbelief – 'denial' is one of the recognised 'stages' of grief that the bereaved are expected to 'work through'. It is especially hard to overcome this sense of denial when you are missing someone who didn't get to live.

I'm a white English person, and we are exceptionally bad at grieving. It's as if sadness isn't an acceptable emotion. We don't engage in the cathartic wailing and beating of breasts that occurs in other cultures; instead we are encouraged to 'hold it together', 'keep your chin up' and not let that stiff upper lip slip. This social prohibition is applied particularly harshly to men ('big boys don't cry'). Your male partner may be trying to 'stay strong' to protect you. This can leave you feeling emotionally worlds apart.

When people in this culture describe traumatic life events, they will tend to emphasise the 'not-so-bad' aspects of their narrative over the 'completely unbearable' bits.

That is why I recommend attending a support group and accessing bereavement counselling. You need a place to tell your story honestly, and to process events without minimising them.

Family and friends can say some stunningly inappropriate things. Make a mental note of the complete clangers:

- 'I know exactly what you're going through.'
- 'It's all for the best.'
- 'You must be glad that it's all over.'
- 'You can have another one.'
- 'At least you have your older child.'

It's part of our social conditioning to encourage each other to be cheerful. This doesn't make for very functional interactions when someone has good reason not to be.

[If you're wondering, a more helpful thing to say in these circumstances is some variation on 'I don't know what to say'(if you don't), 'I can't imagine how hard this must be for you', and 'How are you feeling?', preferably in a context where it's possible for the bereaved person to answer with something other than the lie: 'I'm fine.']

Being in a hard place can dramatically alter the dynamics of your friendships. A slight acquaintance or colleague can really shine, with unexpected acts of tenderness. But you may find a previously close friend doesn't know what to say. It doesn't mean that they don't love you. It's just, some friends are better at sunshine, and others are there for the rain.

It can really hurt to see other pregnant women. Jealousy is powerful, it's poignant, and it's the simplest way for your mind to help you realise your loss. Embrace it. Although I don't advocate snatching somebody else's baby in the supermarket, I can understand why women do.

You don't have to spend any more time around pregnant women or babies than you feel comfortable with, and you don't have to apologise for your feelings.

There is no 'right time' to feel better from this.
When you are deep in the darkness, it's hard to imagine that there will ever be light. But there will. It won't be a steady progression out of grief – you will step forward, and then you will slip back. Certain days will catch you out, such as the day your baby was due, or the anniversary of their death. But eventually, this grief will not be so raw and all-consuming. There will come a day when you can think of something else besides your baby.

Grief tempers your soul. It makes you a better, more compassionate person. Take comfort from the fact that you will never forget your baby. They live on in your heart.

I'm so sorry.

The next pregnancy

It is possible for you to get pregnant again straight away, but it's a good idea to wait a while until you feel physically and emotionally stronger. Sex can be fraught with sadness if you're terrified of conceiving again yet desperately missing a baby. Just be gentle with yourselves, and communicate with each other about how you both feel.

When you do want to try again, see pages 57 to 64 for advice on pre-conceptual care.

In the meantime, you're not pregnant, and the only thread of silver lining in this enormous black cloud is that it gives you the freedom to fill your body with whatever social poisons take your fancy, and eat French cheese.

Will it happen again?

It's not very likely. First-trimester miscarriages, despite being so common, are random where they strike. You are much more likely to carry the next pregnancy to term than to lose another baby.

Reccurrent miscarriage is rare. Only one per cent of couples are unlucky enough to experience three miscarriages in a row. Of these, only a small percentage suffer from an identifiable or treatable condition.

As far as the medical profession are concerned, they don't know why miscarriage happens, there are no drug treatments that reduce the risk of it happening in the general population, there is unlikely to be a discernible cause if it does recur and it probably won't happen to you next time anyway. So keep trying.

This is extremely tough on the (admittedly very few) women who have a treatable blood-clotting disorder which causes pregnancy loss. They have to lose three consecutive babies before they are eligible for medical investigation. This doesn't happen elsewhere in medicine – you don't have to break your leg three times before they'll put it in plaster.

One more word about words. There are highly offensive medical terms in store for women who suffer repeated pregnancy loss. You would think the term 'recurrent miscarriage' would be a reasonable one to be entered on to medical notes, but no! Doctors prefer the term 'habitual abortion'. Words fail me!

And that's not all. One of the principal causes of repeated late miscarriage/early stillbirth is when the cervix comes open as the baby grows, causing very premature birth. The term 'cervical weakness' would be a good description of the phenomenon – not the recognised medical term 'cervical incompetence'. That's adding insult to injury! Who invented this term? Was he suffering from 'Smaller-than-Average Penis Syndrome'?

To be honest, it doesn't matter what your statistical chances are of losing another baby. It feels very different getting pregnant again when it all went wrong last time. Anxiety is another, less well recognised 'stage' of grief, and there may be various triggers in your pregnancy, such as antenatal scans or appointments, that bring back difficult memories.

Women show immense courage in this situation; they do endure, and find a measure of healing in the process. The next baby will not compensate you for the one that died – he or she might poignantly remind you of the lost sibling – but be brave and trust that things will work out better next time.

Good luck.

And fingers crossed.

7 *Blooming marvellous!*

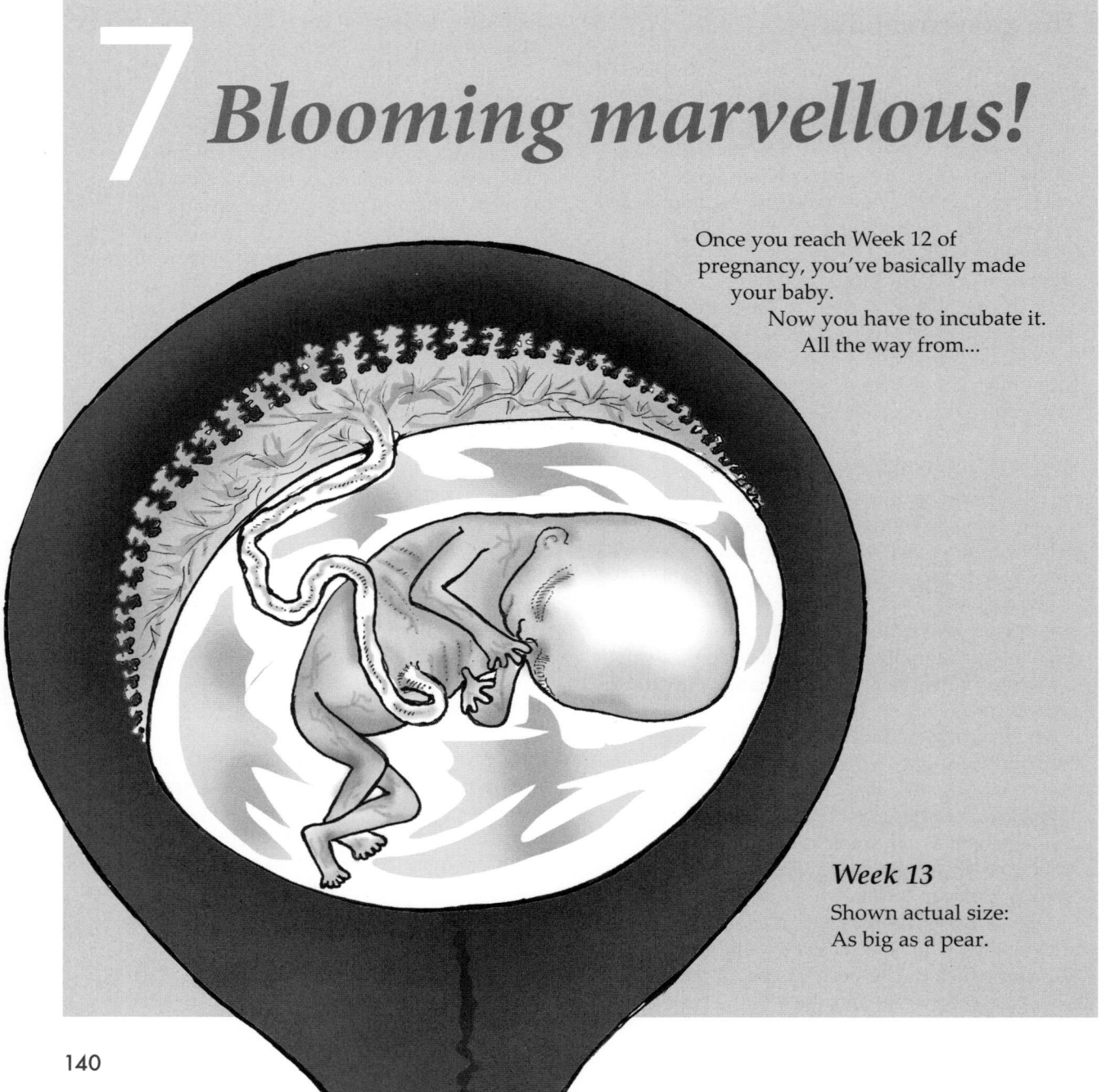

Once you reach Week 12 of pregnancy, you've basically made your baby.
Now you have to incubate it.
All the way from...

Week 13

Shown actual size:
As big as a pear.

...via these edited highlights...

Week 15! Fingerprints!

Week 17! Genitals!

Week 19! Eyelashes!

Week 18! Hiccups!

Week 20! Nerves!

Week 21! A bum hole!

Week 22! Full body fur!
Seriously! We are monkeys.
This usually disappears
by Week 35.

Week 23! Toenails!

Week 26! Thumb-sucking!

Week 27! Eyesight!
Although it's all usually black in there,
with some occasional red,
when you're sunbathing.

Week 28! Baby grease!
Skin becomes coated with a layer
of waterproof vernix caseosa,
Latin for 'cheesy varnish'. Nice!

Week 29! Sleep/wake cycles!
Which don't coincide with yours,
and probably won't for some years.

Week 30! Chubbiness!

**Week 32! Could theoretically
probably breastfeed!**

**Week 35! Fully working, but as yet
untested lungs!**

...all the way up to...

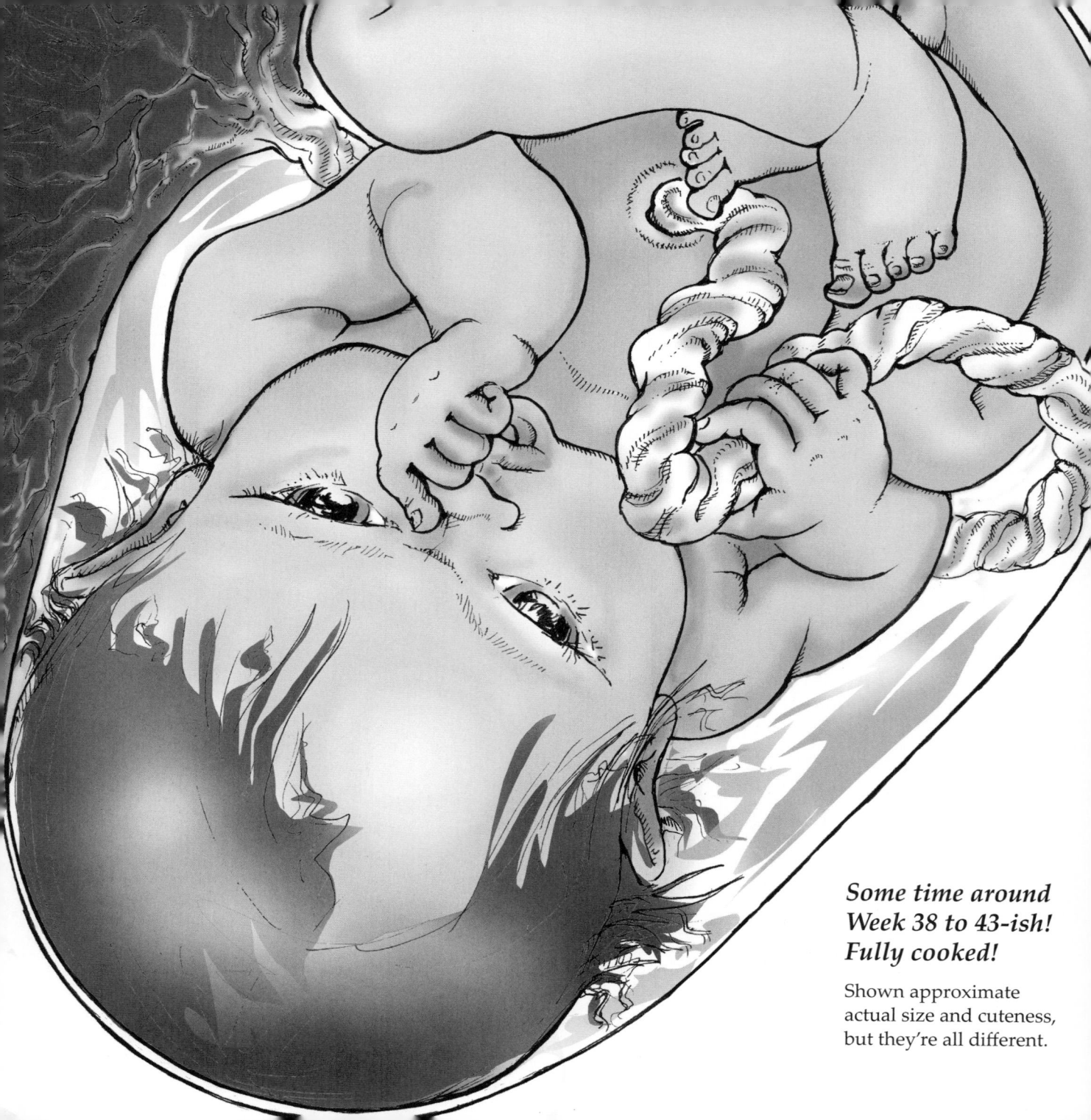

Some time around Week 38 to 43-ish! Fully cooked!

Shown approximate actual size and cuteness, but they're all different.

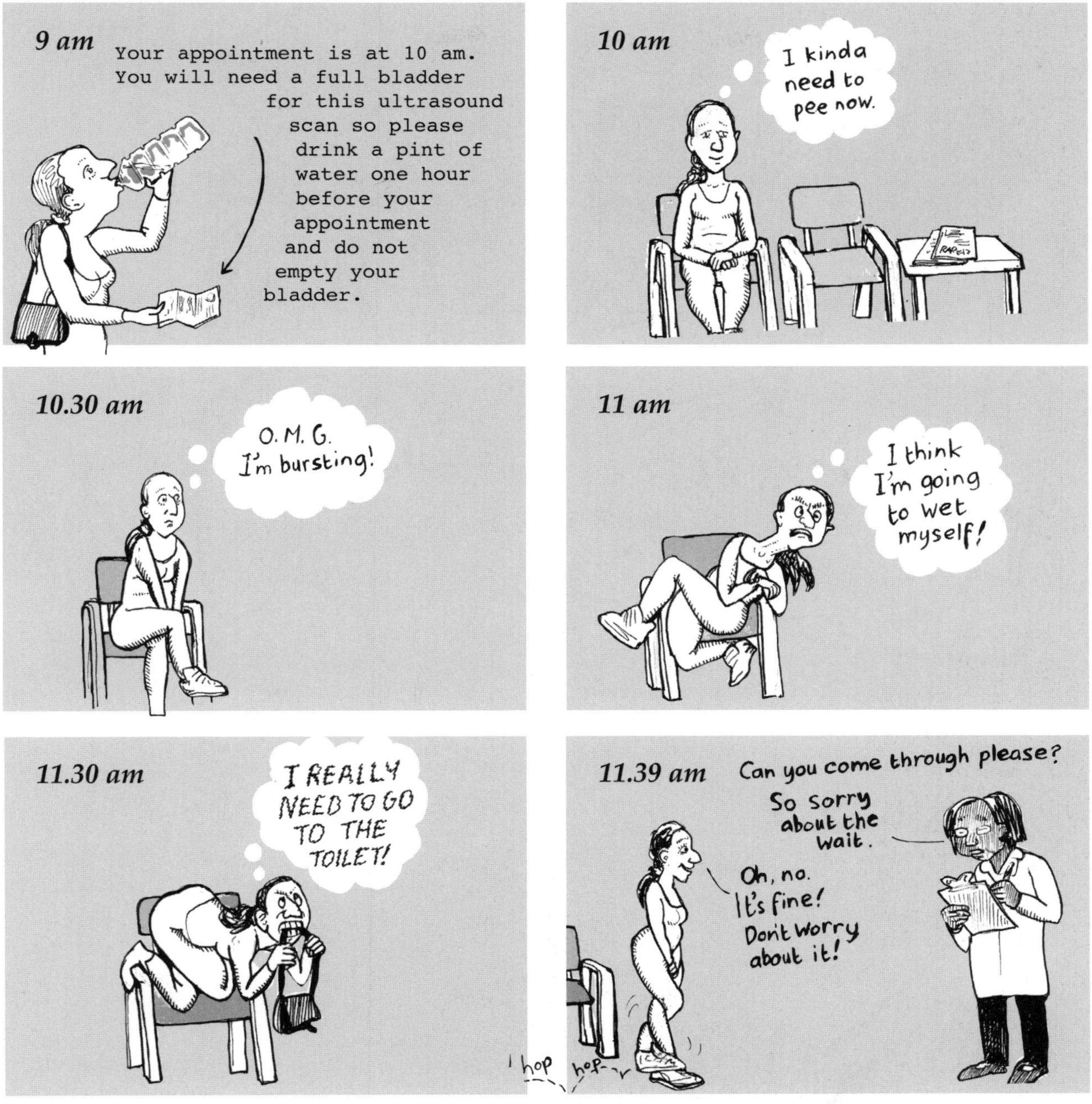
9 am
Your appointment is at 10 am. You will need a full bladder for this ultrasound scan so please drink a pint of water one hour before your appointment and do not empty your bladder.
10 am
I kinda need to pee now.
10.30 am
O.M.G. I'm bursting!
11 am
I think I'm going to wet myself!
11.30 am
I REALLY NEED TO GO TO THE TOILET!
11.39 am
Can you come through please?
So sorry about the wait.
Oh, no. It's fine! Don't worry about it!
hop
hop

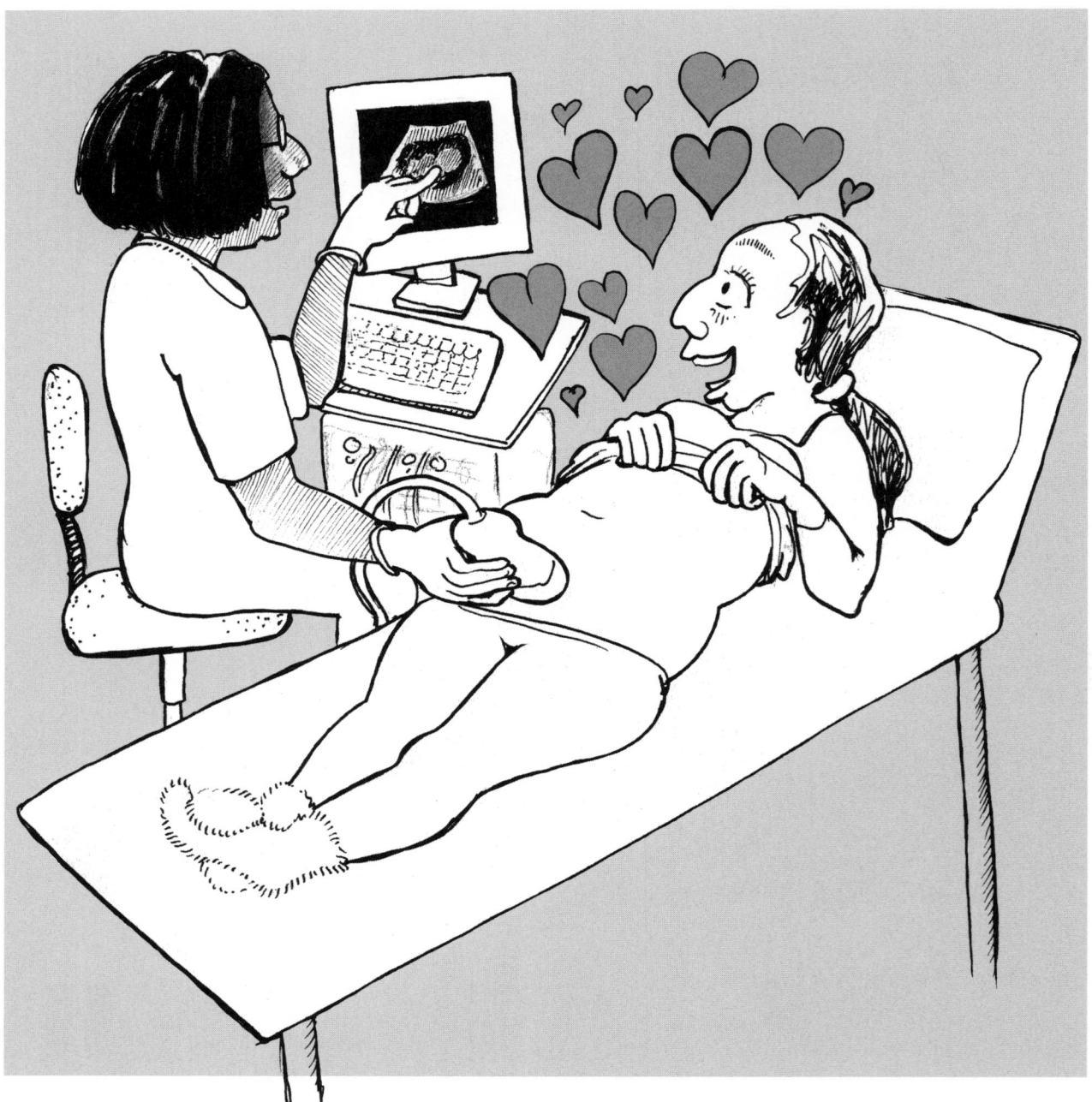

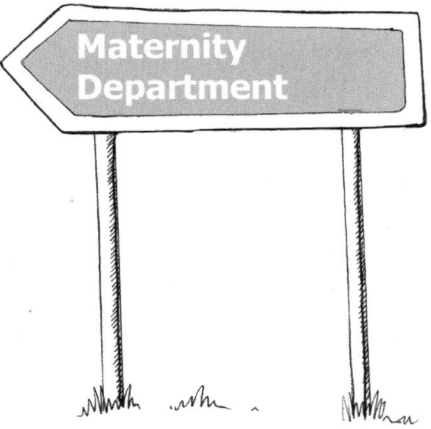

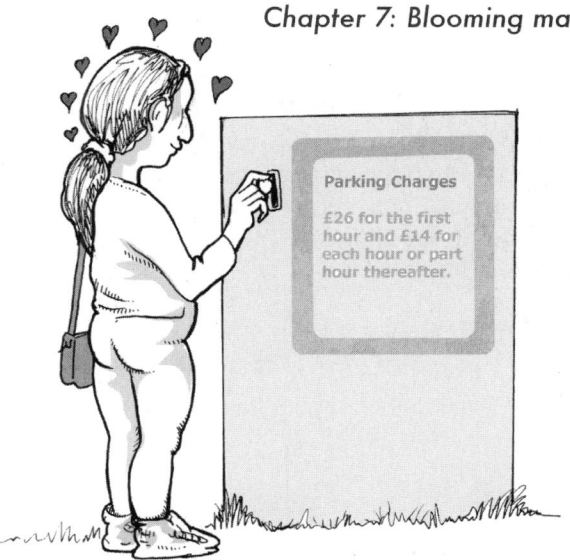

Parking Charges

£26 for the first hour and £14 for each hour or part hour thereafter.

Your pregnancy will be officially measured, monitored and marked by appointments with your midwife. Attend them. They're useful and they're free. You get about ten with a first baby, and seven for a subsequent one, unless you have special circumstances and they want to watch you more closely.

BUT it is the job of the medical profession to look for anomalies, and constantly check you for things that could go wrong. They worry about babies that are too big, and babies that are too small, about maternal blood pressure, and blood sugar levels, about twins and triplets, pregnancies that are too short or too long, about amniotic fluid and placental function. Let them fret.

This is not your job. Your job is to get on with growing your baby and having a fine time.

Here, replicated from your maternity notes, is a checklist of signs for concern:

- abdominal pain;
- vaginal bleeding;
- waters breaking;
- severe headache;
- blurred vision or sensitivity to light;
- persistant itching;
- reduced foetal movements.

If you get any of these symptoms, phone your midwife. If you're worried about anything at all, phone your midwife. Don't ever feel that you shouldn't bother your midwife. If you're concerned about something, she needs to know.

BUT you don't need to be an expert on everything that could go wrong with a pregnancy. That's the midwife's job. You don't need to read medical textbooks. You don't need to Google rare pregnancy disasters. You will not find a long list of disorders of the unborn child in this book. Even if your baby had every one of them, to you it would still be your baby, not a clinical case study.

So, phone your midwife if you need to. Otherwise relax and have fun. Sure, all kinds of horrendous things *could* happen, but the chances are they won't. Why stress yourself out?

145

Because this is the fun bit. You've done the
hard part and you're past the worrying point.
  You'll probably have more energy;
your bump is starting to show.
You can get some credit now,
and some congratulations.

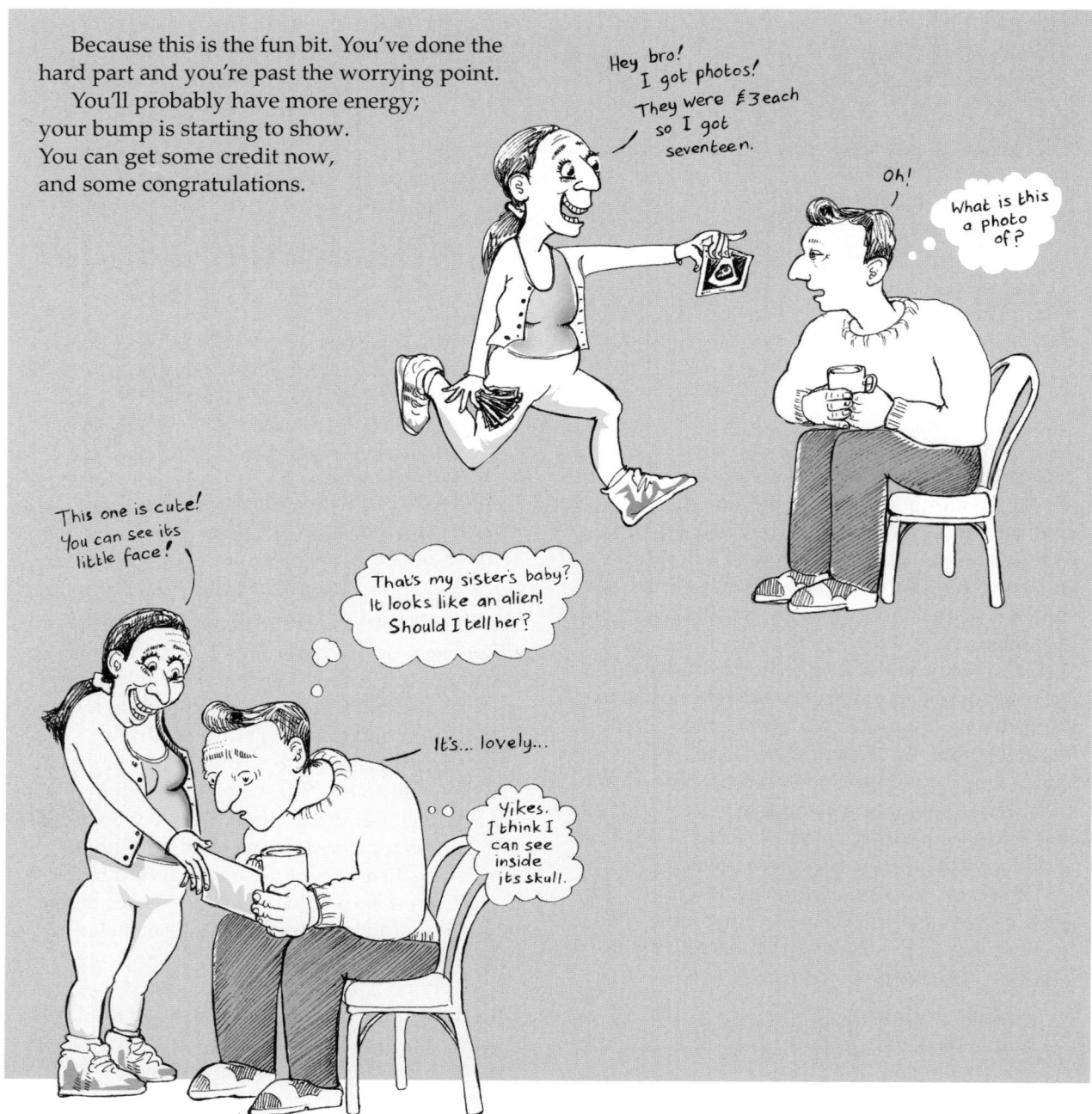

146

Butterfly kisses

Scan photos are the 21st-century baby-bonding ritual, so suitable for our technocratic age. Your baby as a fuzzy grey spaceman, bouncing around in a distant orbit.

You can build your own picture of your baby too. Let your thoughts wander as you chat to your child. Some ideas might come to you about what they're like. And you might just be right.

In one survey[1] of pregnant women, half of those questioned had a strong feeling about their child's gender, and 71% of them were correct. That's spooky. (Mind you, that does mean the other 29% bought the wrong baby clothes.)

Then comes the 'quickening': the first little flutters of movement inside, like butterflies, or burps, or popcorn pops. They're usually unmistakable by the time you're six months gone, but you could feel them much earlier. No, you're not imagining it. They're doing handsprings in there.

Your baby starts to hear you from 16 weeks on. If you or your partner regularly sings them a lullaby, you can use it to soothe them after they're born.

Those butterfly brushes rapidly turn to bumps and thumps, and, just as your day follows a pattern of sleeping and waking, so does your baby's. Just not at the same time as yours.

You are the expert on your baby. From the seventh month (Week 28) onwards you can start to keep an eye on them, starting a process of maternal supervision that will continue until you are very old and dead and buried, and probably, to be honest, won't even stop then.

Once you know the times of day or night when your baby bounces most, take note if the pattern changes. It will change, you don't have to freak out, but be aware of it.

If they get less and less wriggly over a couple of days, phone your midwife. If they're not moving when they normally do, phone your midwife. You can check by snuggling up on some pillows on your left side, putting the telly on and counting the kicks. Have a hot or a cold drink and give them a poke. It is unusual to get fewer than ten kicks in two hours at what's normally bouncy baby time. If you're not feeling this number of movements, phone your midwife. After hours, ring the hospital delivery suite. *Don't wait until the next day*. The medical establishment exists to keep you both healthy. You pay tax. You pay their wages. Bother them.

8 *Better shape up*

I am going to encourage you, now that you have a little more energy, to use it for moderate aerobic exercise. When you get fitter, your body works more efficiently, and that means your placenta works better, and more nutrients reach your baby. Your baby will be less likely to be born early, or to be exceptionally large, or very tiny, and may be slimmer and healthier in later life.[1] You'll also be less likely to develop pre-eclampsia or diabetes in pregnancy.[2] And during labour you'll have more stamina, and you might just need that.

Move! It's the other thing you can do, together with eating well, to help your baby be healthy. Do it! Listen to your body, though. Your ligaments are stretchier at the moment, and, if a move feels wrong to you, don't repeat it.

Some sports are not recommended. Although your baby is beautifully cushioned inside the womb, it makes sense to minimise the risk of falls and hard knocks. So lay off mountain biking, roller derby, showjumping, kickboxing and skiing. (Or don't. You're an adult; it's your baby and your body.) Scuba-diving is definitely out because the unborn baby is vulnerable to decompression sickness, which could potentially cause birth defects[3] (although if you went diving before you knew you were pregnant, don't worry). Don't exercise if it's crazily hot, and, if you go up to altitudes over 2,500 metres, wait until you have acclimatised. Don't do sit-ups with a bump.

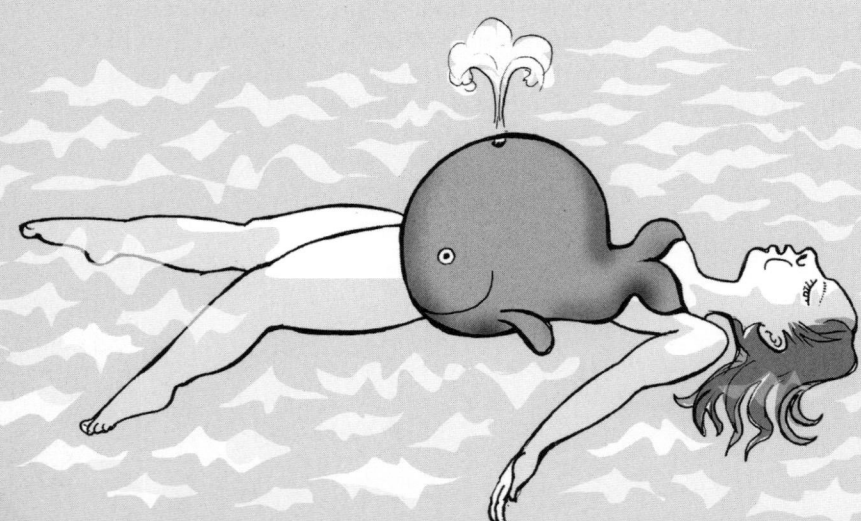

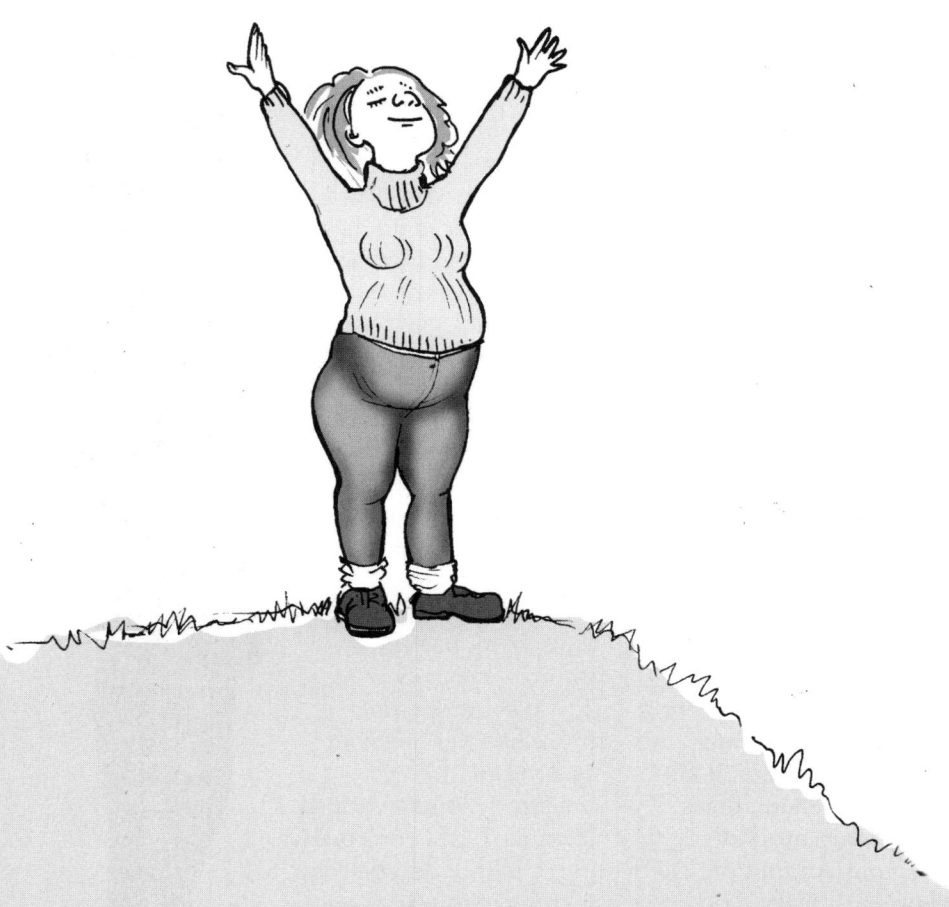

Walk.
It's easy and it's free.
Start with a mile a day.
That's about 20 minutes: it won't take long.
Then build from there. Aim for five miles a day.
That's about how much walking we were designed to do,
before agriculture, then urbanisation, and then cars made us sedentary.
Get a shopping trolley and you can make yourself useful while you're at it.

And squeeze...

There's one particular exercise that you'll be encouraged to do a lot: pelvic floor exercises, also known as Kegels, regularly consciously contracting and releasing the muscles around your vagina. Dysfunctional pelvic floor muscles are endemic in our society. Everyone, women, men, people who give birth vaginally and who birth by Caesarean – we are all at risk of incontinence and organ prolapse. Yikes! And when you're pregnant, your internal organs are heavier, and your ligaments are more stretchy. Double yikes! On the plus side, better pelvic floor muscles give you stronger and easier orgasms.[4] Yay!

If you already know how to do pelvic floor exercises, you're probably already doing them right now. And squeeze! If you don't know what I'm talking about, these are the muscles you can clench around your vagina to grip something pleasurable, or, less romantically, to stop your pee. Have a play around. How long can you hold them for? Try squeezing on one side, then the other, the front, and then the back. Imagine you have an elevator in your ladyparts. Can you make it stop at different floors? Try chewing an imaginary cherry up there, and then spit out the stone. Try squeezing as you exhale,

and picture yourself shunting energy up from your feet towards your baby.

It can be really hard to remember to do these exercises, and there are other things you can do to help your pelvic floor. Try to develop a continual awareness, keeping them engaged *all the time*. By locking the pelvic floor upwards, and pulling the abdomen backwards, you create an internal 'corset' from your core muscles which protects your lower back and improves your posture. Try to stand, sit and move like this as much as you can.

After you have healed from the birth, you could pop a pair of duo balls up there to encourage you to keep those muscles toned. (I'm going to refer you to sh-womenstore.com again to buy these. No, I'm not on commission). It's not a good idea to use internal vaginal devices when you're pregnant.

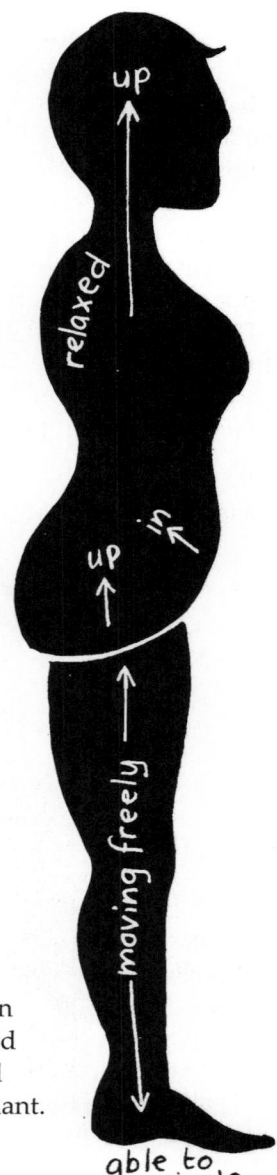

Squat the lot!

But why does everyone in our society have a saggy pelvic floor? Well, we are anatomically designed to squat down on our heels and work at floor level. But instead we have become addicted to sitting on chairs and working at tables. Our hips seize up, our bottoms sag, and all the muscles around our groins lose their tone. Kids can squat easily. But adults seize up and stop being able to. Compare the two pictures below.

The other thing you can do for your pelvic floor is to squat more.

Squatting to use the toilet is particularly beneficial, because it puts you in the most effective position for 'elimination'. Pregnant ladies are at risk of constipation and haemorrhoids, and squatting helps prevent both. You don't have to knock out your toilet with a sledgehammer – you can buy a custom-sized step stool that will lift you to the right height to squat up there comfortably. Do a search for the hilariously named 'squatty potty'. They're not very expensive, and they double as a handy step for your toddler when it's time to toilet train.

Sitting on a gym ball is also good for your pelvic floor. These are less fun around toddlers though – well, actually, lots of fun for the child, but no fun for you and your household ornaments.

This is how my daughter is currently sitting:

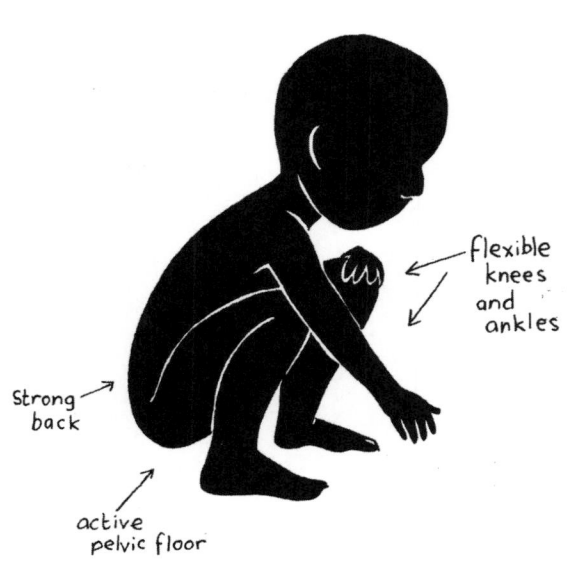

flexible knees and ankles

strong back

active pelvic floor

And this is what I'm doing as I draw this:

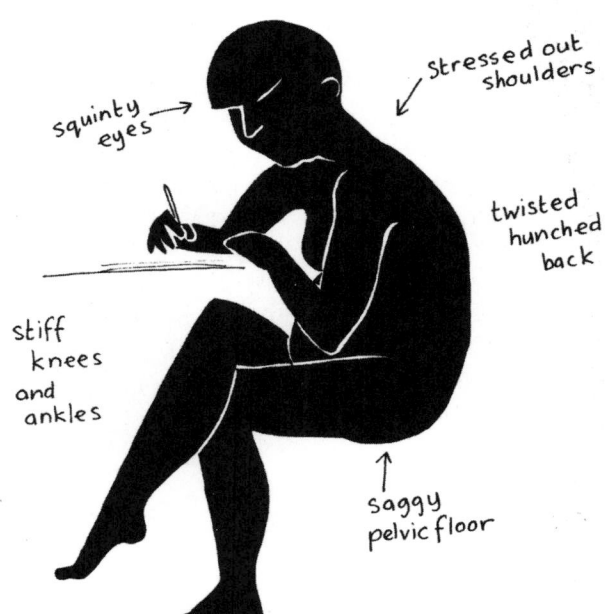

stressed out shoulders

squinty eyes

twisted hunched back

stiff knees and ankles

saggy pelvic floor

If, like me, you are not very good at squatting, you'll need to try some exercises to limber up your hips and hamstrings. This one uses a door knob. You probably have a door at home.

Katy Bowman's app and DVD *'Down There' for Women* is a good resource to revitalise your pelvic floor, helping to build the muscles you've lost by not squatting a lot.

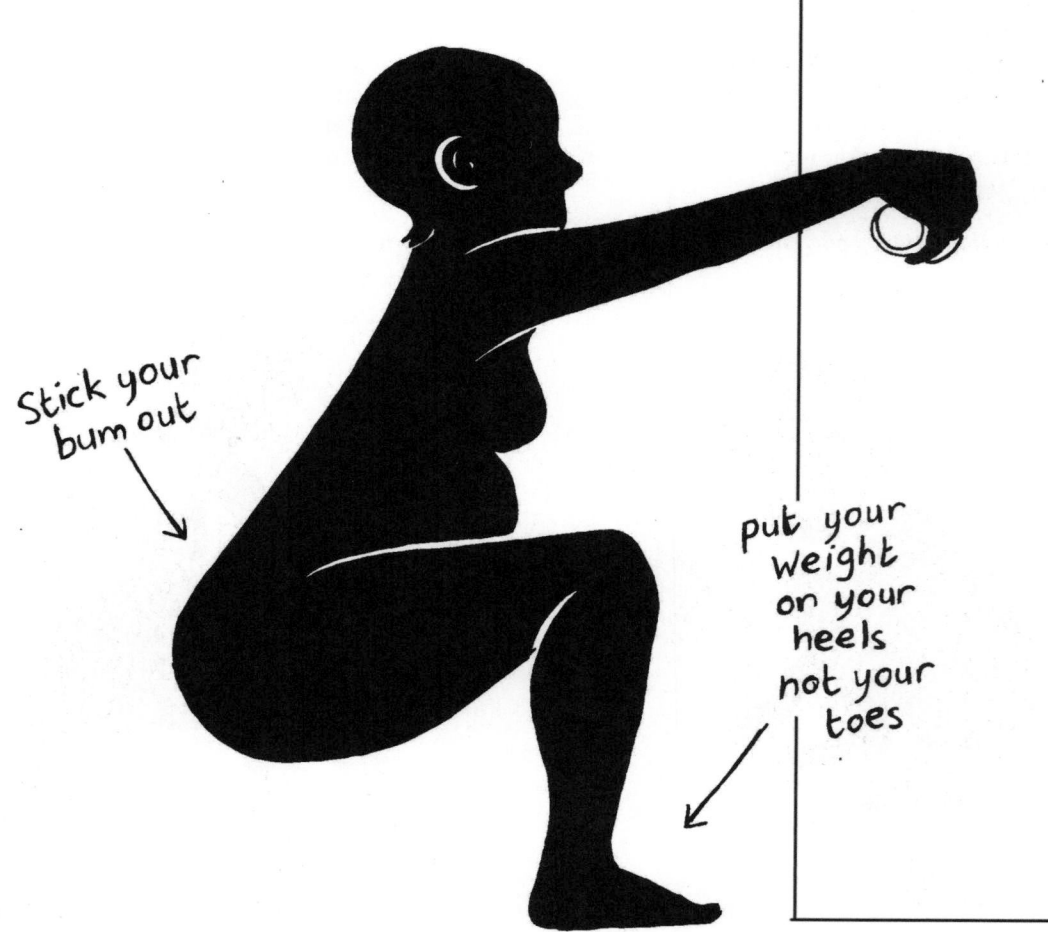

Stick your bum out

put your weight on your heels not your toes

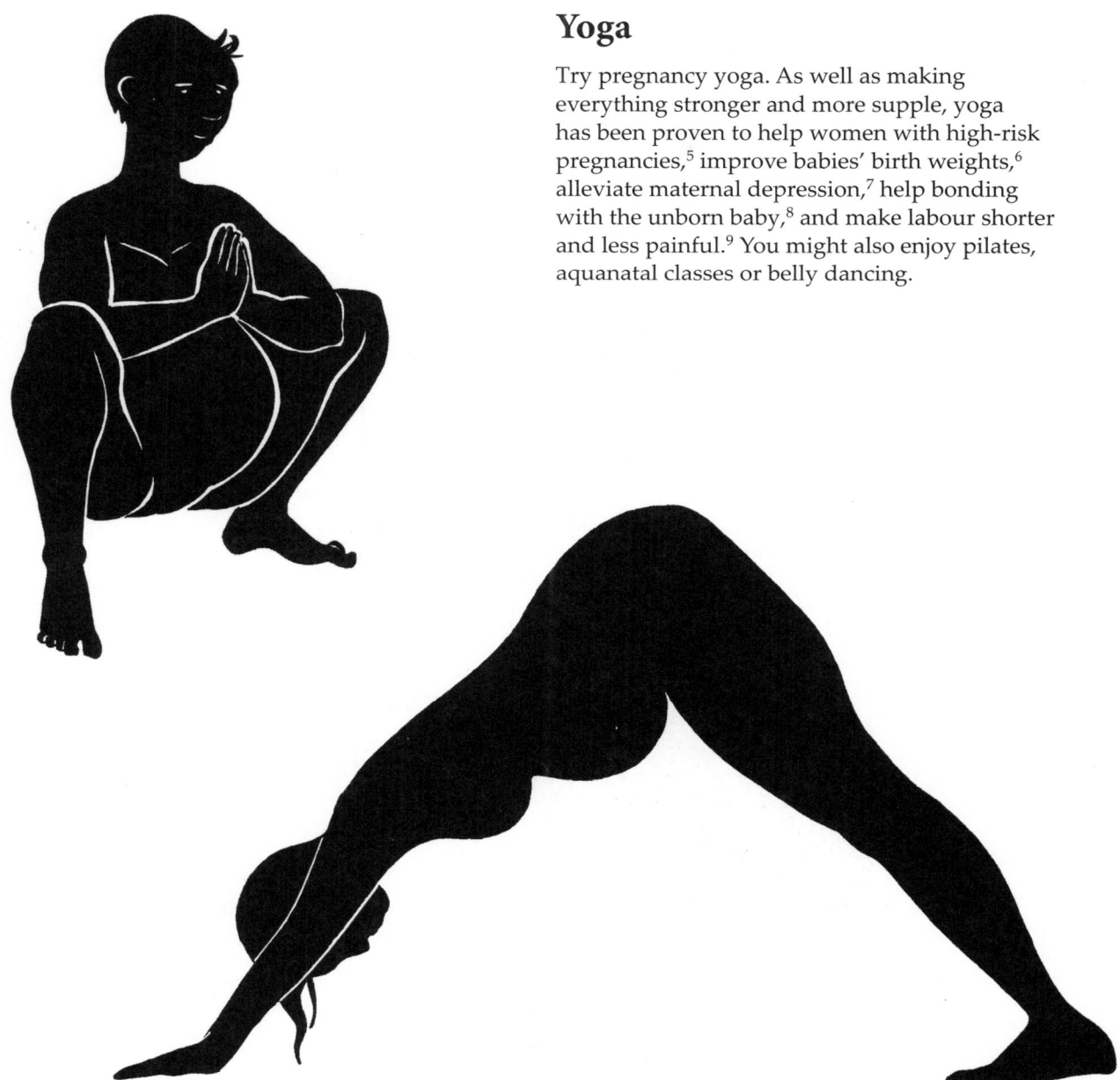

Yoga

Try pregnancy yoga. As well as making everything stronger and more supple, yoga has been proven to help women with high-risk pregnancies,[5] improve babies' birth weights,[6] alleviate maternal depression,[7] help bonding with the unborn baby,[8] and make labour shorter and less painful.[9] You might also enjoy pilates, aquanatal classes or belly dancing.

9 Things that go bump

Once you have a bump, you know you're pregnant...

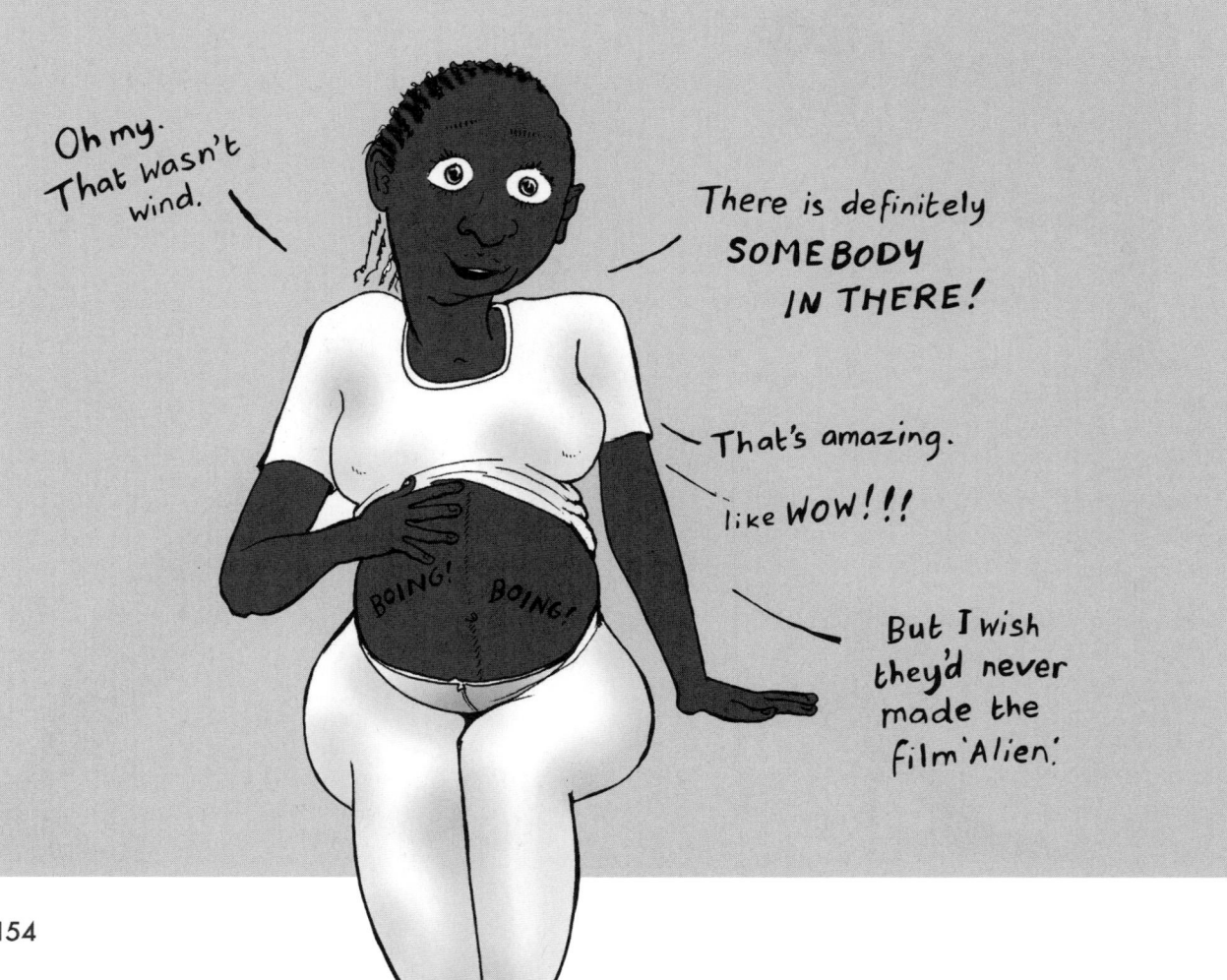

…and the world does too.

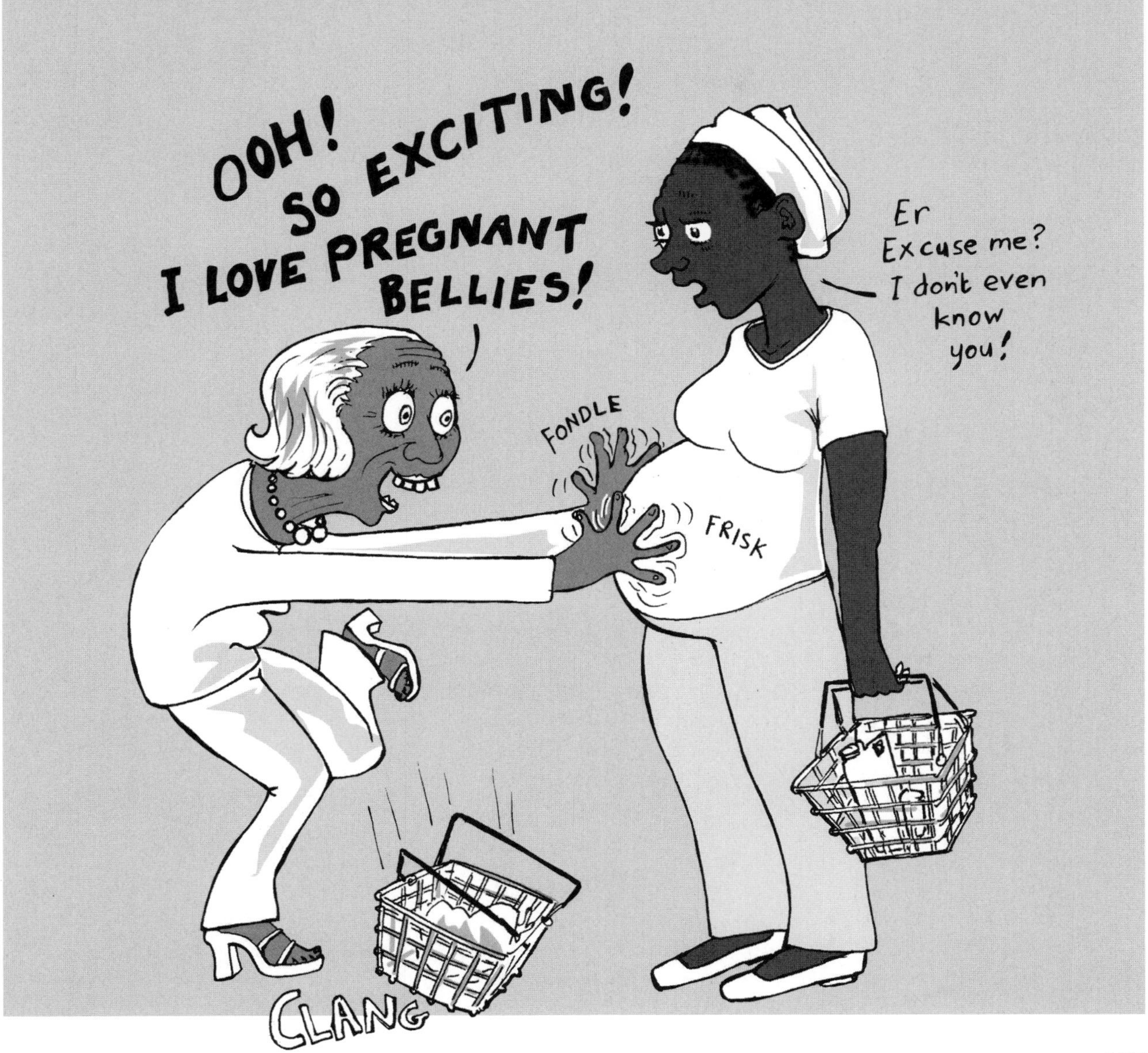
OOH! SO EXCITING! I LOVE PREGNANT BELLIES!
FONDLE
FRISK
Er Excuse me? I don't even know you!
CLANG

Your new shape can take a bit of getting used to.

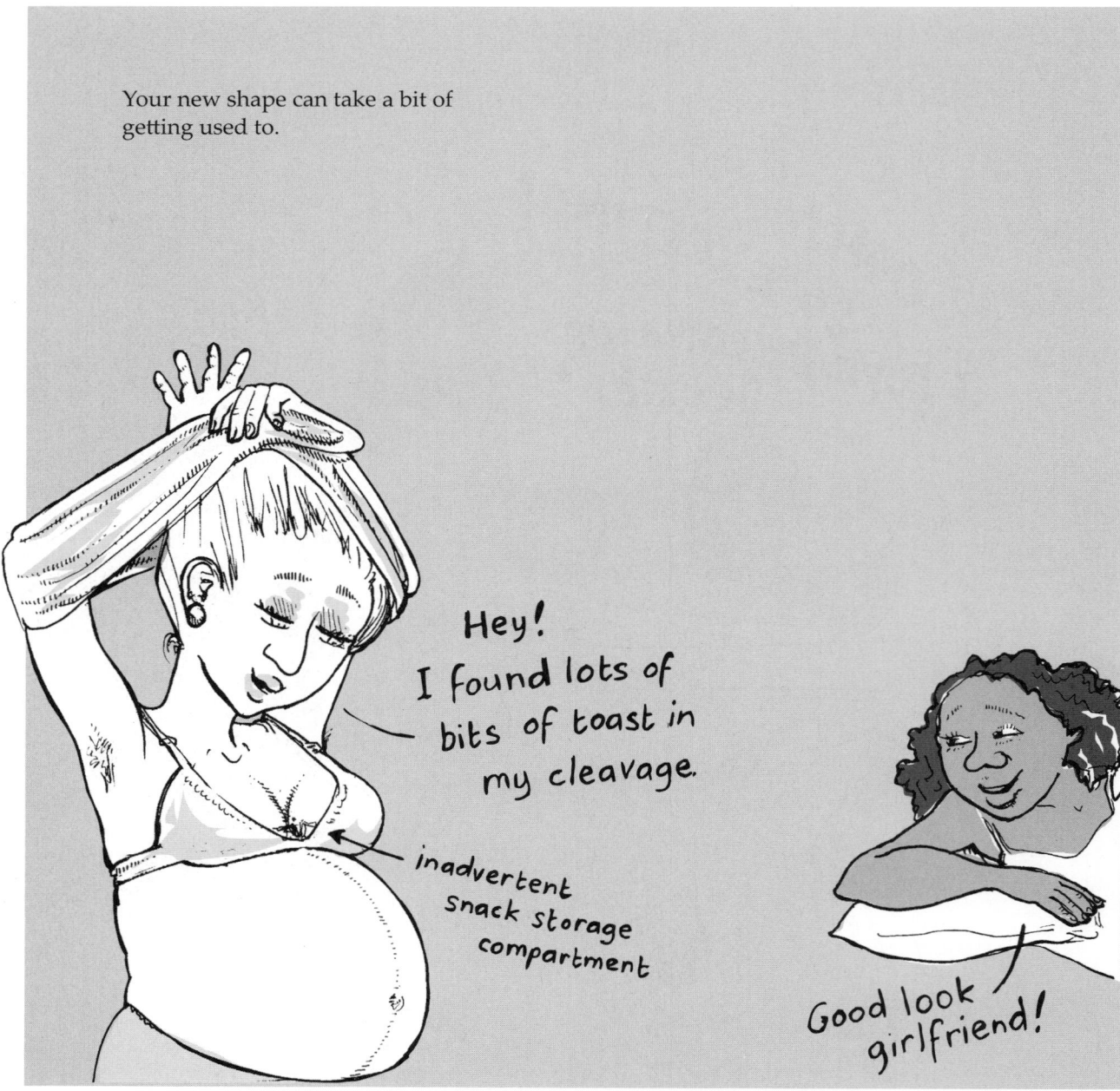

Like the day you turn sideways
to slip through a gap…

…and discover
you are no
slimmer
that way.

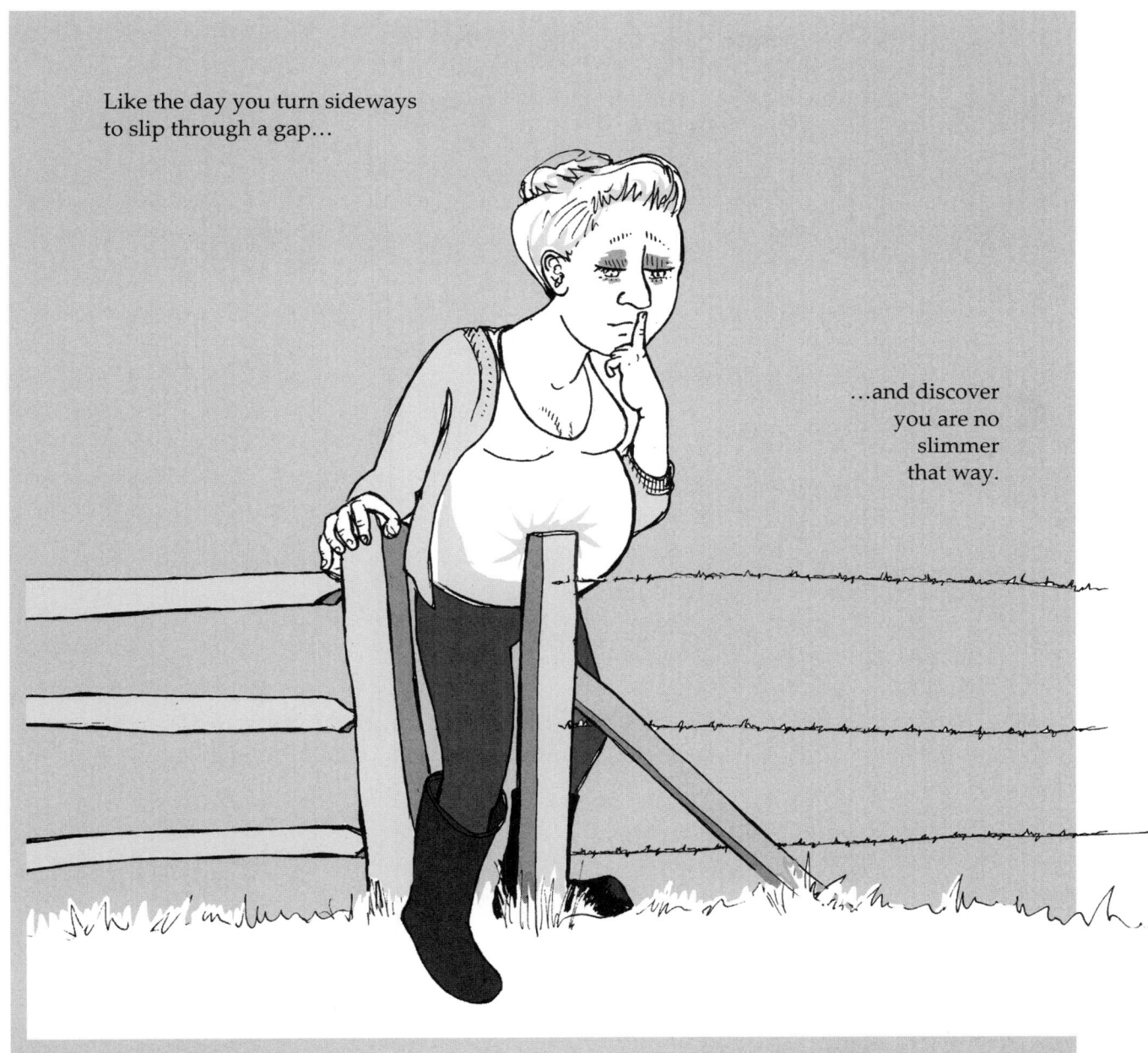

At some point, your stomach muscles give up and wave a little white flag.

As I discovered when I lay down on the floor in the caravan. Big mistake.

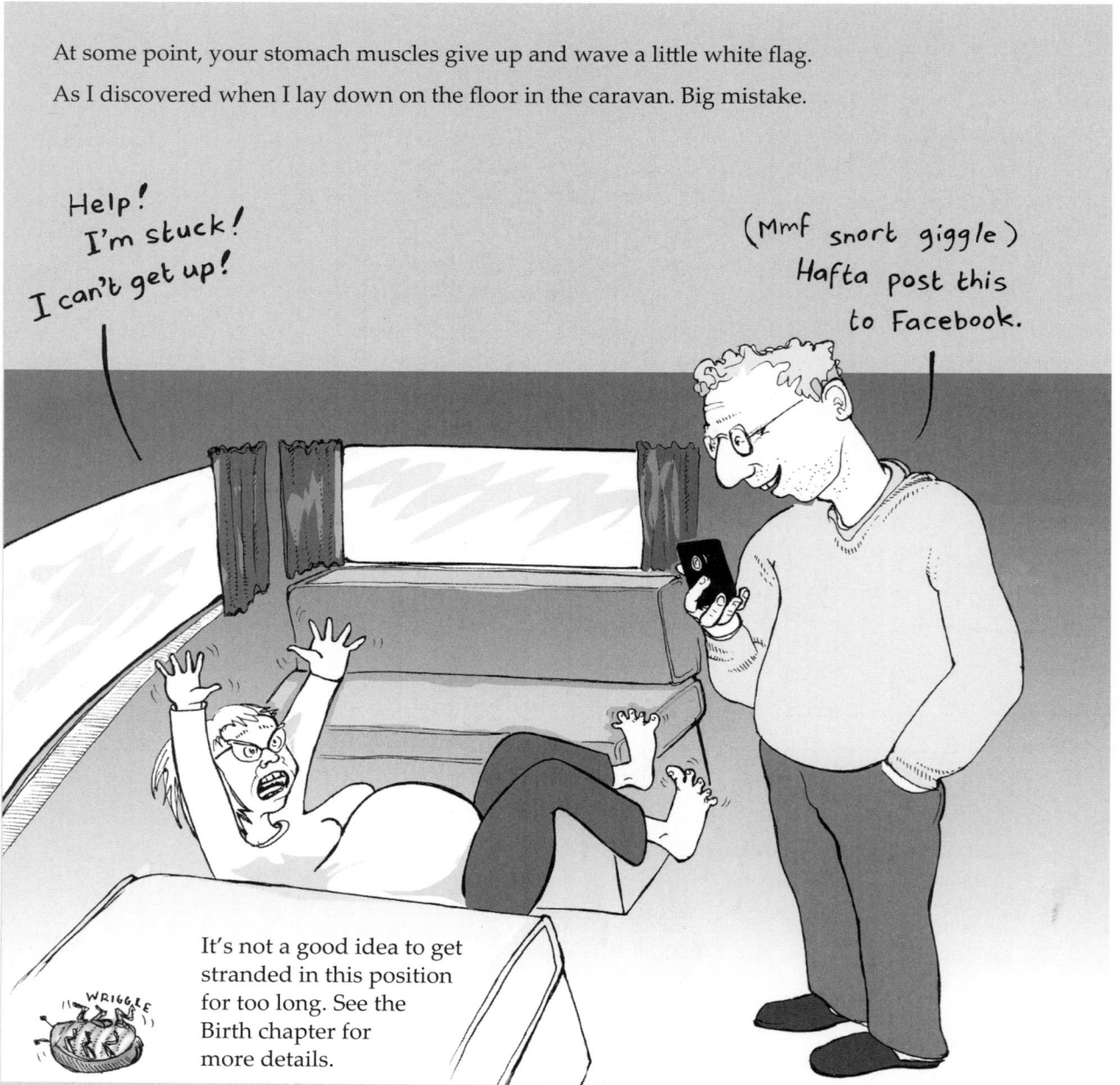

It's not a good idea to get stranded in this position for too long. See the Birth chapter for more details.

And, even though you now look like a sofa, you still need extra padding at night.

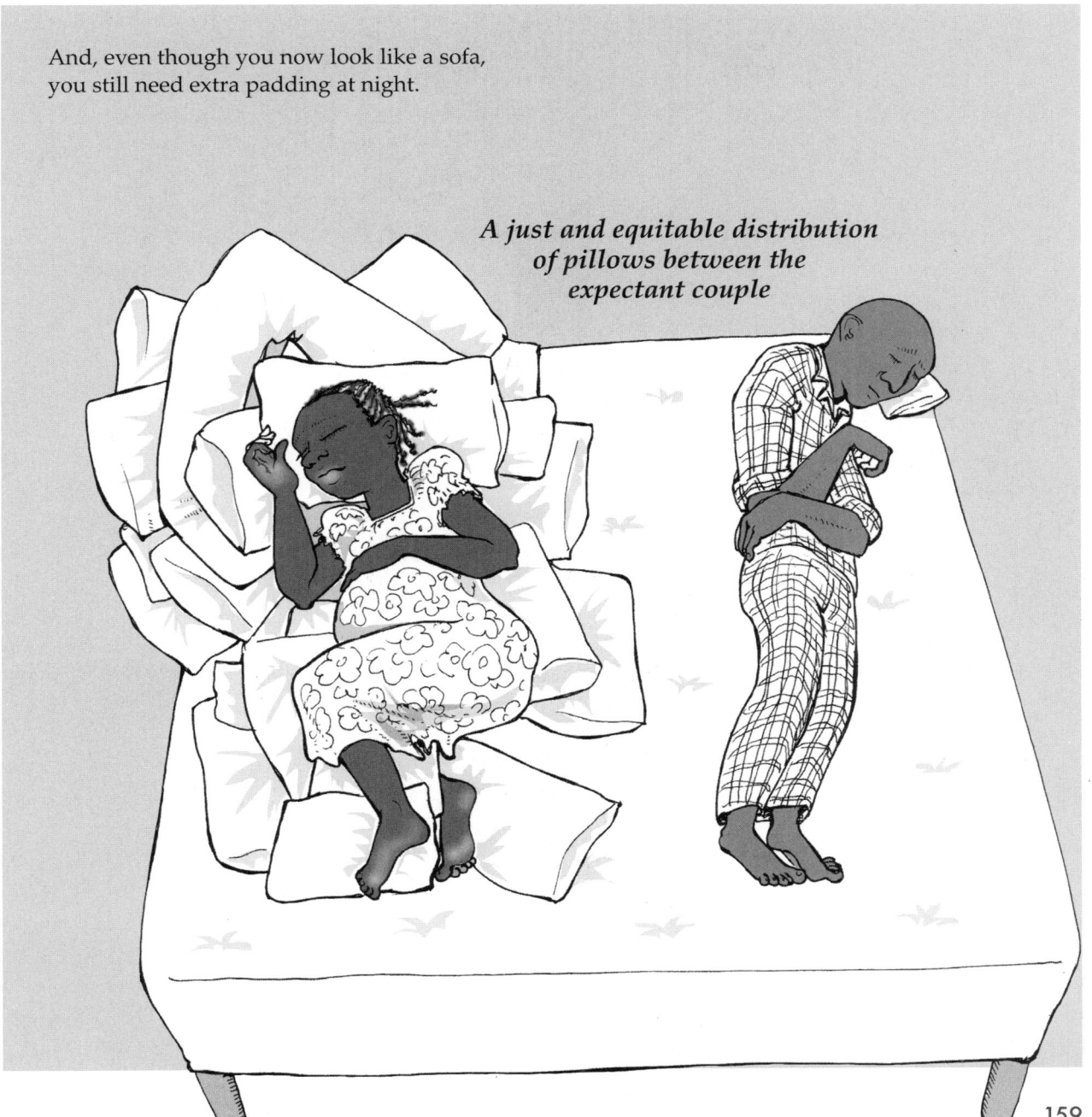

A just and equitable distribution of pillows between the expectant couple

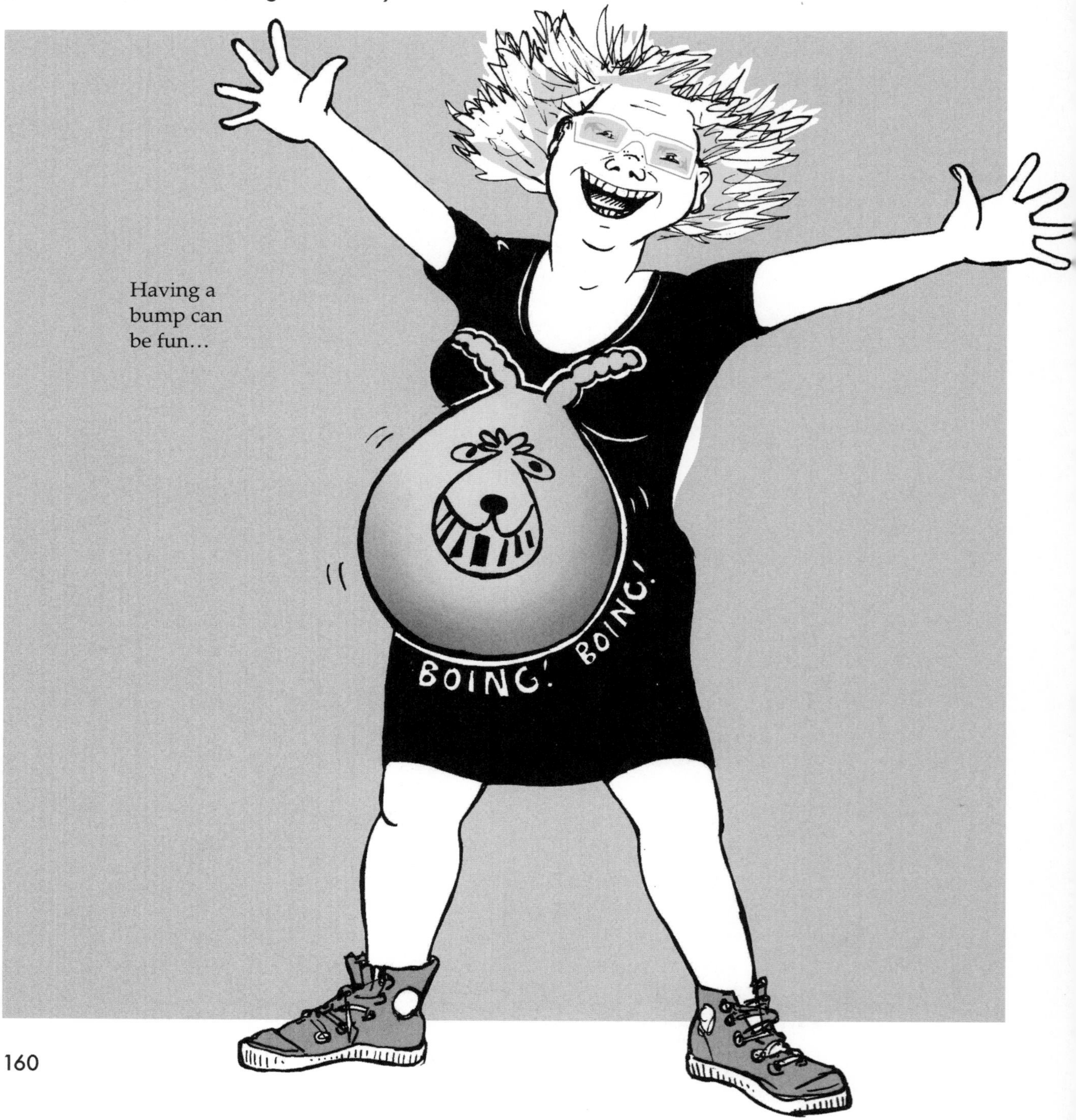
BOING! BOING!

Having a
bump can
be fun…

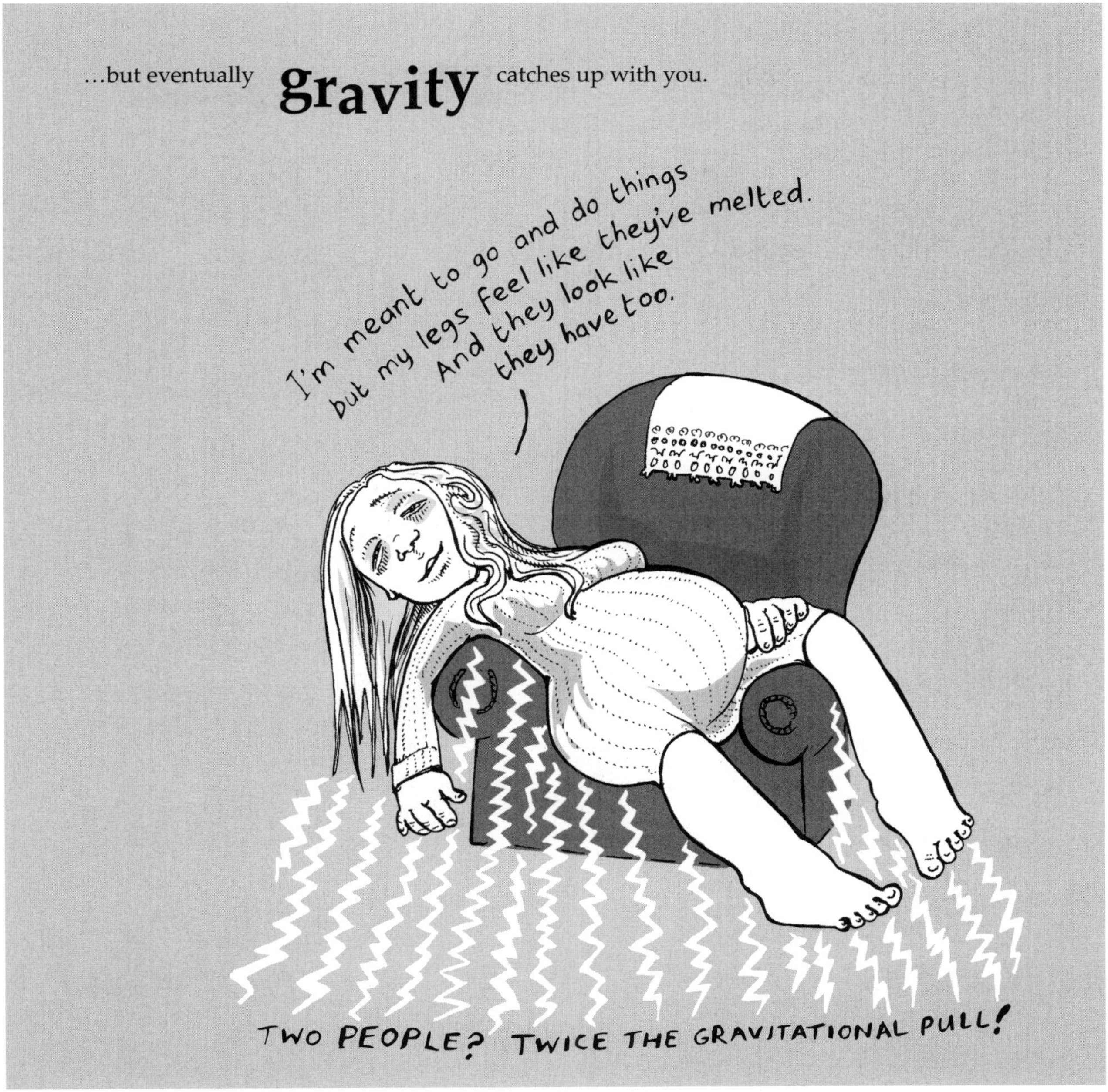
…but eventually **gravity** catches up with you.
I'm meant to go and do things but my legs feel like they've melted. And they look like they have too.
TWO PEOPLE? TWICE THE GRAVITATIONAL PULL!

I, the Divine Being, bestow upon YOU WOMAN! the Greatest Gift of all! You shall BRING FORTH NEW LIFE FROM your LOINS!

With you resides the ULTIMATE POWER! The MIRACLE OF CREATION! The very FUTURE OF THE HUMAN RACE!

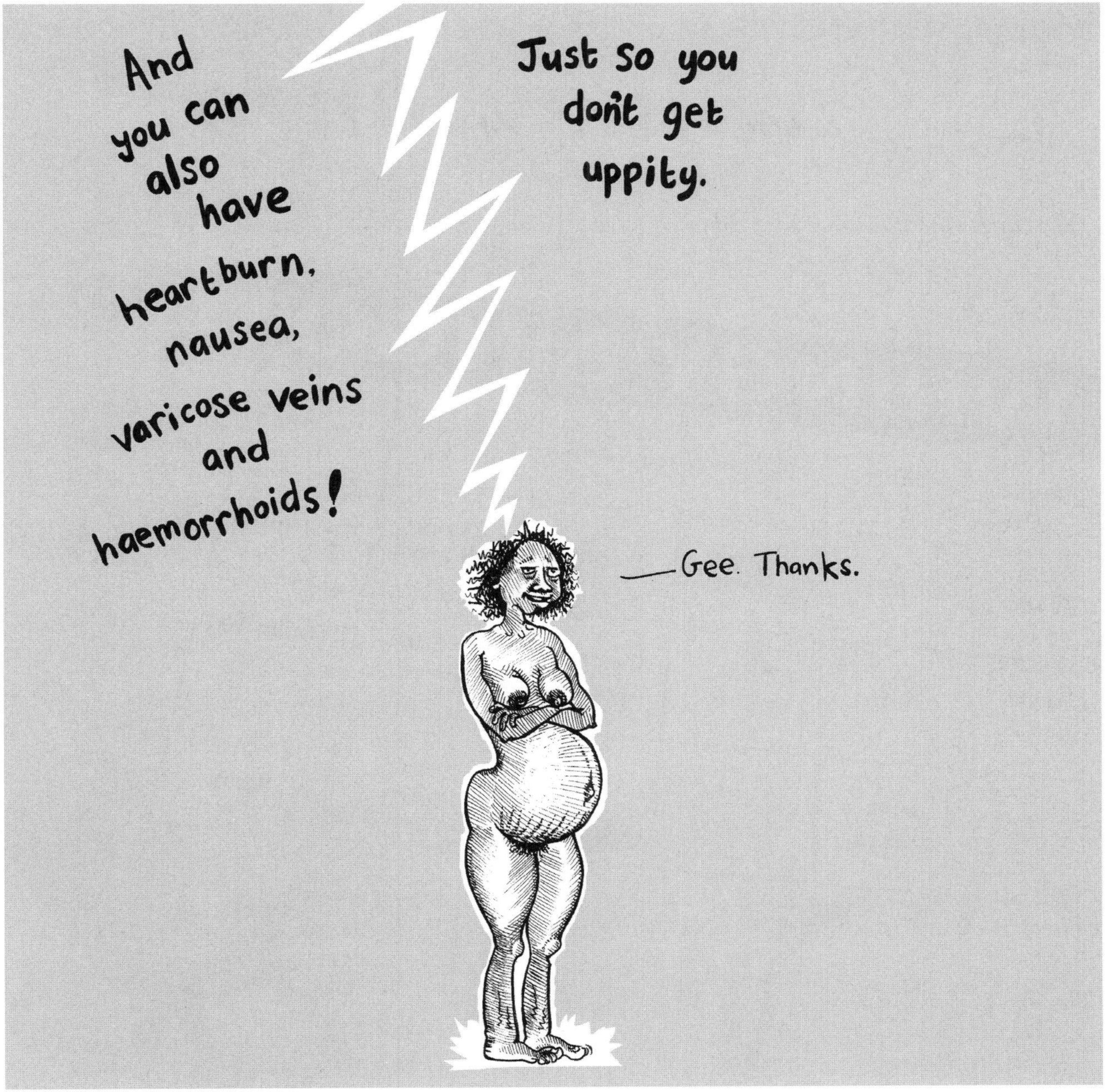
And you can also have heartburn, nausea, varicose veins and haemorrhoids!
Just so you don't get uppity.
Gee. Thanks.

10 *Whingy bingo*

Us pregnant ladies have a lot to moan about.

WHINGY BINGO

Being sick	Bleeding gums	Thrush	Heartburn	Swollen ankles	Cystitis
Piles	Sniffles	Stretch marks	Itching	Crazy dreams	Insomnia
Consti-pation	Cramp	Back-ache	Varicose veins	Head-ache	Breathless-ness
Faintness	Sore wrists	Fat fingers	Peeing yourself	Pelvic pain	Sleepless-ness

How do you score?

Nausea and vomiting

Your levels of hCG, the hormone implicated in morning sickness, decline from the 12th week of pregnancy until the 20th, and then they level off. So you're likely to be less nauseous in later months than you were in the first weeks, but, once you get to 20 weeks, however sick you are, that's how sick you'll stay. Try hypnotherapy or acupuncture treatment, as these can both really help.

Other self-help tips are on page 89.

Have a bonus 50 points if you are inadvertently sick on another person. And another 50 points if you throw up in public and someone gives you a dirty look because they think you're drunk.

Gum health

Your gums, like all the connective tissue in your body, become softer and spongier in pregnancy. Infected bleeding gums put you at slightly increased risk of premature labour, so visit your dentist and get germ-harbouring plaque professionally removed from your teeth.

Dental treatment is free for pregnant women.

- Brush twice a day with a soft toothbrush or an electric one. Floss carefully daily.
- Use mouthwash if your gums bleed.
- Don't brush your teeth immediately after being sick as the acid strips the enamel from your teeth. Just rinse your mouth out to take the taste away.
- If tooth brushing makes you gag, take it slowly and allow more time. An electric toothbrush may be easier to handle.
- Sugary fizzy drinks kill your gums.

Heartburn

This is caused by your softer, more spongy and relaxed oesophagus, and the upward pressure on your stomach from your womb.

- Eat six small meals a day instead of three big ones, and chew your food slowly.
- Don't lie down immediately after eating, and try to eat in the middle of the day rather than in the three hours before bed.
- Drink plenty of water in between meals.
- There is a shiatsu spot to help with heartburn four fingers' width above your belly button. Press this point firmly for ten seconds at a time, intermittently for ten minutes. I'm copying this piece of information out of a standard midwifery textbook, by the way – it's not just random hippy ramblings.
- Things that might trigger an attack for you could include caffeine, chocolate, citrus, fatty or spicy foods.
- Other foods might help: try fresh or crystallised ginger, pineapple, coconut water, a spoonful of plain yoghurt at the end of the meal, chewing gum (though that's technically not food), fresh papaya and papaya enzyme tablets and slippery elm food supplement.
- Consult an acupuncturist.
- Your pharmacist can recommend an antacid for use in pregnancy.
- If it's cripplingly awful, prescription medication that stops your stomach from producing acid can be obtained from your doctor.

Thrush

See page 106.

Swollen ankles and fat fingers

Bigger, spongier, softer and more swollen...
are you noticing a theme here?

It's kinda funny that having a child with
someone, that ultimate act of commitment for
a couple, results in you having to take your
wedding ring off and leave it in a drawer.

- Drink lots of water. This seems counter-
  intuitive, but you want to get fluid moving
  through your body, not lingering around.
- Move, stretch, massage, rest and elevate
  swollen parts.
- Try a massage blend of one teaspoon of base oil
  (olive oil is fine) and one drop each of lemon
  and geranium essential oils.
- Relax in a bath with a cup of Epsom salts in.
- Do these foot exercises. Sit upright on the floor
  with both your feet together in front of you.
  Make big circles with your feet side by side,
  12 times in each direction. Now point your feet
  back towards you while pressing your calves
  into the floor. Arch your foot downwards while
  keeping your toes pulled back. Point your toes
  down, pull them back, and then arch your
  feet back towards you. Repeat 12 times. These
  exercises also help prevent cramps and varicose
  veins.
- Yoga also helps. If you can't make it to a yoga
  class, YouTube has videos of pregnancy poses
  for swollen feet.
- Buy a leafy green cabbage and put it in the
  fridge. When cold, break off a couple of leaves
  and wrap them around your ankles, holding in
  place with a sock, tubigrip or crêpe bandage.
  Leave in place until it's damp and limp, then
  discard and repeat. Your feet now smell of
  cabbage. It will help with the swelling, though.

Cystitis

Guess why you get cystitis? Could it be because
your urethra is softer, larger and more relaxed?
Yes! Coupled with the fact that your bladder is
squashed by your massively enlarged womb.
It can be difficult to get out the last drops of
pee, so sit on the toilet a little longer, and shift
your weight to empty your bladder fully.
Any left behind can harbour bacteria and cause
infection.

If you feel a burning, stinging sensation when
you pee, and unusual urgency that only produces
a trickle, quick, take action!

- Immediately drink a pint of water with a
  teaspoon of bicarbonate of soda in. This is
  the active ingredient in the sachets of cystitis
  relief remedies you buy in the chemist
  (although the flavourings in those make them
  taste a lot nicer.)
- Keep drinking water; at least three litres over
  the next 12 hours. Substitute barley water or
  no-sugar-added cranberry juice if you get sick
  of water.
- Have a hot bath with a cup of table salt or
  Epsom salts in. You can pee in it. This will
  help fight the infection. Stay in it, and keep
  drinking. This gets boring, so take a book in
  there with you.
- If you are feverish and feel horrible, see
  your doctor without delay. You may need
  antibiotics. Remind her that you're pregnant,
  unless that's obvious.
- Don't have penetrative sex until your
  symptoms clear.
- Drinking a glass of cranberry juice every day
  will help prevent further attacks.

Piles, aka haemorrhoids

Bigger, spongier, more swollen bottom veins? Too Much Information!

- Get some pile ointment from the chemist.
- Dilute one drop of geranium essential oil in a teaspoon of olive oil and smooth gently over the affected area.
- Increase the amount of red and black berries in your diet, and eat more garlic. These foods allegedly help strengthen your veins.
- There is a shiatsu point on the top of your head, in the very middle. Press it firmly for about ten seconds three times.
- Drink plenty of water to keep your poos soft – see 'constipation' on the next page.
- Don't strain when you poo. The squatty potty mentioned on page 151 may help.
- You can take paracetamol for severe pain.

Snuffles, snores and nosebleeds

The blood vessels in the lining of your nose can also become enlarged, sometimes alarmingly so. There's not much you can do about this except wait until the baby is born, although the foods listed above could theoretically help.

If you get a nosebleed, sit down, pinch the area just below the bridge of your nose firmly and lean forward so the blood doesn't run down your throat. Frequent nosebleeds could be an indication of high blood pressure.

Stretch marks

Since every other part of the pregnant body is becoming larger, softer and spongier, why can't your skin keep with the programme?

Ninety per cent of pregnant women get stretch marks, and the magic cream that prevents them hasn't yet been discovered (no matter what the adverts for expensive skin care products say).

But what's wrong with them? They're a bit alarming when they first come up – great purple claw marks – but they soon fade to a lovely dappled-silver effect. We don't like them, because they make us look as if we've had babies. Well, that's a stupid ideal of beauty, because having babies is a beautiful thing to do. For several hundred years, freckles and sun tans were considered disfiguring. Not any more. Let's change our thinking, celebrate our bodies, and reclaim our stretch marks.

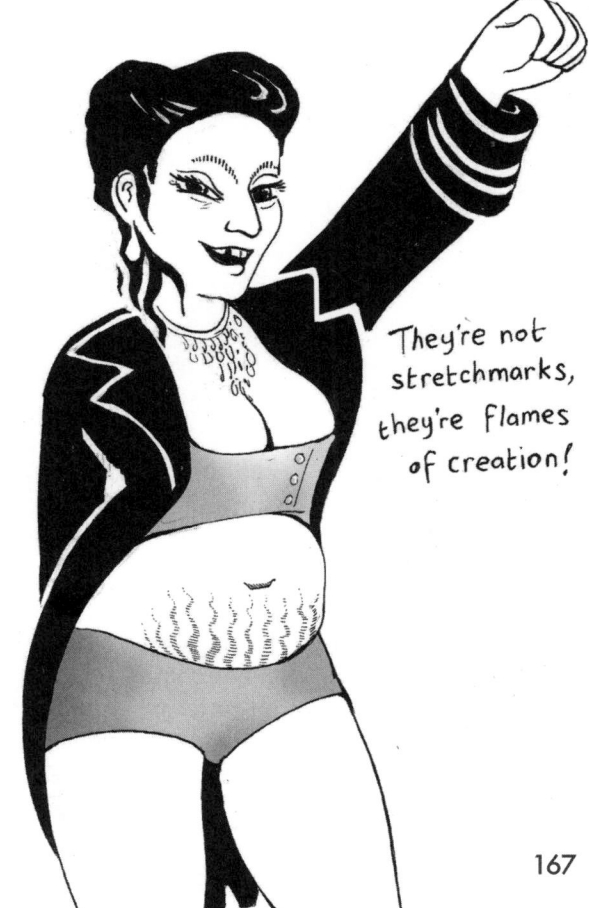

They're not stretchmarks, they're flames of creation!

Itching

Around 17% of pregnant women get itchy skin, particularly on their bumps, the palms of the hands and the soles of the feet. The stresses on the stretching skin, and the hormone oestrogen, could be to blame. You can even develop a rash of bumps, blisters or pustules during pregnancy that then clears up after the baby arrives.

But pregnant women can also develop gestational liver disease, which causes itching and exhaustion and can affect your baby, so definitely mention your symptoms to your midwife.

- Try lukewarm baths with oatmeal in to soothe your skin.
- Stop using perfumed bubble baths or creams in case they make it worse.
- Slap on some plain, unscented E45 cold cream or natural shea-butter moisturiser.
- Wear loose cotton clothes.
- Try not to get too hot.
- Press iced wet cloths over itchy areas.
- Try gently scratching the very tips of your fingers. This fools your brain into thinking you've scratched the itchy places.
- Buy calamine lotion from the chemist.
- Your doctor may prescribe antihistamines or steroid creams if your skin is very sore.
- Acupuncture and hypnotherapy can both help.

Crazy dreams

I had a vivid recurring dream that the baby had been born some time before, but I had been too busy drawing cartoons to notice. I don't know what that was about.

Insomnia

Given the incredible array of debilitating and irritating conditions that you could be suffering from, perhaps it's not surprising that you can find it hard to sleep.

- Increase your exercise. Yoga, swimming and those five miles a day of walking will all help.
- We're meant to go to sleep when it's dark! Blue light from iPads, laptops, TVs and backlit e-readers can fool our brains into thinking it's daytime. The closer the device is to your face, the worse the effect. Banish electronic devices for at least an hour before bed. Read a book instead.
- If thoughts are racing round your head, learn to meditate. Practise this skill during odd moments in the daytime too.
- You can't take sleeping pills, but you can use a hop pillow. Buy fresh or dried hops from a brewers' supplies, and crumble a few into a cloth bag to sniff while you fall asleep.
- Lavender or Roman camomile essential oil may help. Don't use these in the first 12 weeks of pregnancy.

Constipation

Progesterone relaxes the action of the smooth muscle of the gut, and your body also absorbs extra water from your food. This brings on a double whammy of constipation.

- Drink more water.
- Eat more fibre, in the form of bran cereal, fresh fruit and vegetables, wholegrains and pulses.
- Exercise will help. Do that walking!
- Squatting at the toilet helps your bowel action. See page 151.

- Iron supplements can aggravate the problem. Floradix iron tonic may be more easily tolerated.
- Artichoke can help, either eaten as a food or taken in capsule form.
- Massage your belly firmly in a large clockwise circle. This follows the direction of the action of the gut. Use a teaspoon of massage oil with a drop of orange essential oil if you like.
- And you can massage the arches of your feet in a large clockwise circle too. If you can still reach your feet.
- The shiatsu point to help constipation lies on the underside of your bump, halfway between your belly button and the bony part of your groin. Press intermittently for ten seconds at a time for about five minutes.
- Ask your midwife or doctor to recommend a laxative if you are suffering. Stool-softeners or osmotic laxatives are the treatment of first choice. Stimulant laxatives such as senna should only be used under medical supervision in case they trigger premature labour. Liquid paraffin interferes with your ability to absorb vitamins from your food, so is best avoided.

Cramp

Ow ow ow ow ow! This mainly occurs in the legs, at night. OW!

- When calf cramp strikes, push your foot back against the bedstead, nearby furniture or the wall. This will hurt more at first, but will ease the pain.
- Do the foot exercises for swollen ankles on page 166 every night before going to bed.
- Massage your calves before bed. If you can still reach them.

- Lying on your left side increases the blood flow to and from your legs.
- Avoid sitting with your legs crossed.
- Walk a lot. Drink lots of water. (I'm going to keep repeating these two recommendations.)
- If the pain remains constant, or your leg looks swollen in one patch, is red, feels hot or is tender to the touch, seek medical attention immediately, as this could be a sign of a blood clot. This condition is rare.

Backache

You're carrying a lot of extra weight, most of it is in one lump in your tummy, and all your joints have become softer and more stretchy. Back pain is common.

- All pregnant women should get lots of firm lower back massages from their friends and family. (Friends! Partners! Relatives! Offer to do this!)
- When you get up from lying down, first roll on to your side, then push yourself up with your arms. You can strain your back and belly if you try to use stomach muscles that just aren't there any more.
- Wear flat shoes, not high heels.
- Avoid sitting with your legs crossed and pay attention to your posture.
- Before you lift heavy objects or toddlers, consciously engage your abdominal and pelvic floor muscles to protect your lower back, keep your back straight and bend from the knees.
- Pregnancy yoga and aquanatal exercise classes will help.
- If the pain is severe, you can take paracetamol up to the recommended dose.

Persistent backache can be cured completely or improved greatly by a good osteopath or chiropractor. You'll have to pay for treatment, but just a few sessions can make a real difference, so it's money well spent.

Varicose veins

Big, stretchy blood vessels again (see 'Piles' and 'Snuffles'). Big, stretchy, unsightly, painful blood vessels at that. You can also get 'spider veins' – tiny burst blood vessels on the surface of your skin. These usually disappear completely once the baby is born.

- At the first sign of varicose veins, ask your midwife about support garments. You can get unsexy stockings for your legs which should be put on in the morning before you get out of bed. If you get swollen veins on your fanny, you may be given a strange chastity-belt-like garment to wear day and night. (Although it's a bit late for one of those.)
- Lie down on your left side or put your feet up for at least half an hour twice a day.
- If you have to sit or stand for long periods of time, circle your ankles and shift your position frequently. Make time to take breaks to walk around. Ensure that your chair doesn't press into the backs of your thighs – your feet should be fully supported, on a stool if necessary.
- Eat more garlic and berries. Not together.
- Wear flat shoes and unrestrictive clothes.
- Drink more water, walk five miles a day, do yoga. (Shall I just write those recommendations in big fat letters across the top of the page?)
- A herbalist may be able to recommend remedies such as nettle and oatstraw tea or horse-chestnut extract.

Headache

As the blood vessels in your head become enlarged, headaches in the early weeks of pregnancy are common.

- Drink plenty of water.
- Massage your scalp firmly with your fingers, as though you're washing your hair.
- Massage your big toes. Weird, but it works.
- If you need to, take paracetamol, but not aspirin or ibruprofen.
- Talk to your midwife or doctor if your headaches are debilitating.
- Some headaches may be posture-related, in which case an osteopath/chiropractor can help.
- Try cranio-sacral therapy.

Breathlessness

You have a need for 20% more oxygen, and less room in your diaphragm. Do the maths. Episodes of breathlessness can occur at any time, and are sometimes accompanied by pounding heart palpitations. Don't panic. Just take a moment to stop and catch your breath. and change your position. If you are slouched over, straighten your back and expand your ribcage.

- Mention this to your midwife, as it could be a sign of anaemia (low iron levels in your blood).
- Yoga classes will help you learn to breathe more deeply.
- Increase your overall fitness. Are you walking those five miles a day?
- If you experience sudden, severe shortness of breath that doesn't ease off in a few minutes, and/or sharp chest pains, seek immediate medical attention. It is possible (though rare) that you could have a blood clot in your lung.

- Asthma and chest infections can also be serious in pregnancy, as you need all the air you can get. Don't be shy about consulting your doctor about breathing difficulties. They would much rather you see them when your condition isn't serious than that you didn't when it is.

Faintness

The friend of breathlessness. Your body works very hard making a whole new human being. Give yourself some credit.

If you feel faint or dizzy, your immediate reaction should be to lie down on your left side or, if that's not possible, sit down and put your head between your knees (as far as you still can.) If you're driving, PULL OVER NOW, unclip your seatbelt and slump gracefully over into the passenger seat.

Be aware of some triggers of faintness:

- Standing up too quickly. When you get out of bed, move gradually to a sitting position, pause, and then get up.
- Lying flat on your back. In this position, your enormous womb compresses the major artery that returns blood from your lower limbs back to your head. This can make you feel anxious and light-headed. Shift your position. Wedging a pillow under your right hip will tilt your pelvis enough to relieve your symptoms.
- Seeing shocking things, or, strangely, straining to cough, pee or poo can all provoke a reaction in your nervous system, and trigger a faint. This is often preceded by ringing in the ears, yawning, fast breathing, and feeling sick, clammy, sweaty and pale.
- Not eating regularly. You need fuel.

- Getting dehydrated can make you light-headed. How many times must I remind you to *drink lots of water*?
- Overheating makes your blood vessels larger, which causes your blood pressure to fall. If you really like hot baths, keep the window open to cool the bathroom down.
- Anaemia. If your iron stores are low, you have fewer red blood cells to carry oxygen around your body. Your midwife can recommend iron supplements when necessary.
- Being unfit makes dizziness more likely, so, once again, I will nag you to do moderate aerobic exercise. Are you walking five miles a day? Why not?

Tell your doctor or midwife if you ever actually faint, or if you experience dizziness to a worrying degree.

Seek urgent medical attention if the dizzy feeling doesn't pass off quickly, particularly if you have blurred vision, problems co-ordinating your limbs or shortness of breath.

Also seek prompt medical assistance if you have dizziness accompanied by pain in your belly or side in early pregnancy, or if you feel dizzy after a head injury.

If a pregnant woman faints and remains unconscious for more than two minutes, call an ambulance, and put her in the recovery position, preferably on her left side.

Sore wrists and tingling hands

The swollen tissues of pregnancy can compress the nerves of the wrist, causing carpal tunnel syndrome. This is more likely if your job involves repetitive activities such as typing or the frequent use of vibrating power tools.

- Stop any avoidable repetitive activities.
- Personally, I find it helps to stretch out your fingers, rotate your hands fully at the wrists and firmly massage aching areas.
- The backs of your hands should be level with your forearms when you type. Raise your chair so your arms are level, and use wrist supports (socks filled with rice work suprisingly well). An ergonomic keyboard may help.
- The pain is often worse at night. Don't sleep with your wrists bent. If this is difficult, you can get a splint from a physiotherapist to immobilise them.
- Try cold gel packs on your wrists to relieve the pain, and if it's bad you can take paracetamol.
- Acupuncture can help.
- If your wrists are still sore after the birth, you'll need a sling to carry your baby around. A 'pouch' design is probably easiest to use.

Your symptoms should resolve themselves by the time your baby is three months old. If not, get some treatment.

Incontinence

If you pee when you cough, sneeze or jump, you need to improve that pelvic floor tone and mobility. And squeeze! See pages 150 to 152.

If you suffer from sudden urgency, you may also need to retrain your bladder by gradually increasing the length of time between trips to the toilet. Certain foods such as sugar or caffeine may make your bladder more overactive.

Using pads won't help in the long run, as you'll start to rely on them. Ask to be referred for medical help.

Pelvic pain or SPD

This is the only valid excuse that I will accept for not walking five miles a day, and that's only until you get it sorted out.

Pelvic Girdle Pain (PGP) is common in pregnancy, but that doesn't mean that it's normal, inevitable or untreatable. We're talking about pain anywhere in your hips, tailbone or groin area. Symphysis Pubis Dysfunction (SPD) is a particular type of PGP. It feels approximately as if someone has stuck a crowbar in the bone at the front of your crotch and twisted it sideways. I've had it. I know.

You could feel pain when walking, climbing steps, swinging one leg up or turning over in bed. You can't even crawl with severe SPD as you need to keep your thighs level at hip-width to alleviate your symptoms. If you don't get treatment, you could end up using crutches or a wheelchair for the rest of your pregnancy or even beyond.

The pain is caused by stiffness or an old injury to one of your pelvic joints – probably not the one that is hurting. This then puts uneven stress on the rest of your pelvis, which, being extra-stretchy at the moment, starts to flex strangely and become sore. There are no nerve-endings in the joints themselves – the pain you feel is as a result of inflammation in the surrounding tissues. This explains why you can feel OK while you are actually moving, and then be doubled over in agony later that day.

To treat it, someone needs to realign your pelvis. An experienced physiotherapist can do this on the NHS, or you can pay to see a chiropractor or osteopath. Your therapist should assess your movement and then manually move your bones about. This doesn't hurt, and should make an immediate difference. For some women, one session is all they need.

Keep attending manual therapy until you are completely pain-free. This is very important if you ever plan to get pregnant again as you don't want this to recur during the next pregnancy when you also have a hefty toddler to lump around.

You may be given exercises to do between appointments. These shouldn't hurt. If they do, then ask for them to be changed.

While you are waiting for treatment:

- Before you make any unavoidable and potentially painful movement, consciously engage your pelvic floor and abdominal muscles to give your pelvis more support.
- Don't sit with your legs or ankles crossed.
- Keep your hips level in bed by sleeping with a pillow between your legs.
- It's easier to turn over in bed if you wear silky pyjamas or use satin sheets or a slippery sleeping bag.
- Walk upstairs backwards or shuffle up on your bottom.
- You can put a carrier bag on your car seat, then swivel round, keeping your knees together.
- Take paracetamol if you need pain relief.
- Think about positions for labour and birth that don't involve having your legs spread apart in stirrups.

The charity the Pelvic Partnership can give you information, support and recommend a good therapist.

'It'll all be better once the baby is born.'

Score a bonus 100 points if anyone attempts to address your concerns about irritating, painful or debilitating conditions with this trite and unhelpful phrase.

Still, this brings us to an interesting issue – one we have been avoiding thus far. The logical consequence of being pregnant is that… you're going to have to give birth to a baby!

AAAAAAARRRRGGHHHHH!!!

When? What do you need to have ready? And how?

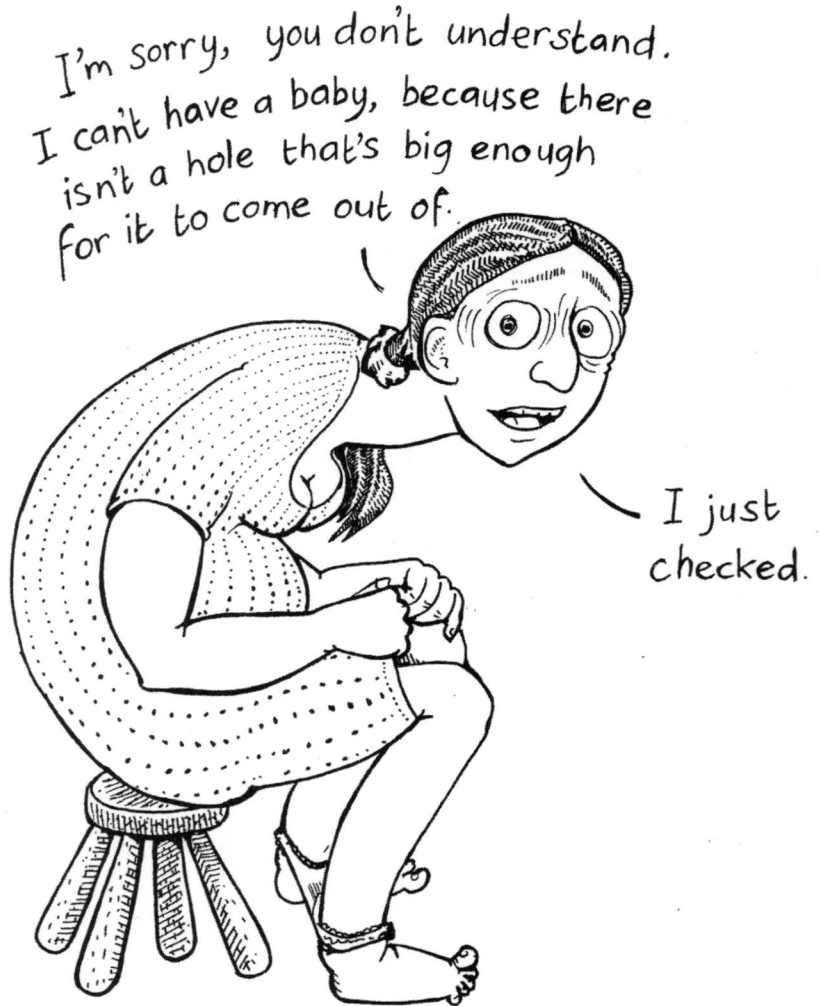

This is an understandable apprehension, but women's bodies are amazing.

Really incredible.

Read on…

Book the Third
How to birth a baby

11 The broke mum's budget baby list

Are you ready to have a baby?

Have you bought enough stuff yet?

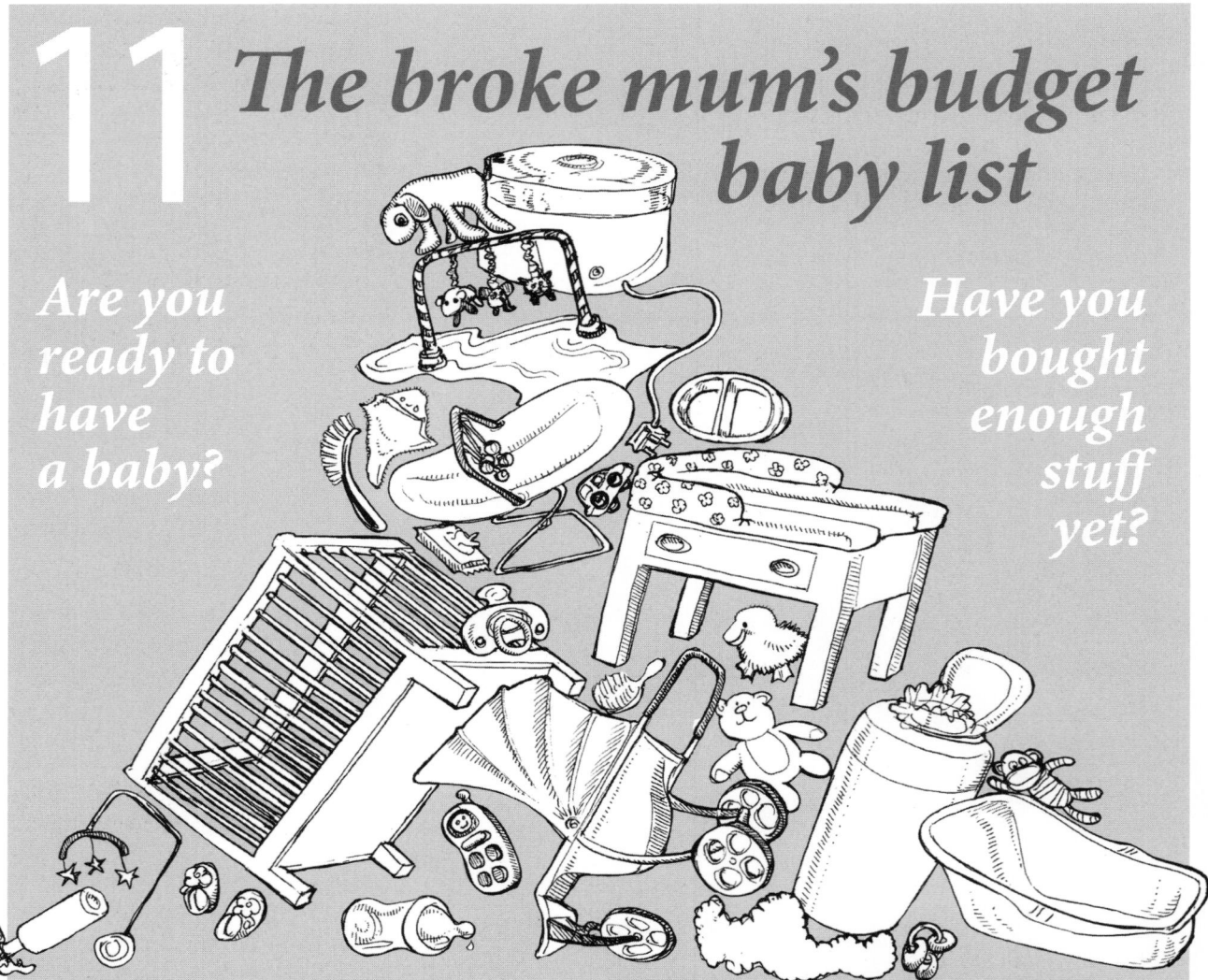

New mum? New consumer!

There's *so much* baby stuff out there to sell you. It could theoretically be useful – it was all invented for a reason – but how much do you actually need right now? Unlike all the pregnancy magazines you read and all the websites you visit, I'm not going to make money out of flogging you baby goods. So let's strip back the marketing speak and isolate the actual essentials.

Somewhere for the baby to sleep

It's normal in our culture to shell out for a cot with all the trimmings, but you don't have to if you don't want to.

If you don't smoke and you breastfeed, you can share a bed with your baby. Like this:

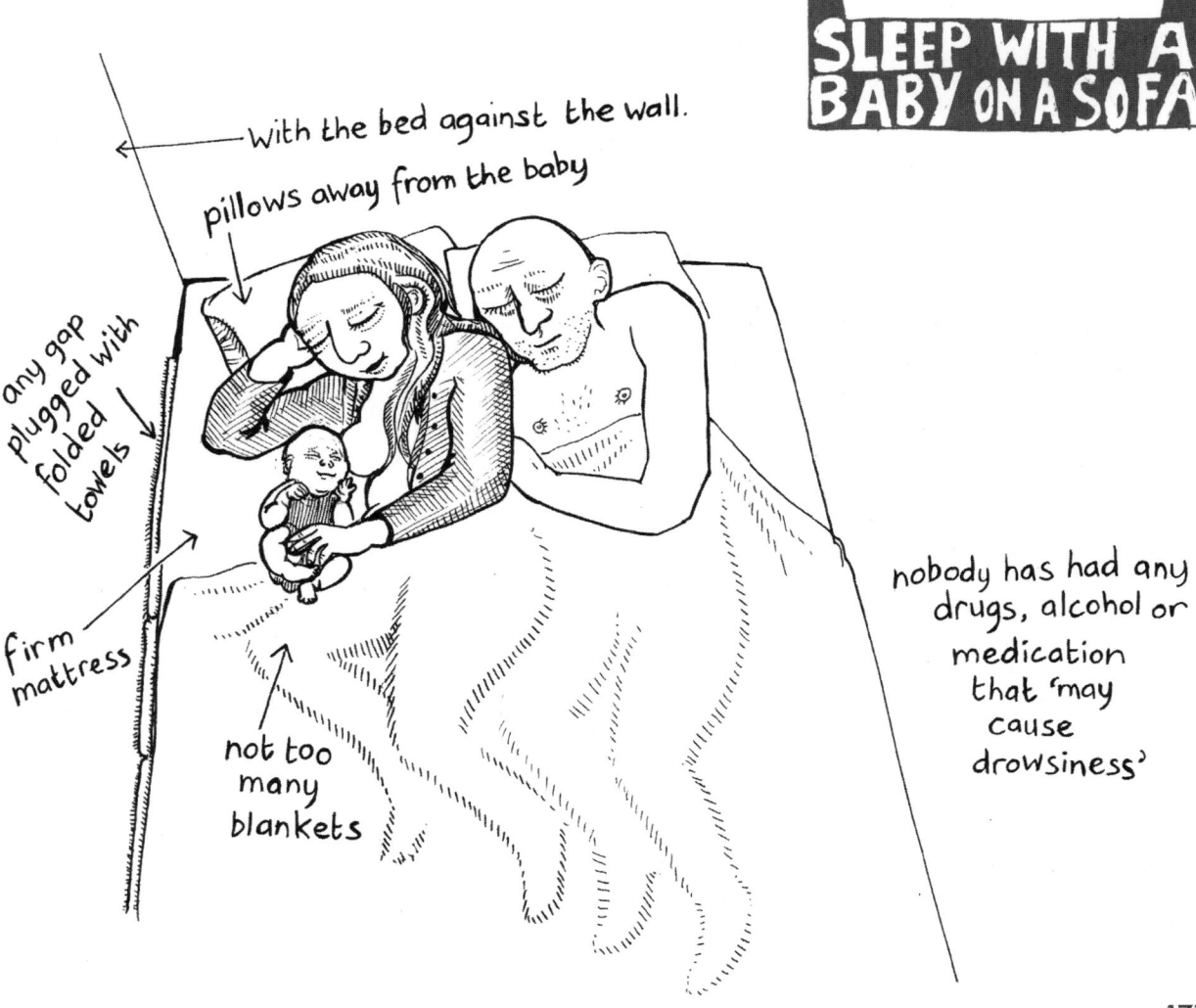

NEVER EVER SLEEP WITH A BABY ON A SOFA

With the bed against the wall.

pillows away from the baby

any gap plugged with folded towels

firm mattress

not too many blankets

nobody has had any drugs, alcohol or medication that 'may cause drowsiness'

If you do smoke or don't breastfeed, your baby is safer in a crib or moses basket. You don't have to buy one. If no one has one spare, you could use a drawer or a cardboard box on the floor by your bed. Seriously! The Finnish government issue all new parents with boxes that their babies can sleep in. Fold up a blanket and cover it with a sheet to line the base.

You don't need

A separate bedroom for your baby. The risk of cot death is reduced if they sleep near you, day or night. This means you won't need a baby monitor yet, either.

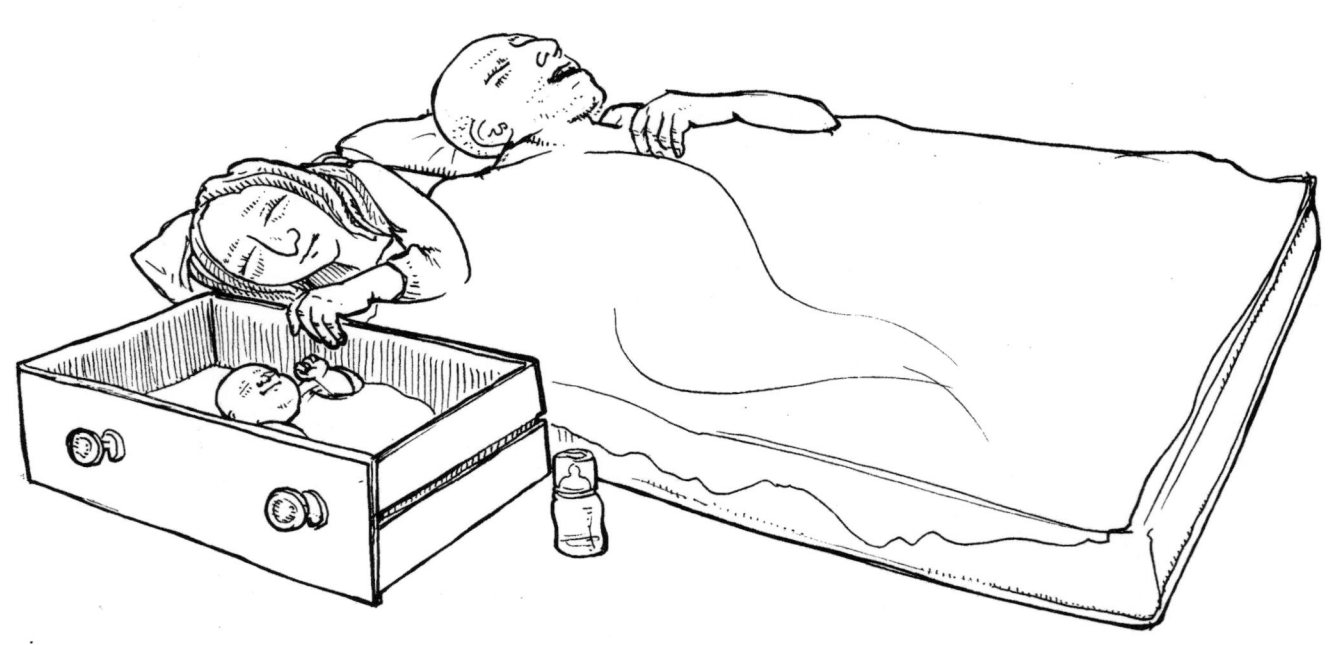

Money spent so far: big fat zero.

Some things to keep the baby warm

Baby clothes will be useful:

You need a couple of baby blankets. My local haberdashery shop sells a metre of fleece fabric for £4. Sorted. No sewing skills required, just chop it off and wrap 'em up.

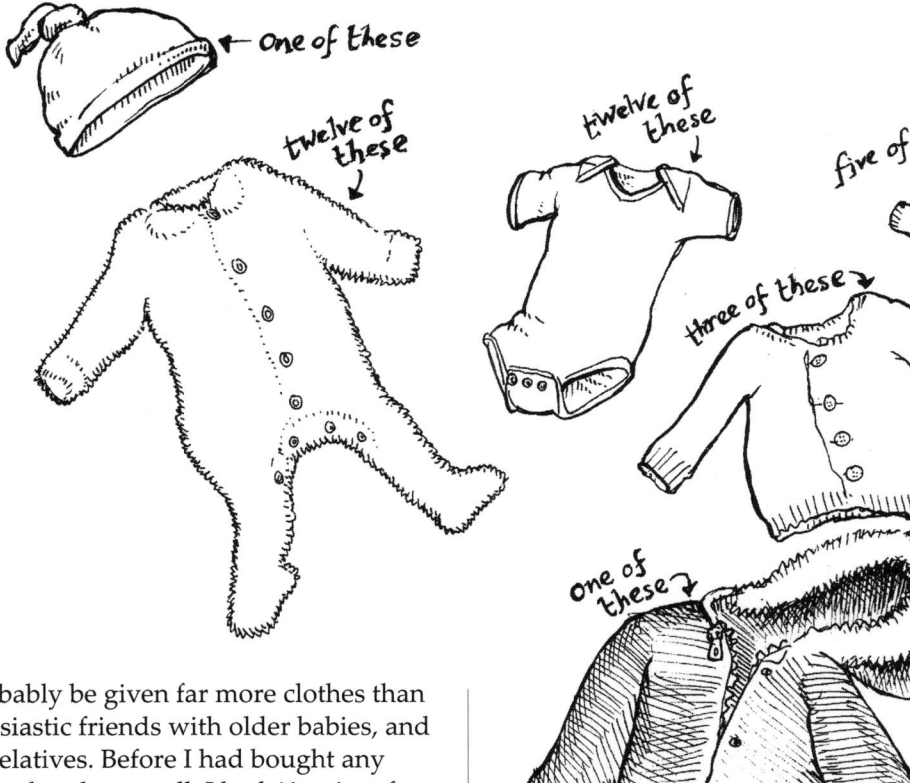

one of these

twelve of these

twelve of these

five of these

three of these

one of these

You'll probably be given far more clothes than this by enthusiastic friends with older babies, and overexcited relatives. Before I had bought any clothes for my daughter at all, I had 41 pairs of trousers in newborn size. Feeling this was a little excessive, I whittled it down to 26.

Failing that, charity shops sell perfectly serviceable baby clothes for 50p. Even if you find it unacceptable to dress your child in second-hand clothes and you'd rather get new ones made in a Bangladeshi sweat shop, you can buy everything you need from a supermarket for less than 40 quid.

Something to mop the baby up with

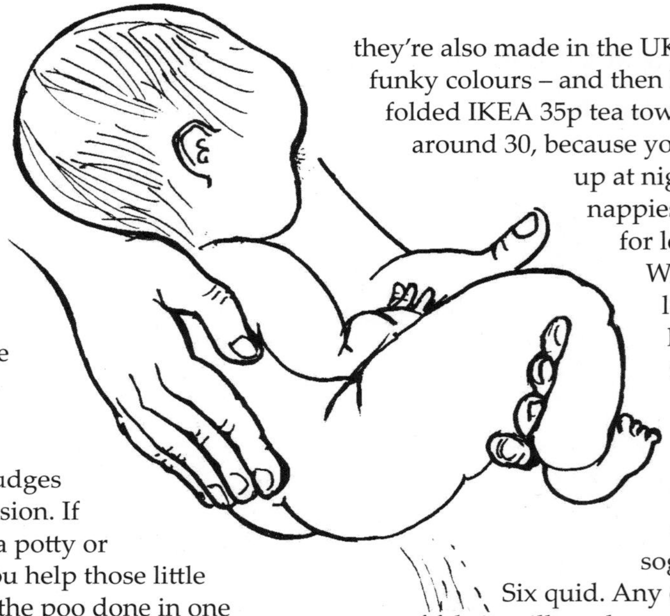

Technically, you don't even need nappies. Google 'elimination communication' if you don't believe me. I tried this for a while with my newborn and it was, er, interesting. I'm not sure we saved on washing, but it did give me some useful skills.

Small babies tend to poo frequently, splotting little smudges on to lots of nappies in succession. If you hold your baby out over a potty or sink at nappy change time, you help those little bowels to work better, get all the poo done in one go, and save yourself a lot of effort.

Assuming you want nappies – which I did in the end – your choice is washable or disposable.

Two packets of newborn disposable nappies are easy to use and won't break the bank. Having a brand new baby is so overwhelming that you don't need lots of washing, so buy some for the early weeks.

If you want to save money, in the long run washables work out cheaper, especially if you're planning more than one child. They're much better for the environment, particularly if you don't tumble-dry them. Check out TotsBots Easy Fit All in Ones. They're made in the UK, they line dry really quickly, and they'll fit your baby from newborn to toddler. You can buy ten for £130 if you shop around.

But we're on a budget, so, for a totally no-frills cloth nappy package, buy four first-size nappy covers – I rate 'Nature Babies' wraps because they're also made in the UK and come in funky colours – and then line them with folded IKEA 35p tea towels. (You'll need around 30, because you double them up at night.) That's all the nappies for your baby for less than 40 quid. Wash them in a full load on 60°C and line-dry them and they'll cost you less than 50p a week.

Get some calendula nappy cream for that soggy-nappied bot. Six quid. Any odd square of waterproof fabric will work as a change mat.

You don't need

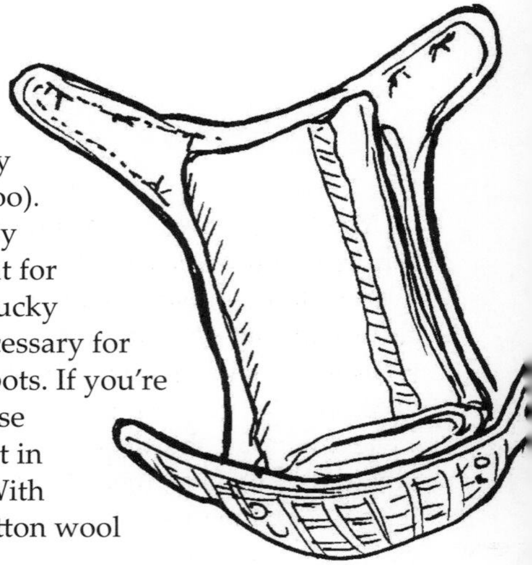

A baby bath. You can bathe with a new baby. It's really nice (unless they poo). You don't need baby wipes. They're great for scrubbing down mucky toddlers, but unnecessary for delicate tiny baby bots. If you're doing washables, use a cloth, and chuck it in with the nappies. With disposables, use cotton wool and water.

Brand-new baby poo is black and sticky: smear a little olive oil on that bum to make it easier to clean.

...and for the other end

You have to mop the top end too. Some babies are sicky after a feed. Invest in a packet of muslin squares: about seven pounds. Wash these and the nappies before use to increase their absorbency, and never use fabric softener on them.

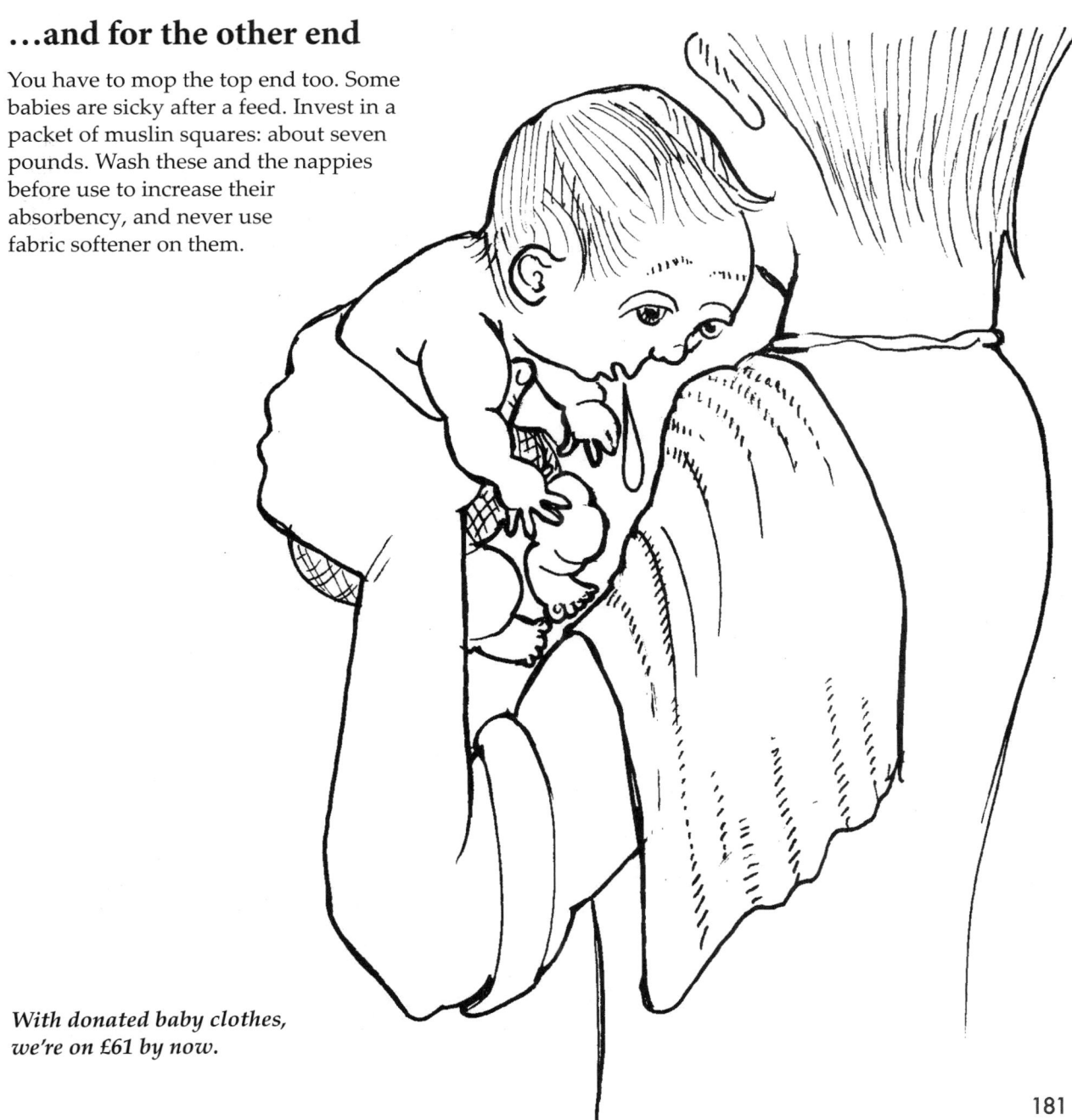

With donated baby clothes, we're on £61 by now.

Something for the baby to eat

Fortunately, you come ready-equipped with two convenient free food sources, right there in your bra.

Unfortunately, connecting baby to breast is not always straightforward, particularly if you've never seen it done before and have no-one around to show you how. I recommend you buy a book on breastfeeding. Which one? Ooh, let me think... How about the one I wrote? *The Food of Love: your formula for successful breastfeeding?*

Here's a picture from it.

However, since we're on a total zero-spending trip, I should also mention that there are good free 'how-to' breastfeeding videos on the Best Beginnings website. (My publishers are going to kill me! Where are the book sales in telling you that?)

Maybe you don't want to breastfeed. Perhaps your breasts are for your boyfriend, not your baby? I still think you could try it, not because it's healthier, or because you 'should' or because 'it's best'. Try it because you might like it. It can be really nice. Just do it for three days and see what you think. If your boyfriend loves you and your baby, he won't mind sharing your breasts for a while.

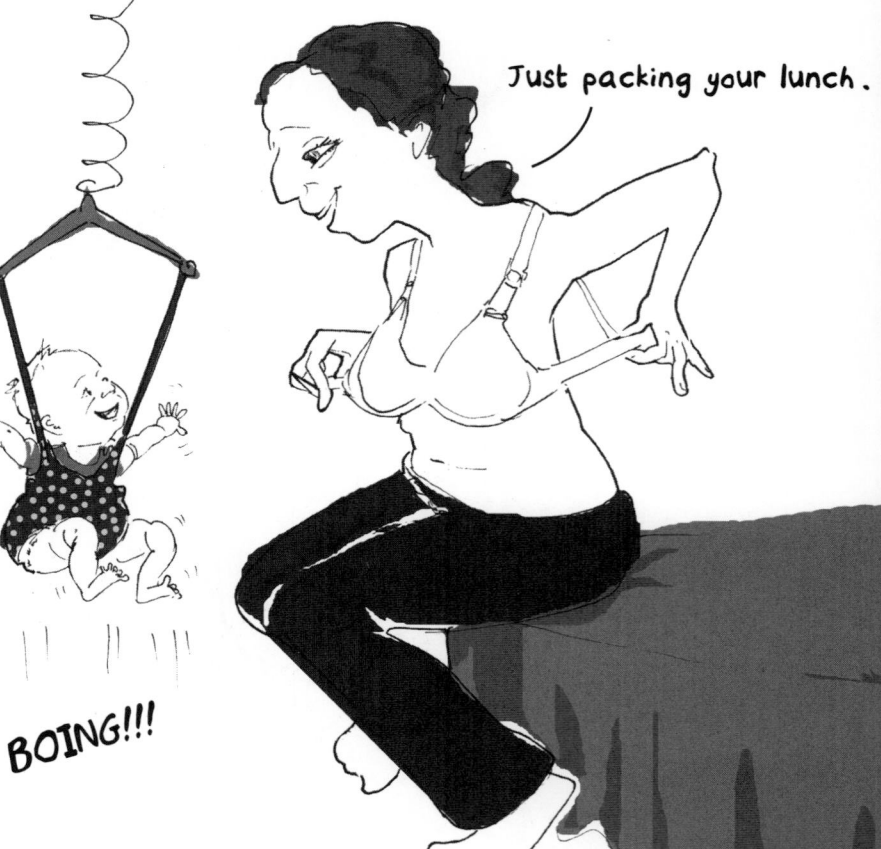

Just packing your lunch.

BOING!!!

Something to carry the baby in

While you're in the haberdashery shop, buy five metres of stretch cotton jersey (T-shirt fabric) that doesn't have Lycra in it. Cut it down the middle lengthways. You now have two wrap-style baby slings: one to wash, one to wear. Enter 'baby-wearing' into YouTube and you'll find videos showing you how to use them.

If you have a car, you'll need a car seat. Buy this new, because a second-hand seat could have been damaged in an accident. Once you've bought it, strap it into the car and leave it there. Learn from my experience, and do not try to fit it for the first time at two a.m. in a hospital car park, with a four-hour-old baby in it.

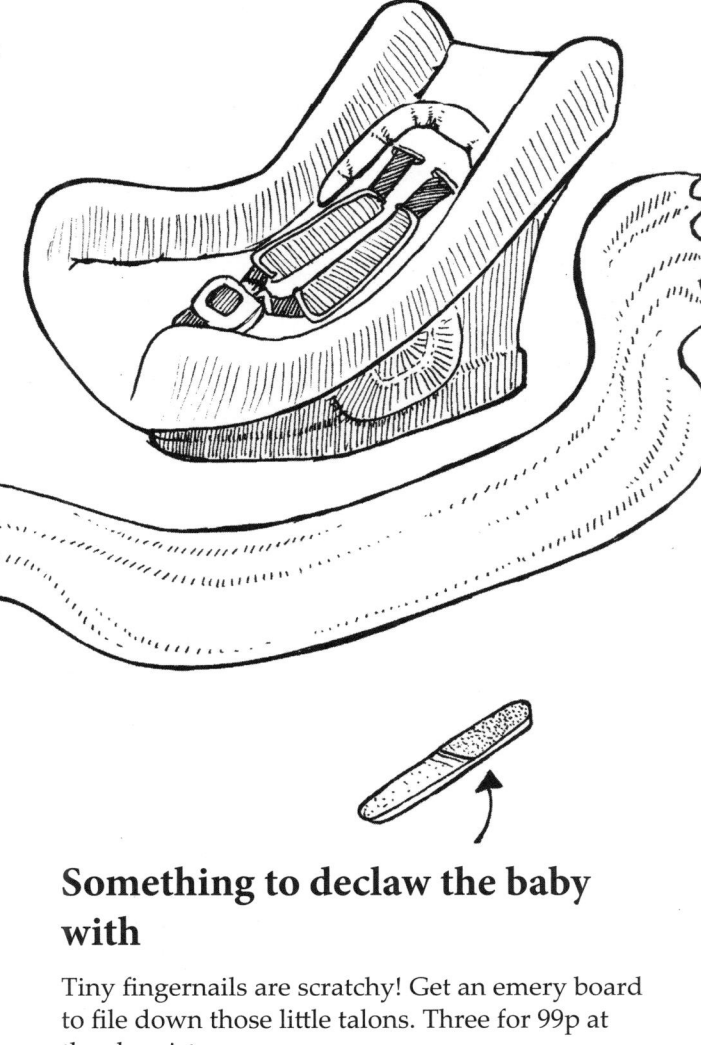

Something to declaw the baby with

Tiny fingernails are scratchy! Get an emery board to file down those little talons. Three for 99p at the chemist.

There. That's baby care sorted for a little over a hundred quid. This book just paid for itself.

Some things to birth the baby with

While we're in the mood for making lists, let's itemise what you need for the birth. There are two lists here. Read both. If you're planning a home birth, you could still choose to transfer quickly to hospital. And babies that are scheduled to be born in hospital sometimes arrive unexpectedly at home.

Home birth

- Two clean warm towels, the first to dry the baby and the other to cover mum and baby. If the heating's on, keep them on the radiator.
- Tea and biscuits for the midwife. Very important. She has to have tea.
- Plastic to protect your furniture. Two cheap 'value' shower curtains, a big towel and an old sheet should have it covered.
- Biological washing powder to clean anything you missed with the plastic sheet.
- Bin bags for laundry.
- Hairbands if you have long hair.
- Mega monster maternity sanitary towels.
- A soft side light to give birth by.
- A bright side light or torch in case you decide to have some 'embroidery' afterwards.
- A bucket could be useful.
- An extra cardigan and fluffy socks.

Optional things:
- Ice cubes to suck.
- A gym ball to rock on.
- A water spray to cool you down.
- A hot water bottle for pain relief.
- A sports bottle for drinking water.
- Aromatherapy electric oil diffuser: if the midwife needs to use oxygen cylinders, you can't have candles.
- A hired water-birth pool, plus lots of towels.

Hospital birth

Pack a bag with:

- Three babygros, three vests, ten nappies, a hat and a blanket for the baby. If it's cold, add a fleecy oversuit for going home. (Ooh, just think! This could be the first time you leave home with an exceptionally large bag of baby accessories! Get used to it.)
- Mega monster maternity sanitary towels.
- Comfy pants. If you have a Caesarean birth you need massive granny knickers.
- Two stretchy nursing bras.
- Toothbrush, hairbrush, travel-size toiletries, hairbands if you need them.
- Some T-shirts and leggings. These are more practical than nighties and easier to cuddle your baby skin-to-skin in. Wearing your own clothes helps you feel like yourself, not a patient.
- Fluffy socks and cardigan or dressing gown.
- Camera, phone, charger, money. Nothing else of value.
- Snacks. Hospital food is rank, and the portions are tiny.
- Don't forget the car seat.

Optional things (but remember, you have to lug them with you all around the hospital):
- A soft side light to give birth by.
- A water spray to cool you down.
- A hot water bottle for pain relief.
- A sports bottle for drinking water.
- Mp3 player.
- Aromatherapy electric oil diffuser and essential oils.
- A favourite pillow.
- Pack something to celebrate with! Cheers!

That's the practicalities sorted. Now for the emotional side.

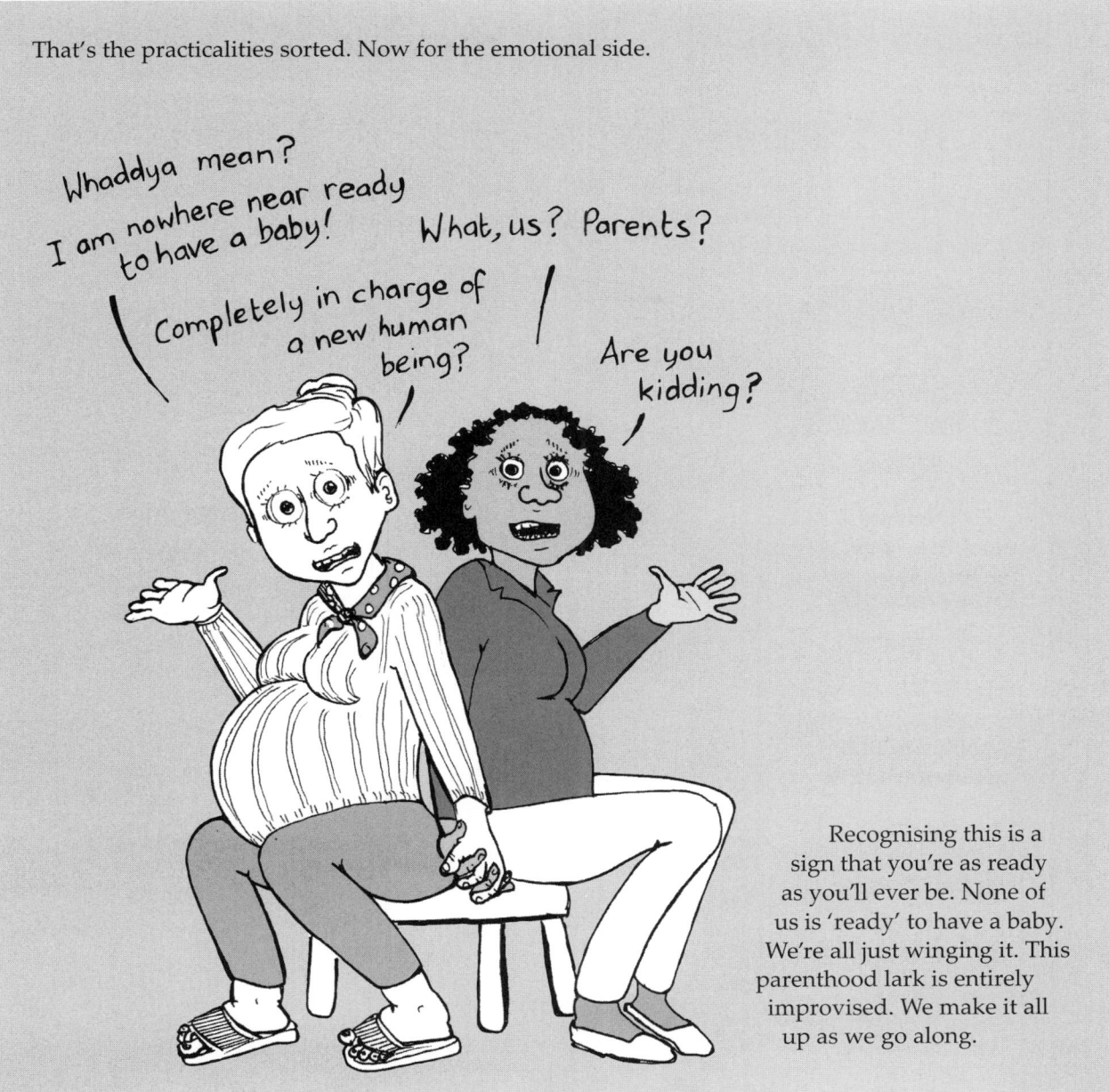

Recognising this is a sign that you're as ready as you'll ever be. None of us is 'ready' to have a baby. We're all just winging it. This parenthood lark is entirely improvised. We make it all up as we go along.

PICK YOUR OWN ADVENTURE MOMENT!

There's more than one way to birth a baby, in fact there are as many different birth stories as there are people that have ever lived.*

There's more than one good way to birth a baby. We are so lucky to live in an age and a nation where life-saving surgical techniques are available for babies who need them.

Are you about to avail yourself of them?

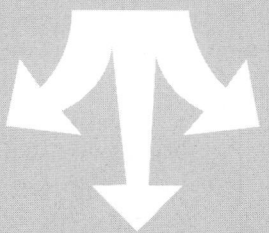

YES!

I'm having a Caesarean birth, and the reasons for doing so are rock-solid and crystal-clear.

You can skip the next 98 pages of wittering about uncertain birthdays and learning to love labour.

Go straight to the 'Caesarean section'. Turn to page 284.

Er, probably.

A doctor has told me I have to have a Caesarean, but I don't know how I feel about that.

Read 'Birth Rights' on page 270, then come back and read the rest of the book.

It will help you take control of your care.

Probably not.

I can't think of an obvious reason to have major surgery, but we'll see how it pans out in the end.

Read on...

* Not true! There are slightly fewer. Twins and multiple births only get one birth story between them. Just fact-checking my statistics. Sorry for the pedantic interruption. As you were.

12 *Baby, get down!*

Have a look at this picture. Study it intently. And instruct your baby to take note.

This baby is in prime position for a natural birth: **'left occiput anterior'** ('occiput' = back of the head – their head, and 'anterior' = front – your front).

Here's why.

You want your baby to be born with the top of the back of their head first. It's like when you put a T-shirt on someone: you find the top of the back of their head to pull it over, because that's the smoothest and smallest circumference.

(If you don't currently have any experience of putting T-shirts on other people, you're about to start years of practice.)

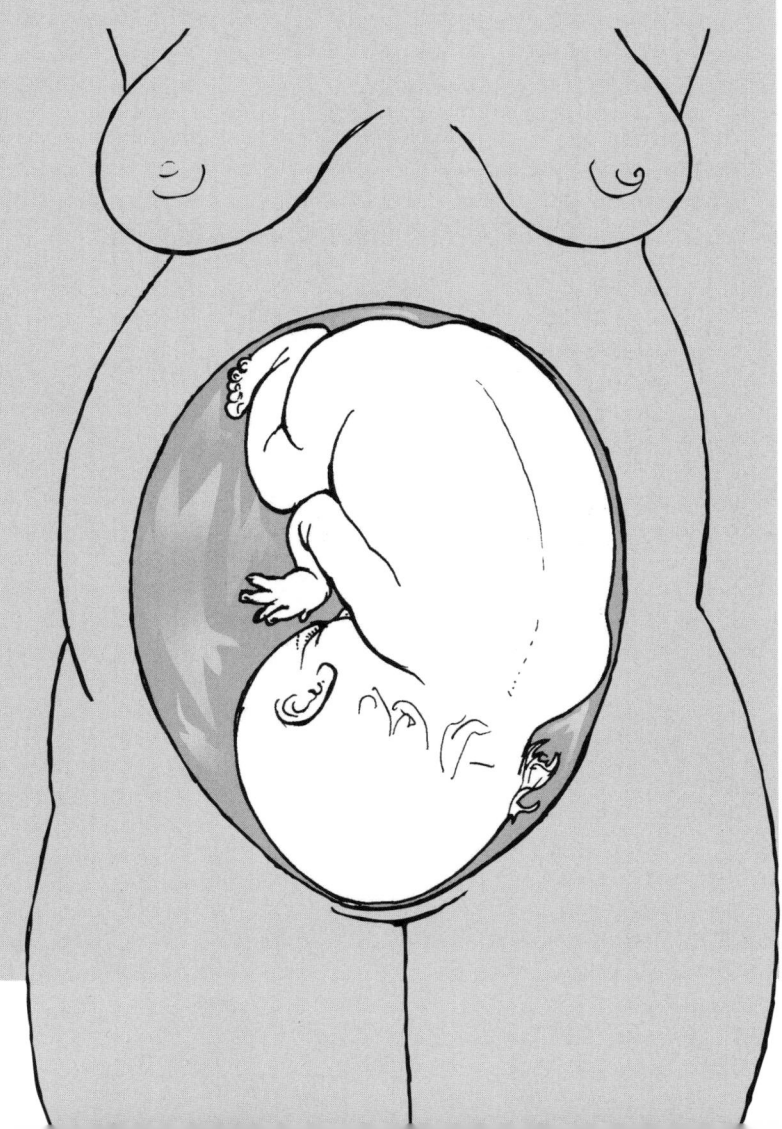

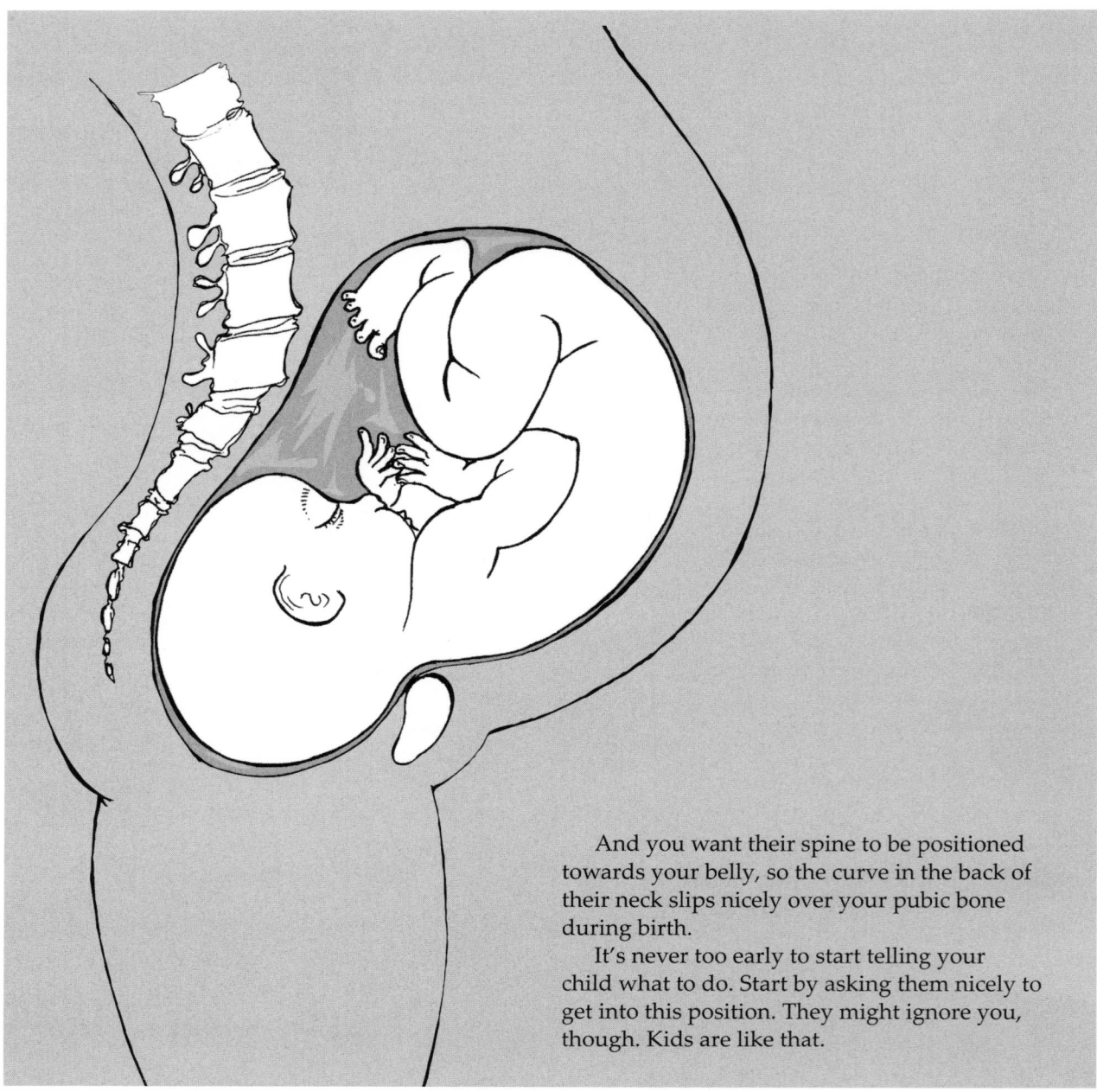

And you want their spine to be positioned towards your belly, so the curve in the back of their neck slips nicely over your pubic bone during birth.

It's never too early to start telling your child what to do. Start by asking them nicely to get into this position. They might ignore you, though. Kids are like that.

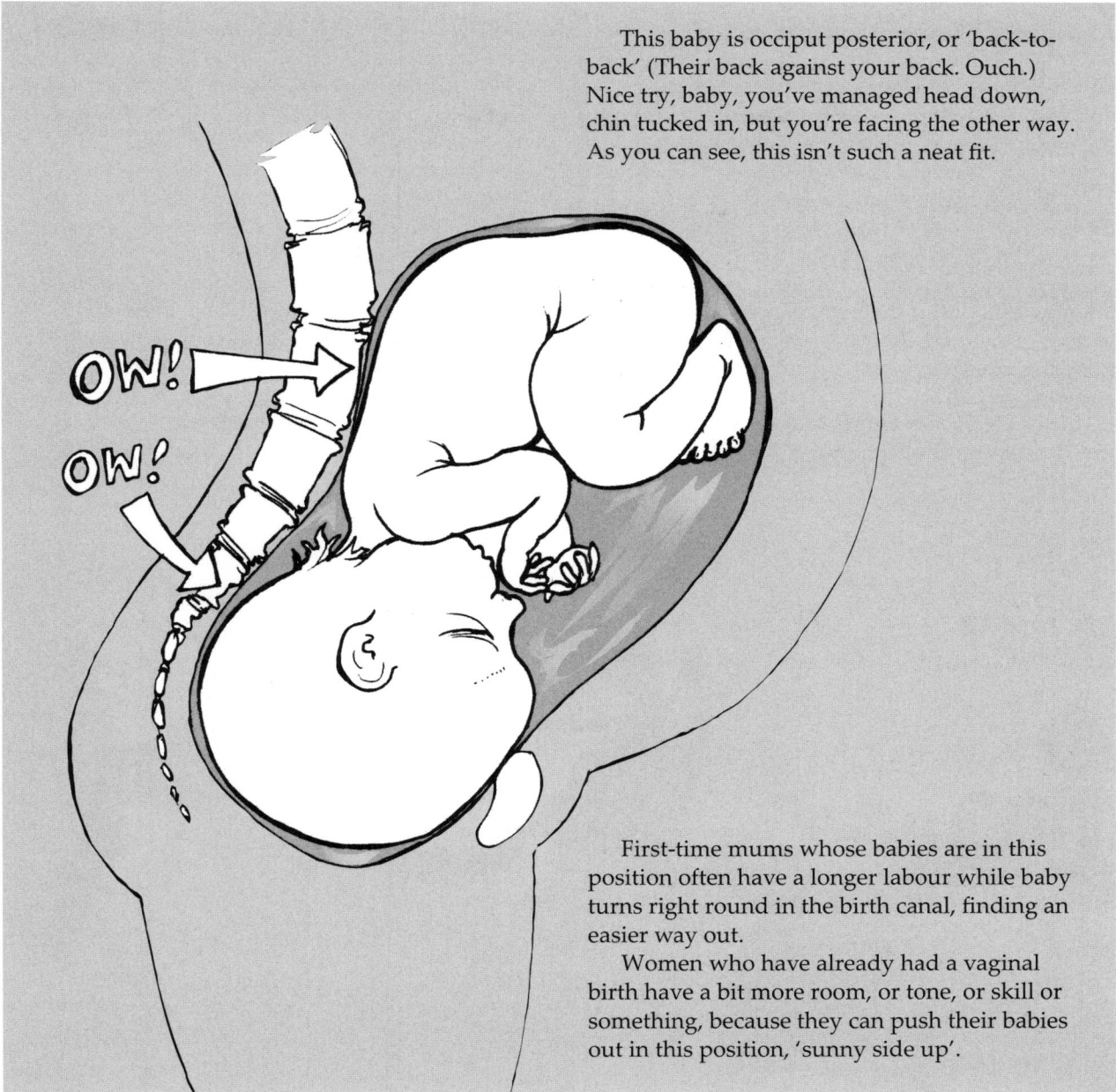

This baby is occiput posterior, or 'back-to-back' (Their back against your back. Ouch.) Nice try, baby, you've managed head down, chin tucked in, but you're facing the other way. As you can see, this isn't such a neat fit.

First-time mums whose babies are in this position often have a longer labour while baby turns right round in the birth canal, finding an easier way out.

Women who have already had a vaginal birth have a bit more room, or tone, or skill or something, because they can push their babies out in this position, 'sunny side up'.

Optimal foetal positioning

Given a choice between a baby that's occiput anterior and occiput posterior, you want to choose the 'not hours and hours of backache labour' option, right?

There is a theory that you can affect the position of the baby in late pregnancy. It's called 'optimal foetal positioning'.

First, work out which way your baby is facing. You can ask your midwife to tell you how your baby is positioned – she'll be an expert in 'belly mapping', as it's known – or you can have a feel yourself.

Lie down flat on your back for a minute, and give your bump a prod. If your belly feels nice and firm, your baby's back is probably lying up against it. You can also tell where their spine is, because it's the opposite side to where you feel the main kicks and punches. So you're wanting firm belly, and kicks towards your back, yes?

If, instead, the area around your belly feels squishy and can be easily pressed in, and you feel big kicks towards the front of your belly, your baby could be occiput posterior.

If your baby is occiput anterior, aka 'the right way round', then everything's fine. If they're back-to-back, you can encourage them to turn. Their spine is heavier than their arms and legs. If you adopt forward-leaning postures, gravity will encourage them to snuggle round and use the front of your belly like a hammock.

Not like that...

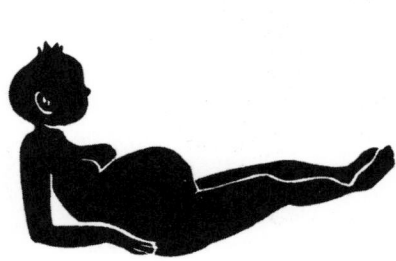

This position, which has probably been one of your trademark postures in pregnancy thus far, is not a good one when you're heavily pregnant.

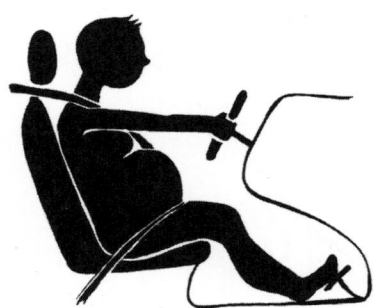

The 'Porsche' position. Don't drive the Porsche. You'll never be able to get a baby seat into it anyway.

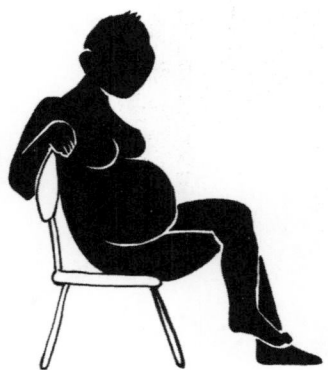

Sitting with your legs crossed makes your pelvis smaller at the front, which is not what we're wanting.

...like this!

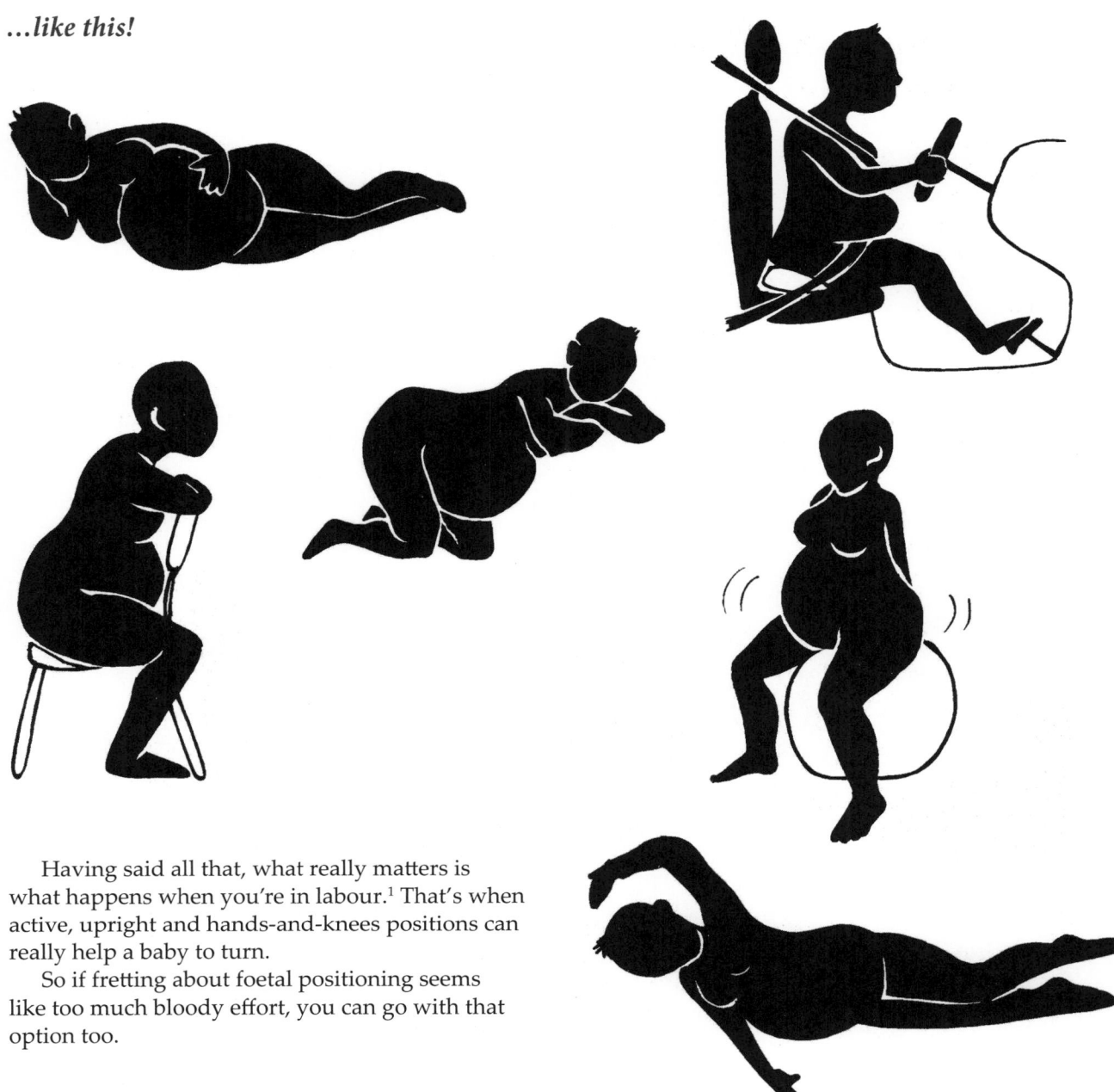

Having said all that, what really matters is what happens when you're in labour.[1] That's when active, upright and hands-and-knees positions can really help a baby to turn.

So if fretting about foetal positioning seems like too much bloody effort, you can go with that option too.

These positions alarm obstetricians

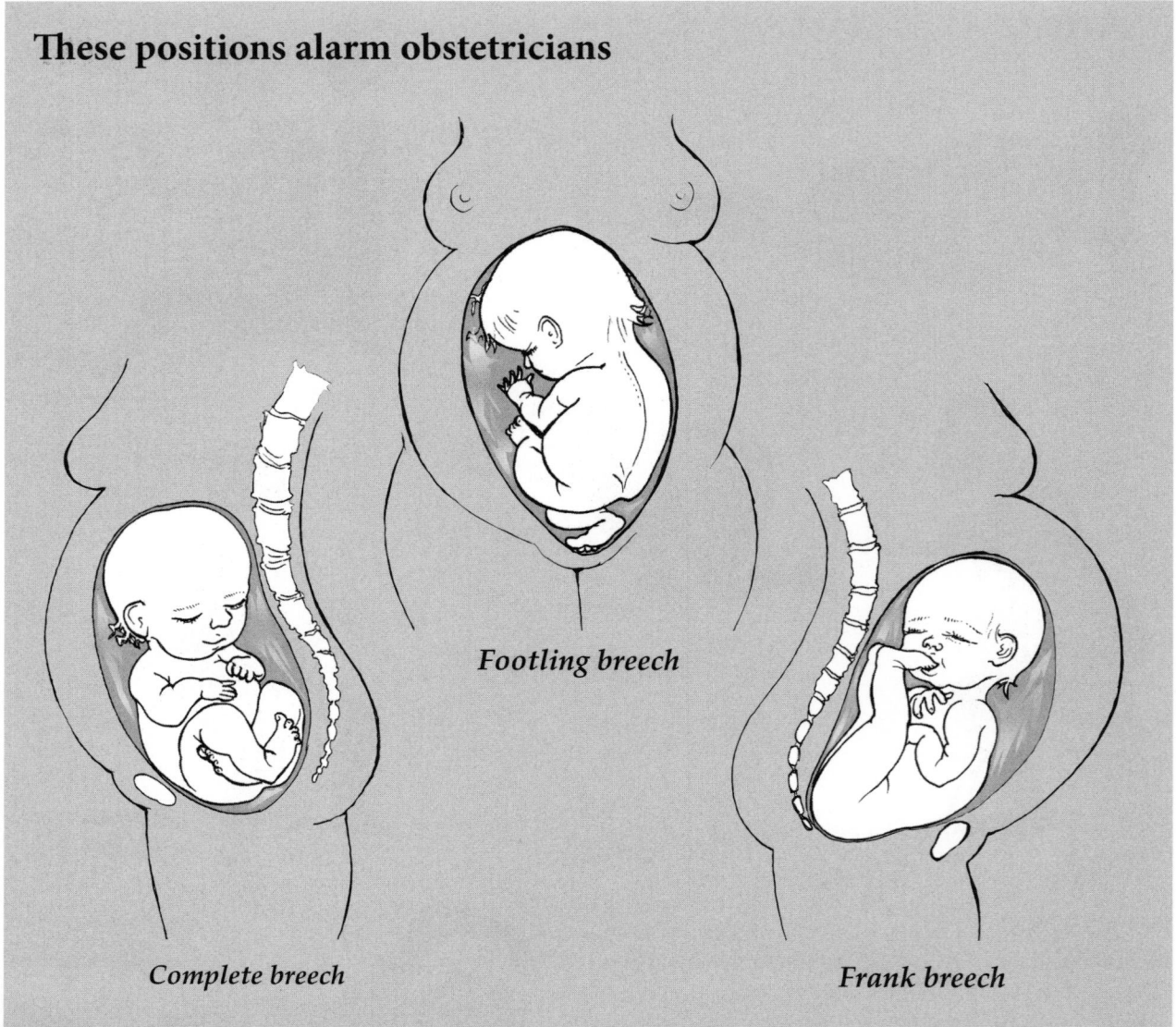

Footling breech

Complete breech

Frank breech

These babies are the other way up. They are breech. About 3-4% of babies are this way up at 38 weeks' gestation, though it's more common when babies are born early.

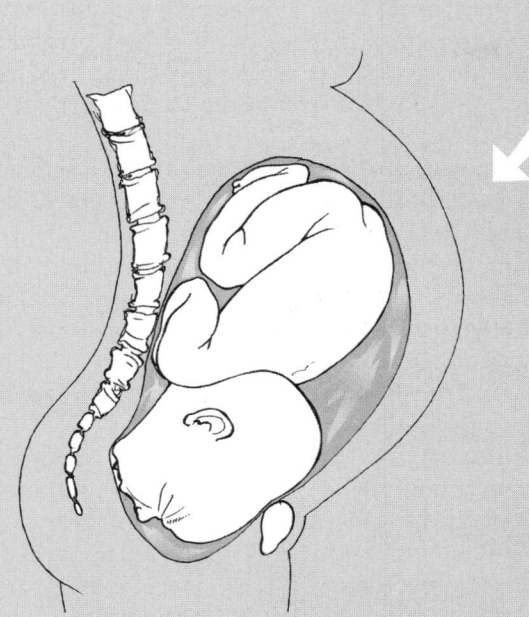

Here we see why your baby was meant to keep their chin tucked down. This is called 'face presentation'. Naughty baby!

'Brow presentation' is even tricker. That's where the head is slightly less tilted, and its widest circumference enters the birth canal. Really, baby, no. I'm not even drawing a picture of this one. I don't want to give your child bad ideas.

It is possible for babies to be born vaginally in all these positions, but it's not straightforward. We're wanting 'straightforward'. That's our desired aim.

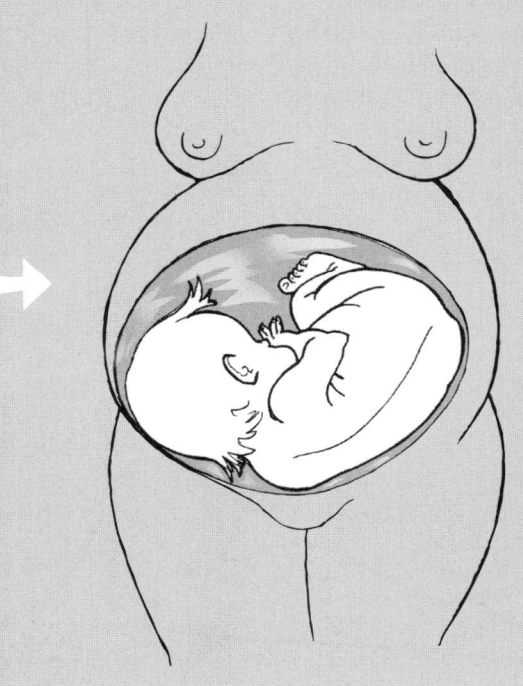

This baby has totally lost the plot and is lying sideways – 'transverse lie' or 'shoulder presentation'. If she stays like this, there is just no way she is coming out via the traditional route. Skip to page 284 for a gentle Caesarean birth.

Transverse lie happens in about one in five hundred pregnancies, which means it's 99.95% likely to not happen to you. Face or brow presentations are even rarer.

In the last few weeks of pregnancy your baby moves further down in your pelvis. This is called 'lightening' because it gives you a little more room in your lungs, to breathe (although consequently, less room in your bladder).

So, if your baby is still sitting breech or transverse in late pregnancy, you need to counter the effects of gravity to give it some wiggle room.

Do this:

Spread your knees wide and rock your hips around a little. Listen to some relaxing music, and, if you like, waft some aromatherapy oils around. Pick a time in the evening when older children are asleep, so they don't come in and ride you like a donkey.

Stay like this for two hours, or until the baby moves round, or you are incredibly bored and have terrible heartburn. Give up, go to bed, and lie on your left side.

Also try running a torch slowly down your belly, or

playing music through headphones at the bottom of your bump – maybe your baby will turn head-down to investigate. Try putting a packet of frozen peas on the top of your bump so they wriggle their face away.

An acupuncture technique called 'moxibustion' has been proven to help turn breech babies,[2] and this procedure involves applying heat, rather than using needles, so it's fine if you're phobic.

Also see a chiropractor or osteopath. They will be able to examine your pelvis and see if they can work on it to create more room.

And 'birth' plus 'more room in pelvis' sounds like a good equation to me.

You may also be offered 'external version' by your midwife or obstetrician. This is where a trained professional manipulates your belly to manually move your baby around. The procedure carries some risks.

If your baby stubbornly stays breech, I recommend you contact the Association for Improvements in the Maternity Services at www.aims.org.uk. They have excellent information on all your options for birth.

13 *Ask Aunty Katy*

To enhance your emotional preparedness for the arrival of your child, I have assembled the answers to all the questions about natural childbirth that you're too shy to ask. Think of me as like an agony aunt. Except we're not going to talk about agony. Whoops! We just did!

Will my lovely, sensitive lady-parts tear?

It's possible. There are things you can do that make it less likely. But it won't matter.

What do you mean? OF COURSE it matters!

No, it really doesn't. That's how overwhelming it is having a baby. It makes something that would ordinarily matter a lot (really a lot) seem utterly insignificant.

Will I poo myself?

Maybe a tiny bit, but midwives are handy with a hygienic wipe. You're actually meant to! There's a reason for the anatomical proximity of anus and birth canal. Your intestines contain billions of good digestive bacteria, and, when a tiny trace of poo gets mixed up in the birth process, your baby's digestive system is primed with them. Babies born by Caesarean miss out on the good bacteria they are meant to receive, their gut flora is different, and this could be why they are more prone to allergies and obesity.

Really, don't worry about your body doing whatever your body needs to do. There was a point when I was in labour where I was sick over myself and peed myself simultaneously in a hospital car park. Ordinarily, I would feel a modicum of embarrassment about this, but its significance was eclipsed by the memory of giving birth to my daughter later that day. So forget about a smudge of poo. If you can get through the birth of your child without simultaneously throwing up and wetting yourself, you're doing better than me.

Will my partner still fancy me?

Yes. My experience is with men. Men fancy everything.

Will my fanny ever be the same again?

It will be better! It will still be the lovely sensitive flower that you have always enjoyed, but you can also be proud that it has done something useful.

Seriously?

Well, it might change shape a bit. Post-birth vaginas tend to be a little different from pre-birth ones, but neither sort is more beautiful or functional than the other.

Let's apply the 'what would it be like if men could do this' test to genitalia and childbirth. Imagine if, when a man fathered his first child, his balls dropped a couple of inches. Would men be rushing off to plastic surgeons for uplift surgery? Hell, no! They'd be boasting about it! They'd all be wearing MC Hammer trousers and claiming they could swing theirs into their socks.

OK, I'm not helping. Don't worry. Nothing's going to drop a couple of inches! But what's important about your pleasure garden is not how it looks, but how it feels.

Will that be different after birth? Here's a selection of quotes from an astonishingly frank internet chatroom:

- 'Way better. Way, way better.'
- 'It feels so incredibly good. The sensitivity has heightened.'
- 'I have more control over my vaginal muscles.'
- 'The best sex we had as a couple was trying for our second child.'
- 'A good lube will help.'
- 'I can't recommend Kegels [pelvic floor exercises] highly enough.'
- 'Your body parts are elastic. Your free time after having a baby, not so much.'

And from the men:

- 'There has been no real change in terms of tightness or cosmetic appearance... [but] now when my wife has an orgasm it feels about ten times stronger than it used to.'
- 'My wife had a Caesarean. Sex is somewhat different. She reports that certain positions are more pleasurable.'
- 'Forceps delivery with stitches, but sex now is not noticeably different. Just considerably less of it.'

The consensus here seems to be that your lady parts are likely to recover just fine from the rigours of childbirth. The passion-killing part of having a baby is having to look after a baby. All the time. Still, what you miss out on in sex, you make up for in love and cuddles.

Will labour hurt?

Hmm. There are two ways I could answer this question. I could tell you that there are documented cases of women giving birth without pain. I could even mention that women can orgasm during birth. I could explain that there is a theory that fear and tension in labour produces pain, and so telling you it is going to hurt could make it more likely that it will.

Or I could give you the honest answer.

Yes.

Probably.

But, uniquely among your life experience, this is good pain. You want this pain. This pain is doing something incredible.

So maybe 'pain' isn't the right word. In our society, we treat painful feelings as inconveniences, to be erased by the judicious use of painkillers. We use the same words, 'painful feelings', to describe negative emotions. Birth is a time for positive feelings, not negative ones.

This pain isn't something you can pop two paracetamol for. It's a marathon to run... a mountain to climb... an ocean to cross...

So labour hurts. So what? This is labour, girl! This is work! This is where your body goes to places you've never been to before and you will be all you can be. It's not fun. It can be hard. It can push you past what you thought you could endure. But, in the extremes of the experience, a new person is forged.

A mother.

Bring it on!

14 *The waiting game*

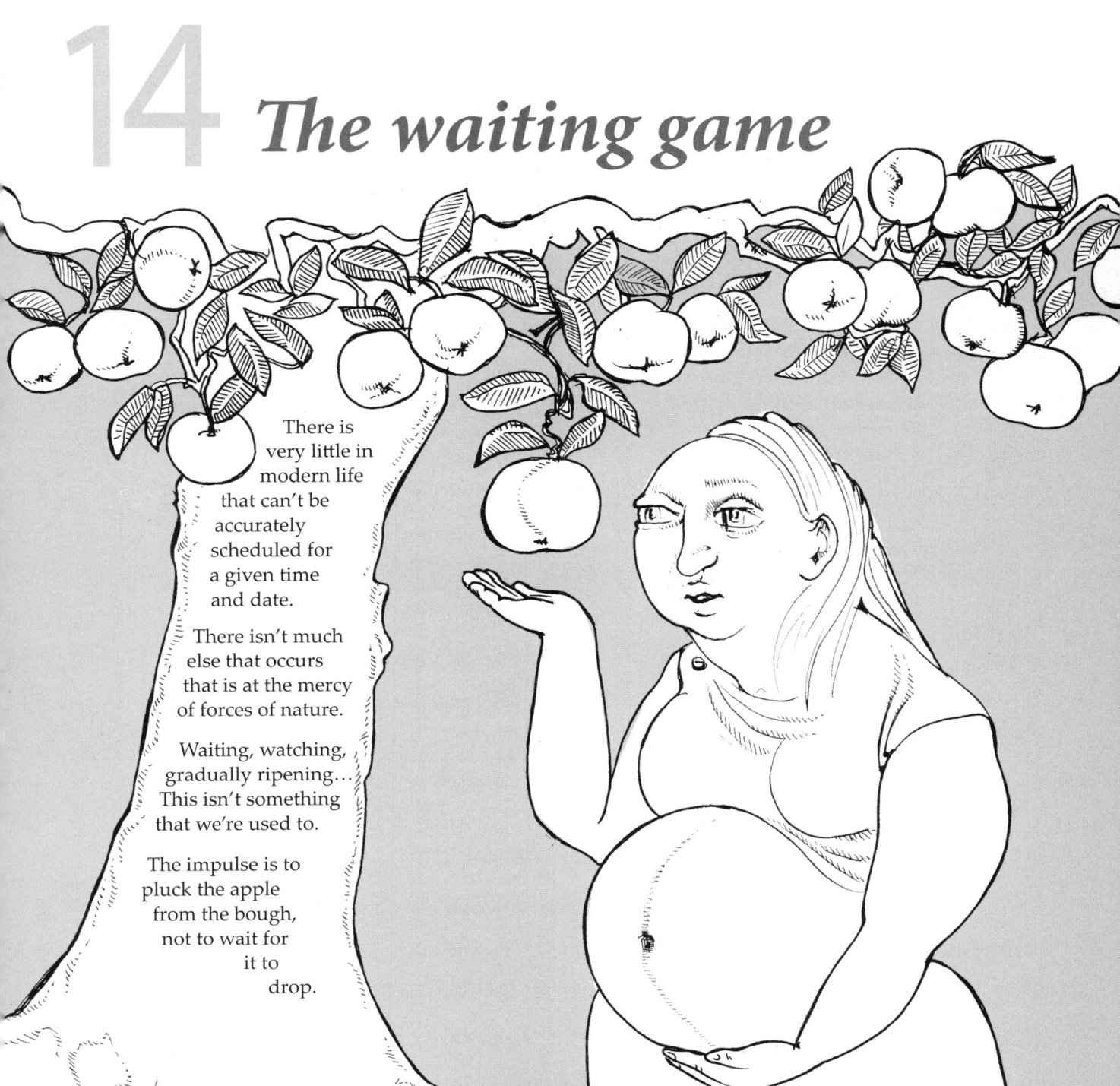

There is very little in modern life that can't be accurately scheduled for a given time and date.

There isn't much else that occurs that is at the mercy of forces of nature.

Waiting, watching, gradually ripening… This isn't something that we're used to.

The impulse is to pluck the apple from the bough, not to wait for it to drop.

When is this baby going to arrive?

PICK YOUR OWN ADVENTURE MOMENT!

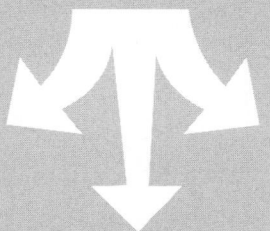

When you really weren't expecting it at all yet.

Nearly 8% of babies are born before 37 weeks' gestation.

Chances are 'having a baby' was not on your list of things to do on the day you became a mother.

Exactly on the day the doctors said it would.

About 5% of babies are born on their 'due date'.

Feel smug.

But don't get too used to your baby doing exactly what's expected of it. Parenthood's not usually like that.

Not for ages and ages and ages.

And 10% of first-time mothers are still pregnant two weeks after their 'due date'.

This is a very long time when you are the size of a hippopotamus.

Read on…

What to do if you're overdue?

Dammit. The doctors lied to you. They said the baby would arrive last Tuesday but, as yet, there's no sign. This is worse than waiting in for the washing machine repair man.

What do you do? Wake up, get dressed, spend time not having a baby, hang out all day not having a baby, eat the biscuits you bought for the midwife, waddle to the corner shop to replace them, waddle home, get into your pyjamas, go to bed, wonder if you'll have a baby tomorrow.

And the next day?

Welcome to Groundhog Day!

Groundhog Day can be very dull. Your friends and family don't want to phone you in case you're

in labour. You don't want to ring them because you can't be bothered to preface your conversation with the phrase, 'No, I haven't had the baby yet.'

There is a physical limit to the number of meals you can make and freeze to eat after the baby's born.

The deadline

Part of what you need to go into labour naturally is a sense that you're safe, calm and supported. And what you get is a midwife standing over you with a stopwatch saying, 'If you haven't had it by next Monday, we'll do a load of medical things to you to make it happen.'

Whether this alarms you depends on your attitude to the birth itself. If you're a 'gimme the epidural' kind of girl, you might be quite relieved. But, if you are eagerly awaiting the unfolding of the natural rhythms of your body, it's the last thing you want to hear.

Firstly. Do you feel safe? Are you supported? Now is not a good time for random people to come to visit. Protect your privacy, and only allow people into your home who you love and trust.

Next, if you want to be 'doing something' to make the birth happen, here are some things that women have tried to move things along:

* Keep walking. It'll bring that baby down.
* Get a gym ball and sit on it as much as you can. Rock or bounce – whatever feels good.
* Your hormones and your emotions feed off each other to make labour happen. Watching a weepy movie and having a good cry, or seeing a comedy show that makes you laugh uncontrollably, are both good things to do.
* Dancing and singing with other people is also recommended. If only for the comedy potential.

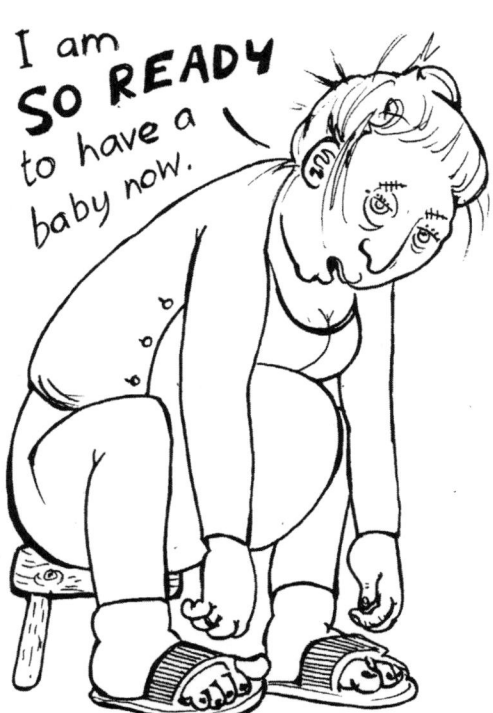

I am SO READY to have a baby now.

- Oxytocin, the hormone that controls labour is released when you make love, so indulge in kissing, tenderness and orgasm. If you don't have a sexual partner, you can take matters into your own hands.
- Semen contains prostaglandins, which ripen your cervix and also help speed up labour. So, if your sexual partner is a man, that's a bonus.[1]
- While you're delving around in the vaginal area (having washed and dried your hands throughly first!), how does your cervix feel? If it is hard, long, and high up at the back of your vagina, it's not ripe yet. But if it's soft, wide and further forward, that's a good sign. Does it feel like big, fat, slightly open lips? It's ripe.

NB. *If your waters have broken, don't have vaginal penetrative sex – though orgasm is fine – and don't check your cervix. See page 276.*

- Firmly massaging a cervix helps it to ripen.
- There is an unproven theory that the enzyme bromelain, found in fresh pineapple, will help ripen the cervix. Buy a load of pineapples, wait for them to smell nice and pineappley, and then make them into smoothies, including the woody bit in the middle. If you like pineapple. If you don't, don't bother.
- When your cervix is ripe, rubbing your nipples has been proven to help bring on labour.[2] Get comfy. Choose a selection of good romantic, weepy or funny DVDs. Ask friends and flatmates to leave. Massage and twiddle each breast alternately for about 15 minutes, or 'a while' each side, for at least three hours. Play around and see if you can find some drops of milk. Your partner might enjoy helping you. Get creative. There is a direct connection between the nerves of the breast and the womb, so stimulating one wakes the other one up a bit.
- Your midwife may offer you a 'stretch and sweep', where she pushes her finger into the cervix and runs her finger around the inside to separate it from the amniotic sac. It can be painful, but that's because it stimulates natural wound-healing prostaglandins which can trigger labour. It works well for women who've had a baby before.
- Everyone will tell you to eat curry. The theory behind this is that 'looseness' in the bowels can stimulate the womb.
- A dose of castor oil has the same effect. It tastes disgusting. Ask your midwife's advice before using castor oil.
- Try acupuncture.
- Drinking raspberry leaf tea from 32 weeks onwards will help to 'tone up' your womb. (Don't drink raspberry leaf earlier in pregnancy.)
- The herb blue cohosh is a strong uterine stimulant. Do not use herbs to induce labour without first consulting both your midwife and a qualified herbalist, because you are effectively giving yourself a drug to start contractions.

But do you know what? You don't have to do *any* of that. You don't have to fret or stress or take any externally imposed deadline to heart. You don't have to try to make it happen. Just be here now, still with your baby inside you, and savour every moment that you're nourishing them to that moment of perfect ripeness. The birth will happen. Just wait. It will.

15 Crossing the sea

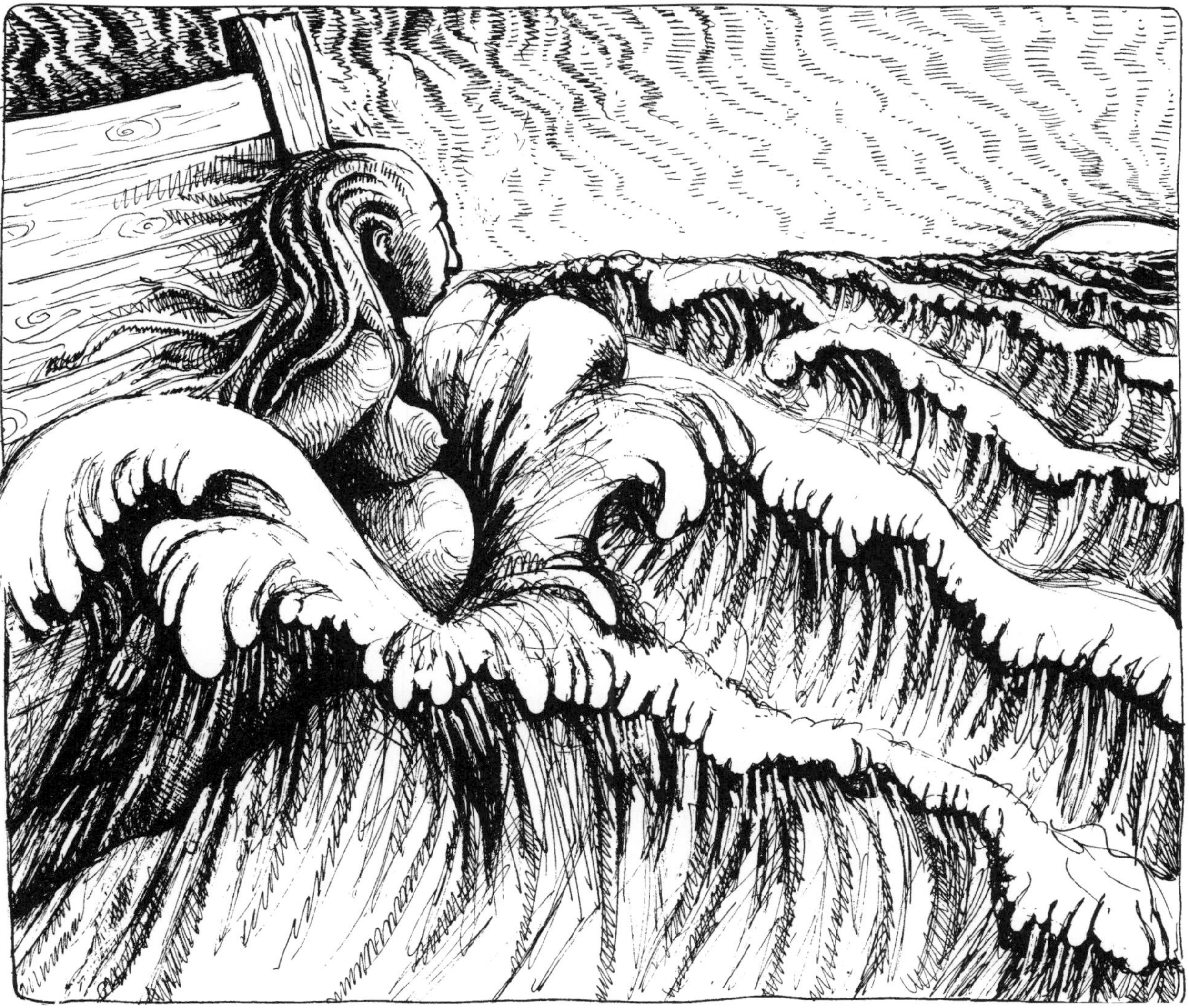

I can't tell you how you'll know you're in labour.
I'm not you, and there's no one feeling that all
women feel.

Watch out for an increased urge to clean things
That's a good sign.

Go with it. You won't get
another chance for quite a while.

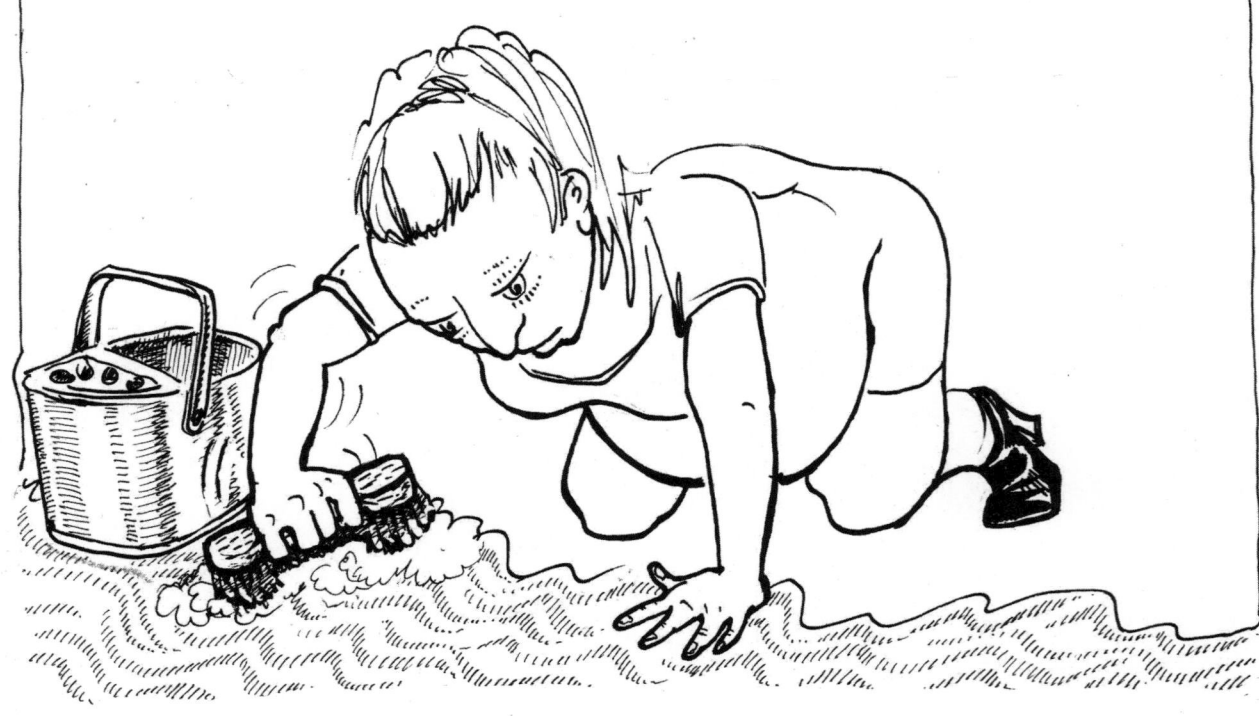

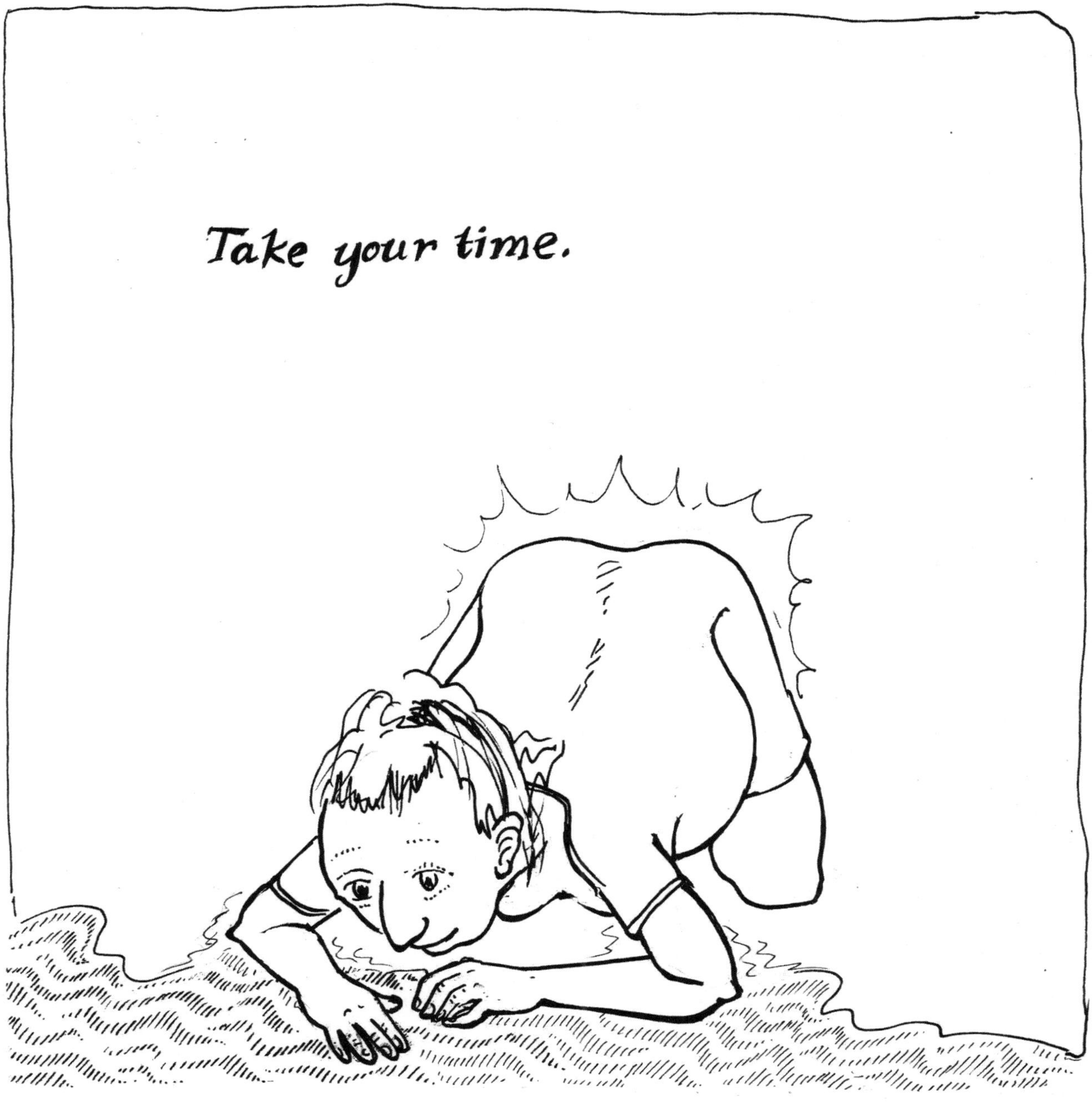
Take your time.

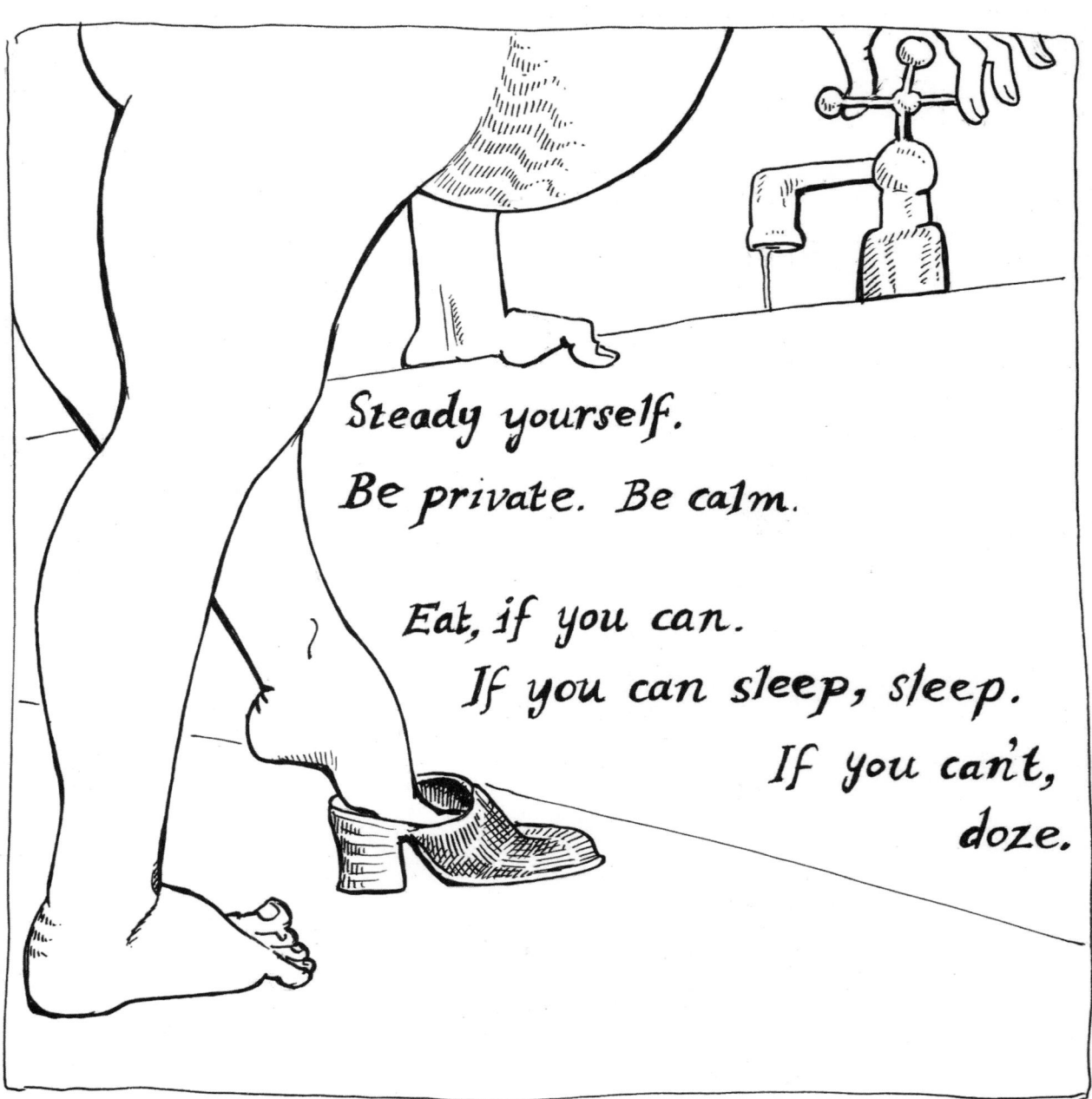

Steady yourself.
Be private. Be calm.

Eat, if you can.
If you can sleep, sleep.
If you can't,
doze.

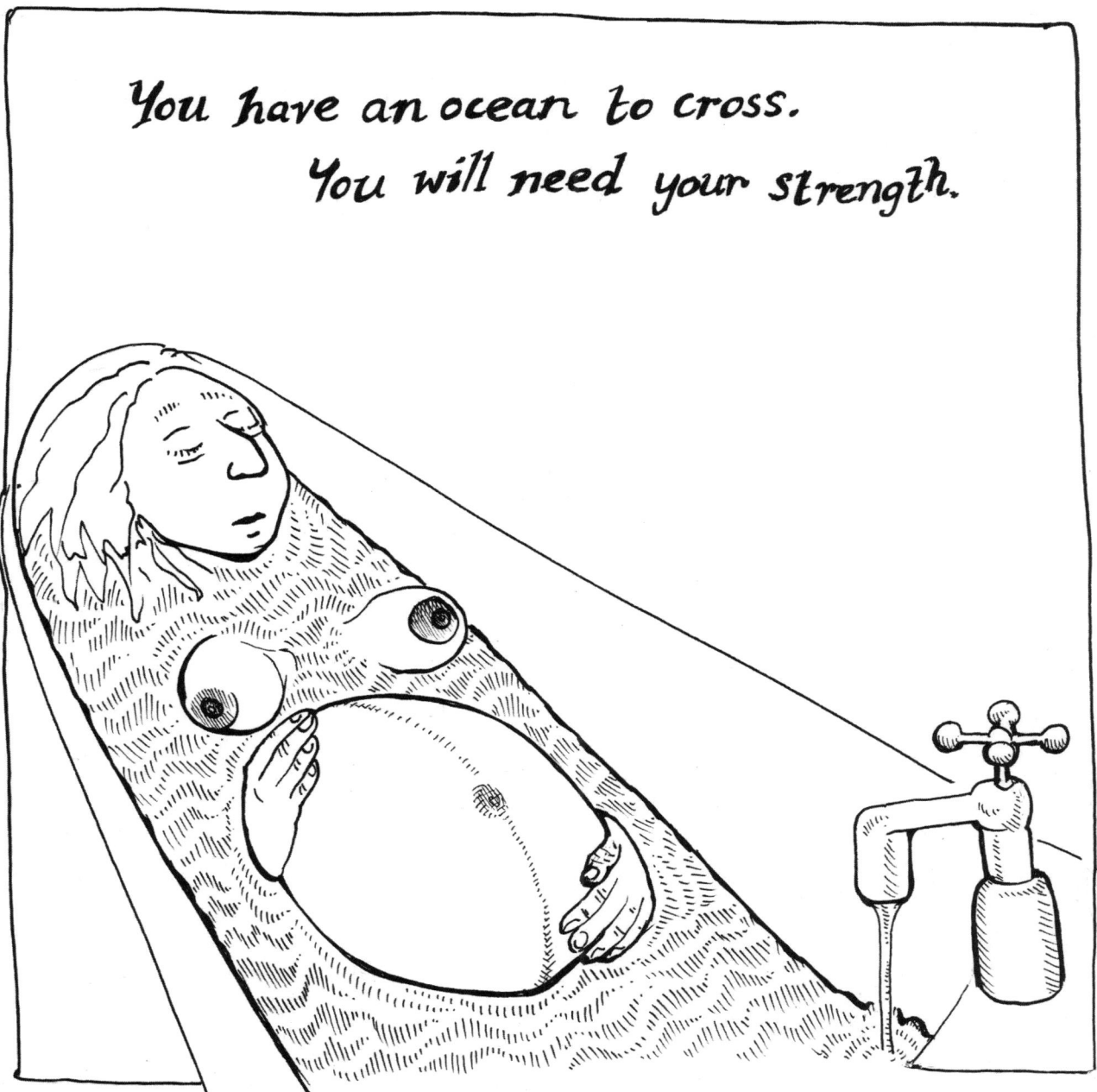

You have an ocean to cross.
You will need your strength.

So now you are standing on the shore of your labour, and the waves are swelling through you. There are things you can find within yourself that will help you...

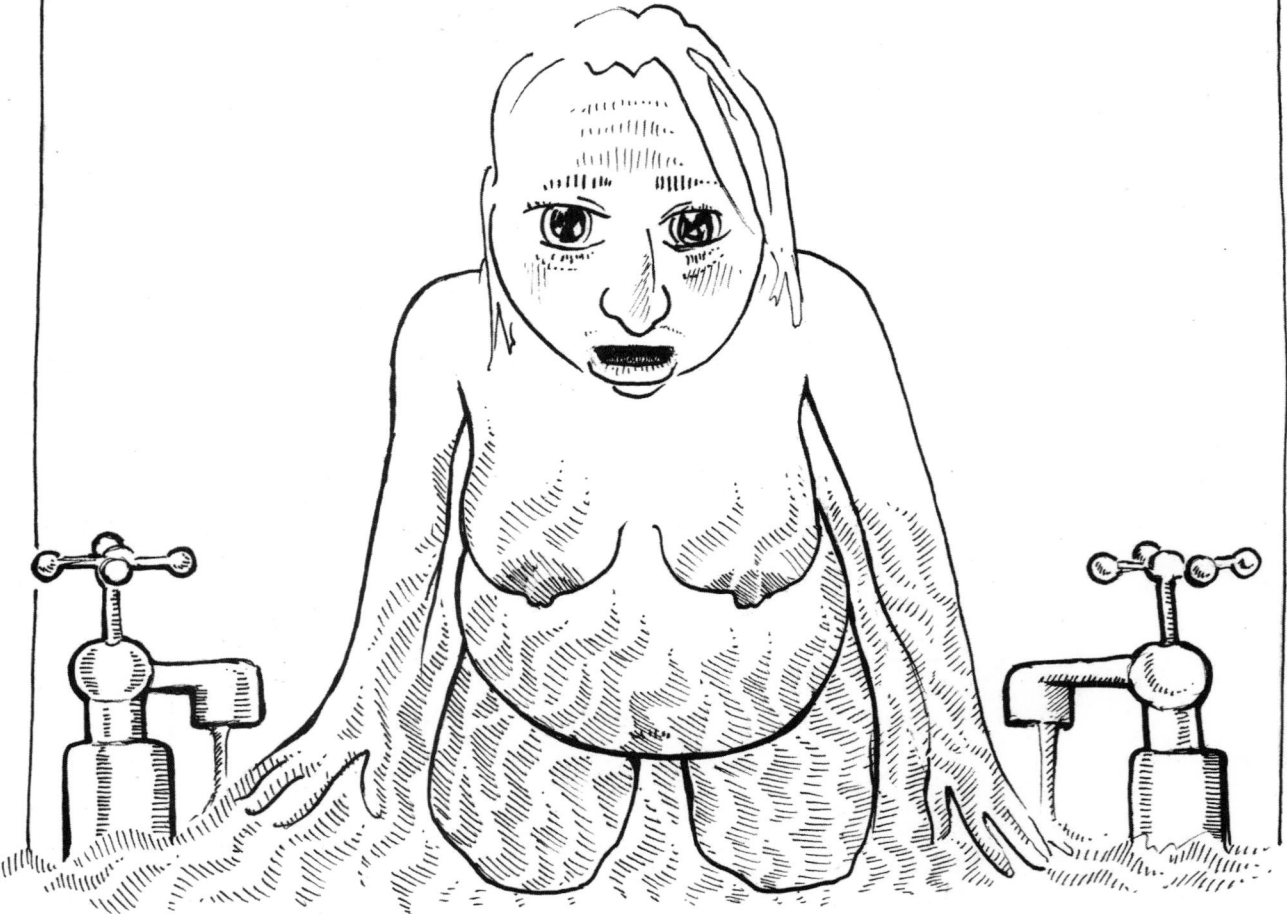

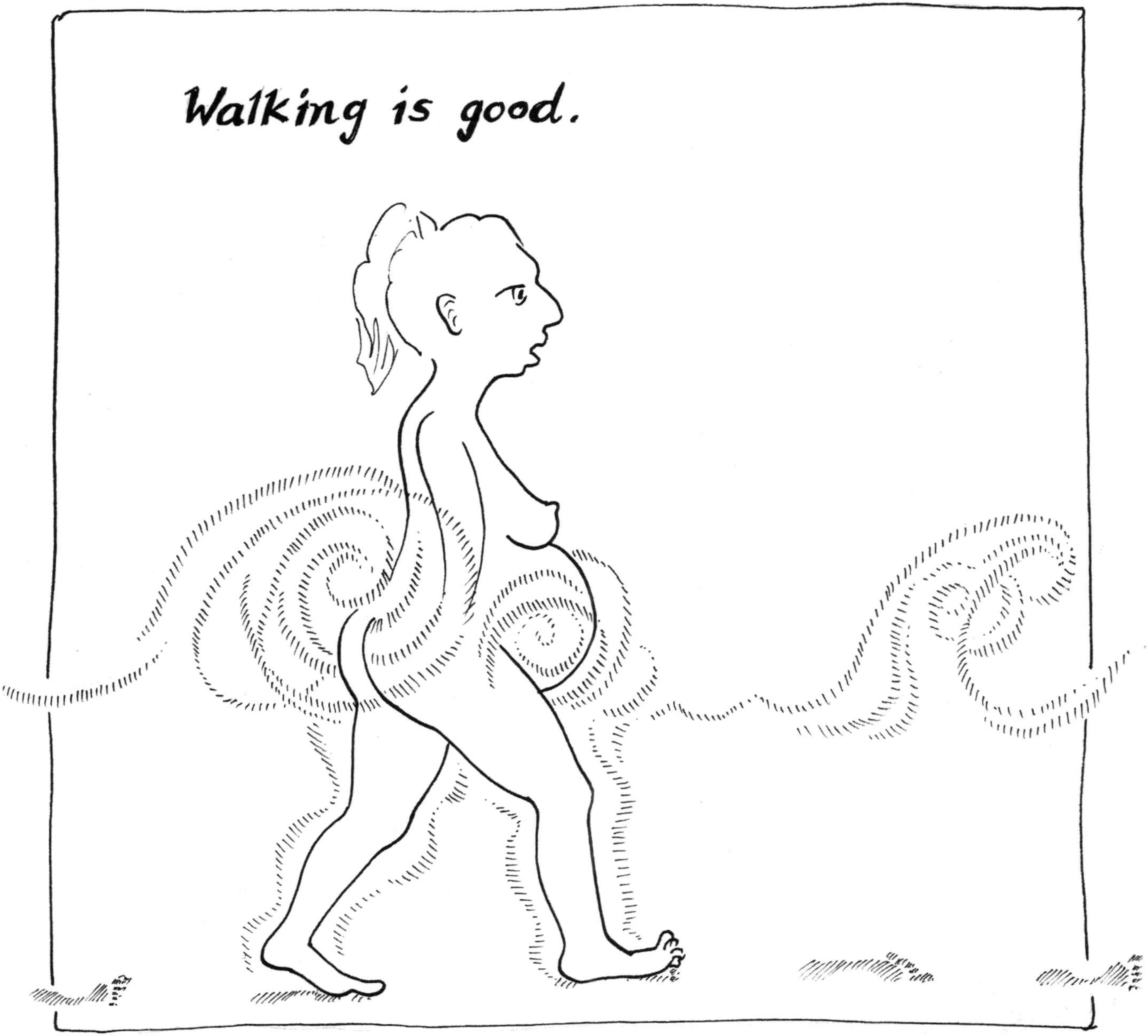
Walking is good.

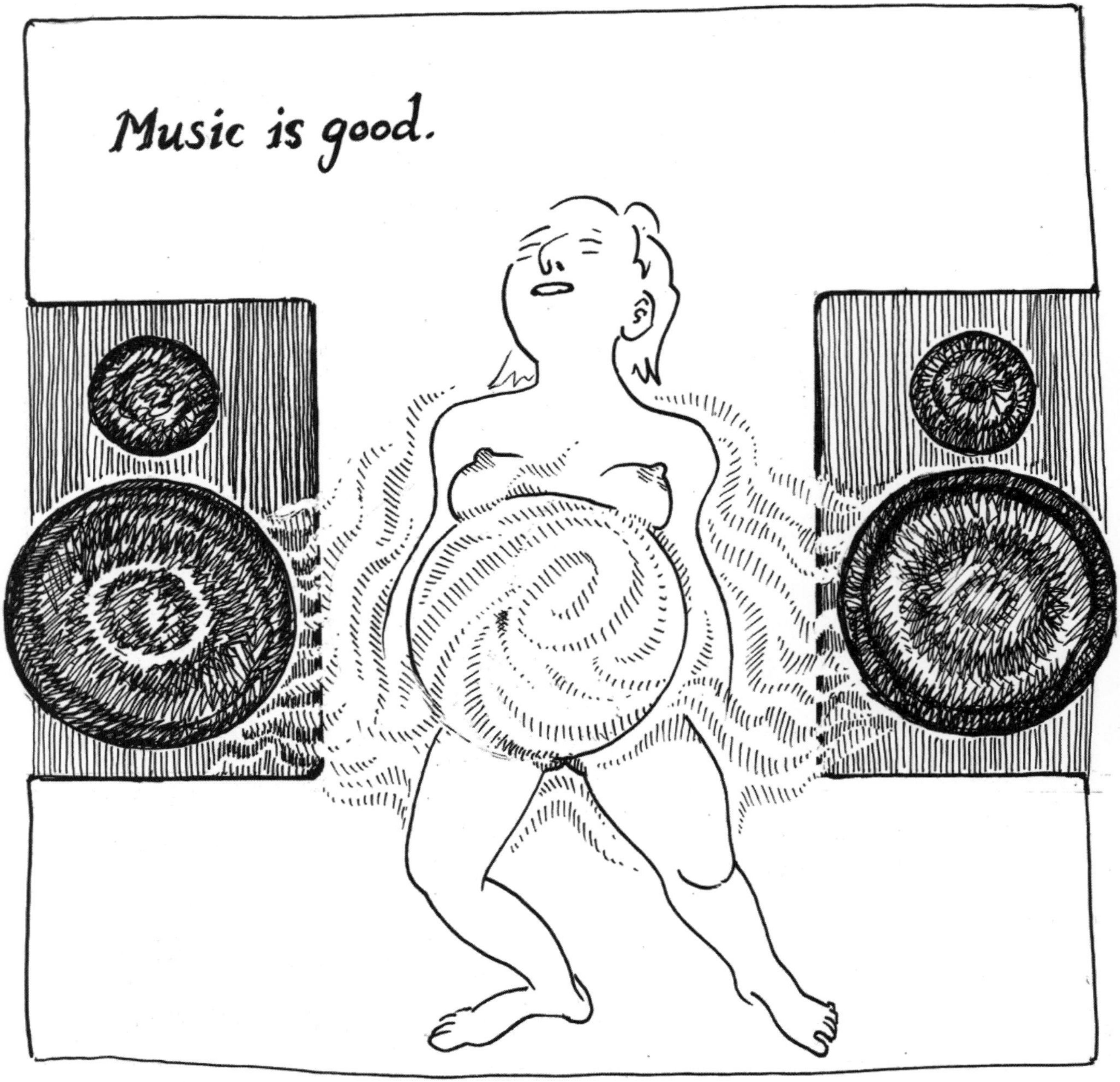
Music is good.

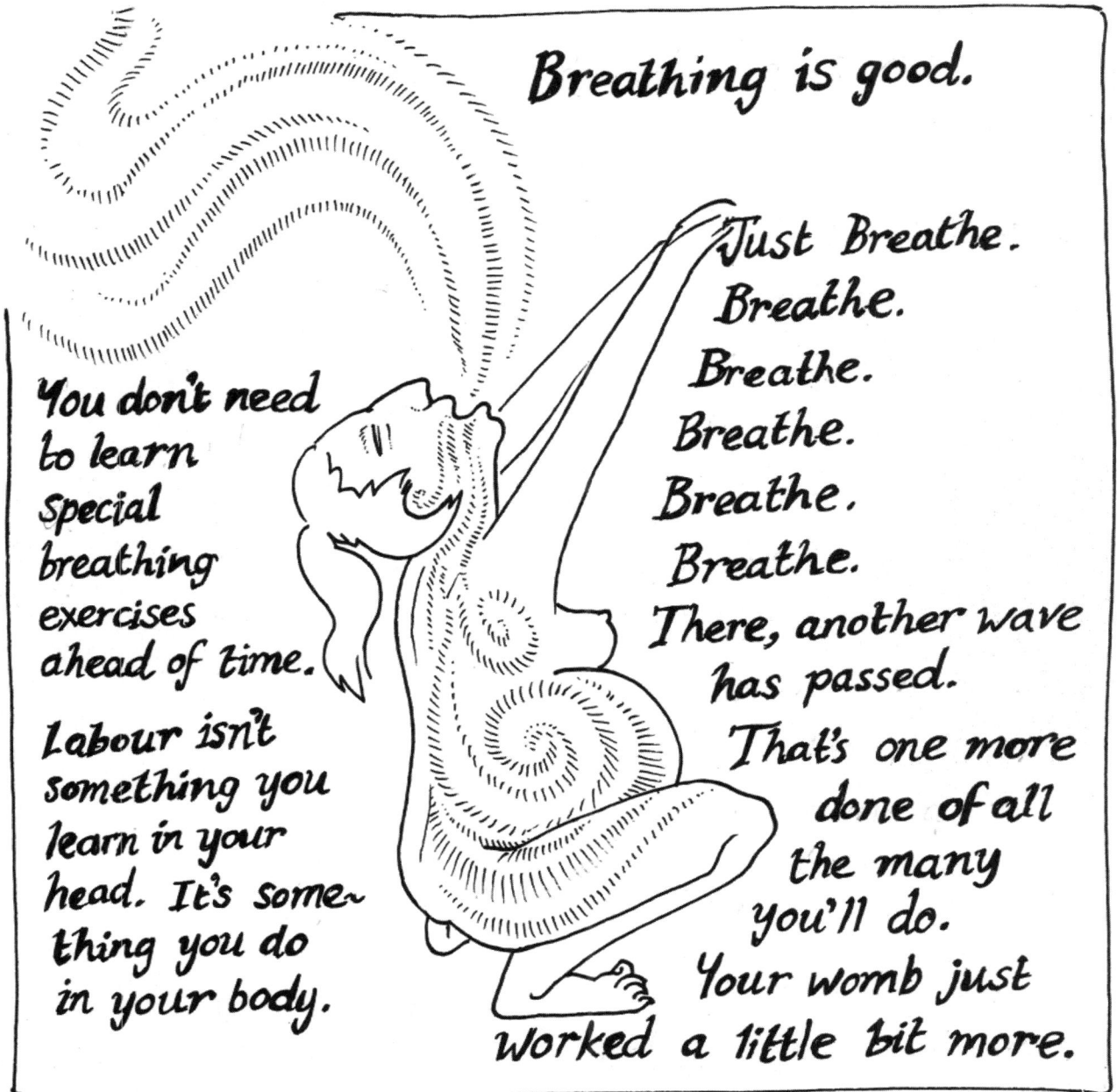

Breathing is good.

You don't need to learn special breathing exercises ahead of time.

Labour isn't something you learn in your head. It's something you do in your body.

Just Breathe.
Breathe.
Breathe.
Breathe.
Breathe.
Breathe.
There, another wave has passed.
That's one more done of all the many you'll do.
Your womb just worked a little bit more.

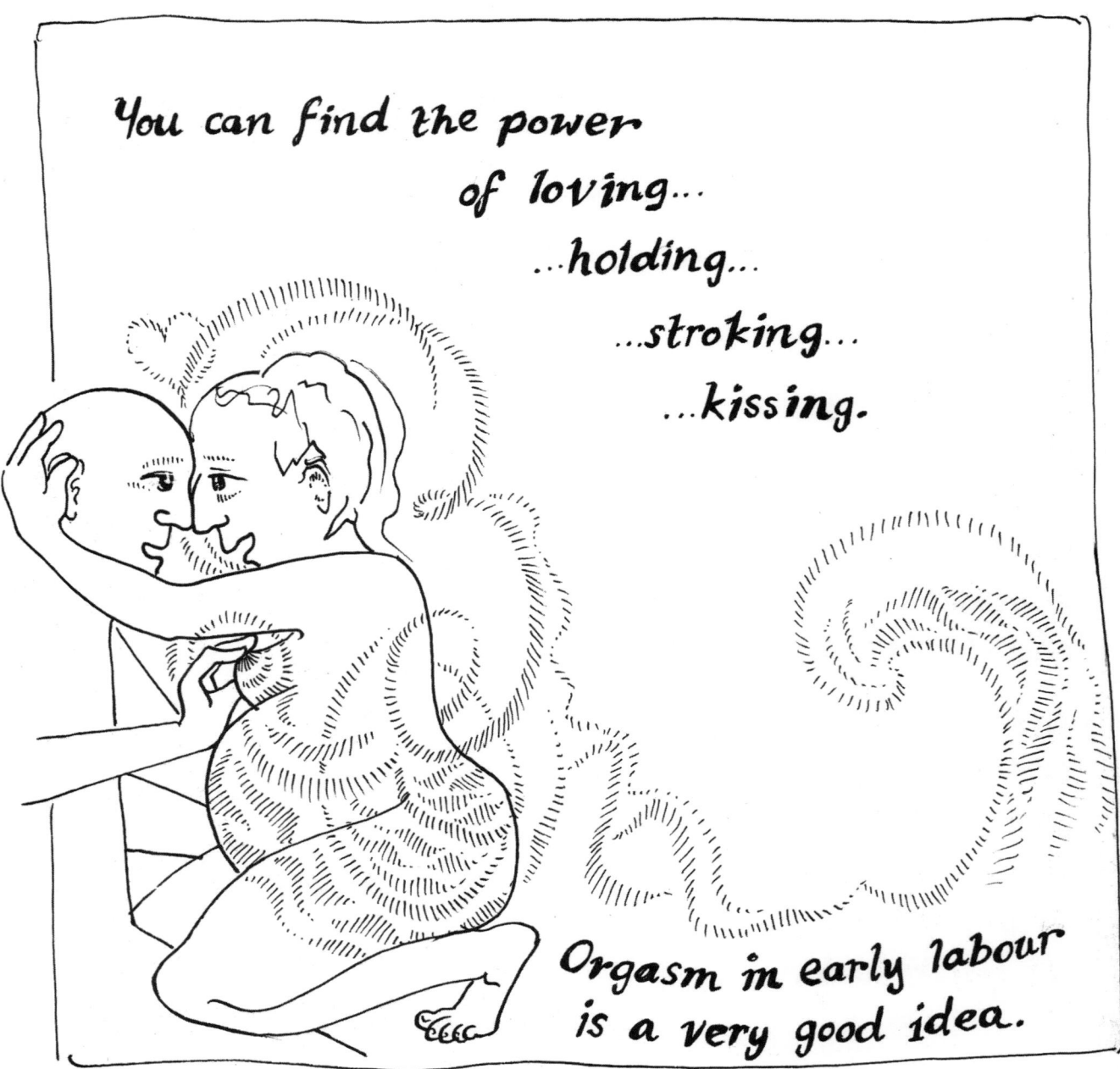

You can find the power
of loving...
...holding...
...stroking...
...kissing.

Orgasm in early labour
is a very good idea.

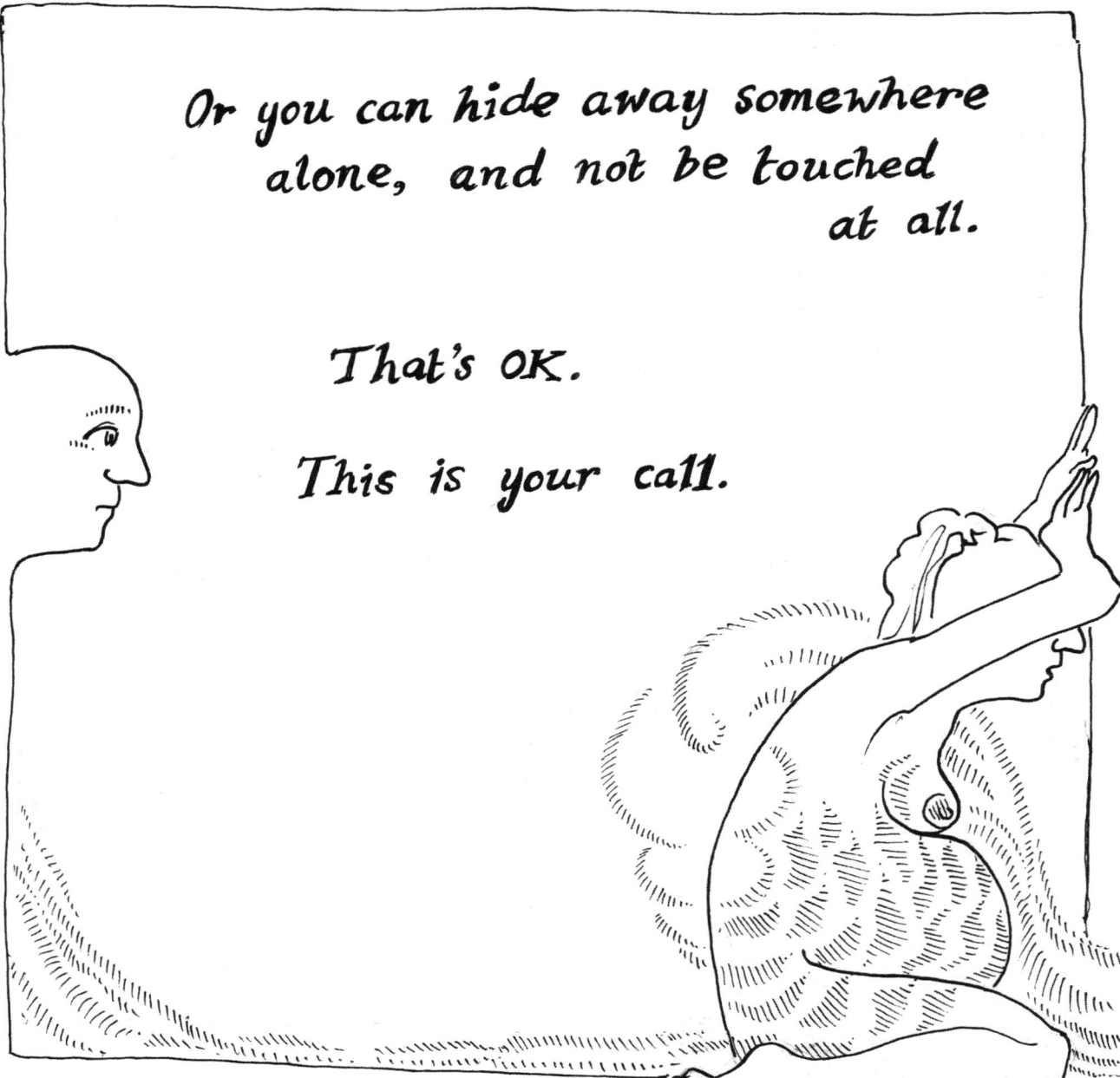

Or you can hide away somewhere alone, and not be touched at all.

That's OK.

This is your call.

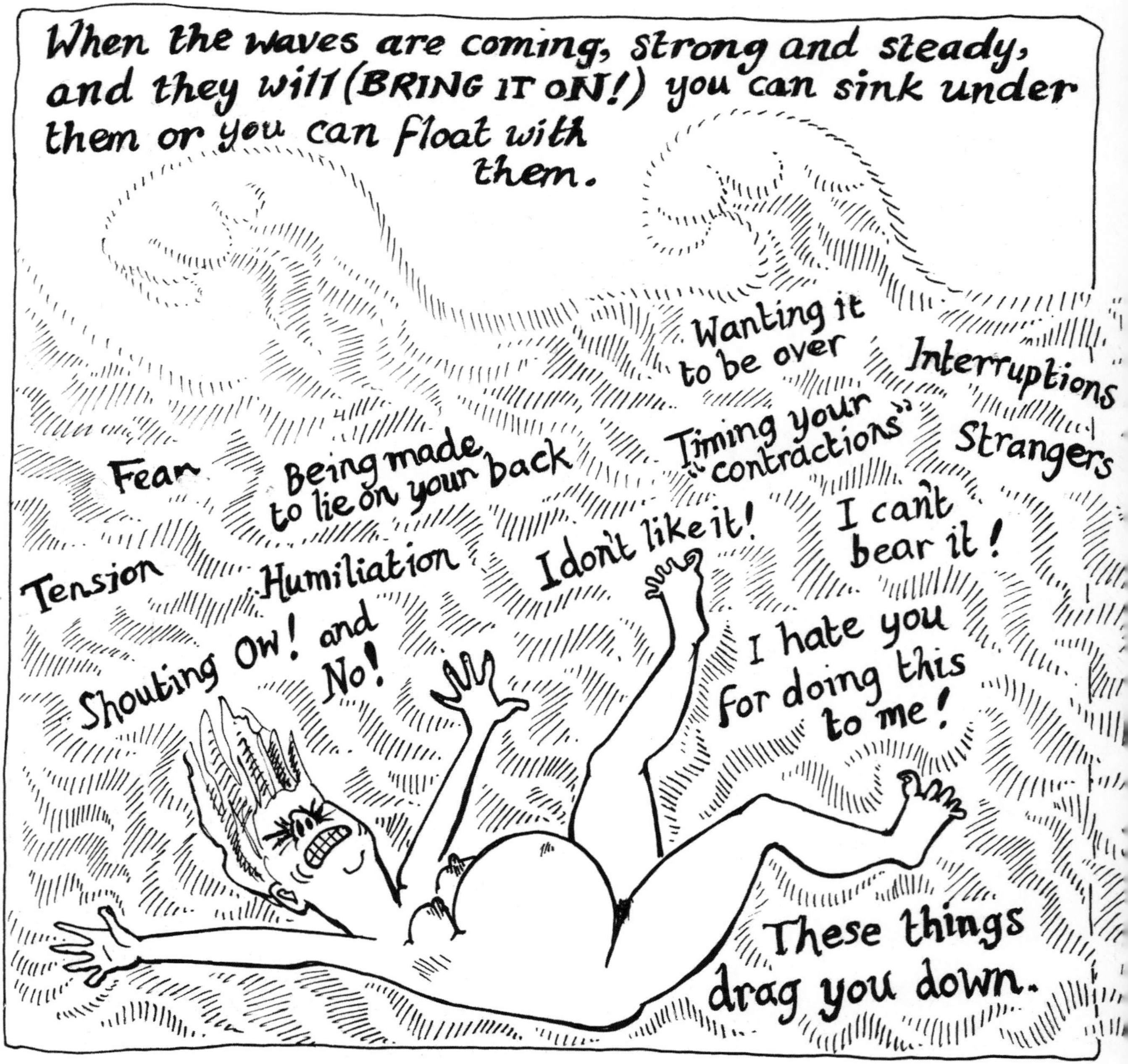
When the waves are coming, strong and steady, and they will (BRING IT ON!) you can sink under them or you can float with them.
Wanting it to be over
Interruptions
Timing your "contractions"
Strangers
Fear
Being made to lie on your back
I can't bear it!
I don't like it!
Tension
Humiliation
Shouting Ow! and No!
I hate you for doing this to me!
These things drag you down.

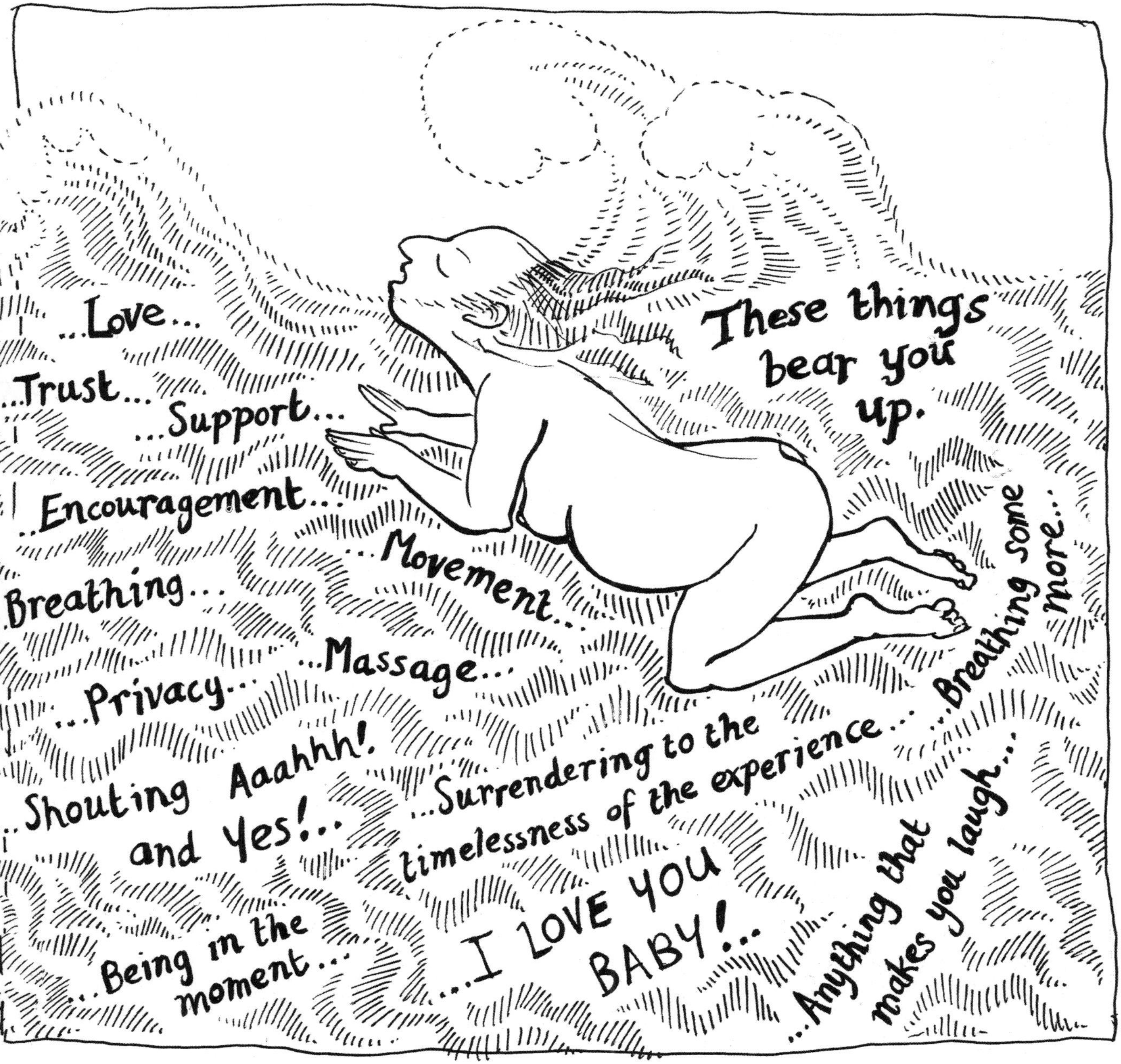
...Love...
...Trust...
...Support...
...Encouragement...
Breathing...
...Movement...
...Privacy...
...Massage...
...Shouting Aaahhh! and Yes!...
...Surrendering to the timelessness of the experience...
...Breathing some more...
...Being in the moment...
...I LOVE YOU BABY!...
...Anything that makes you laugh...
These things bear you up.

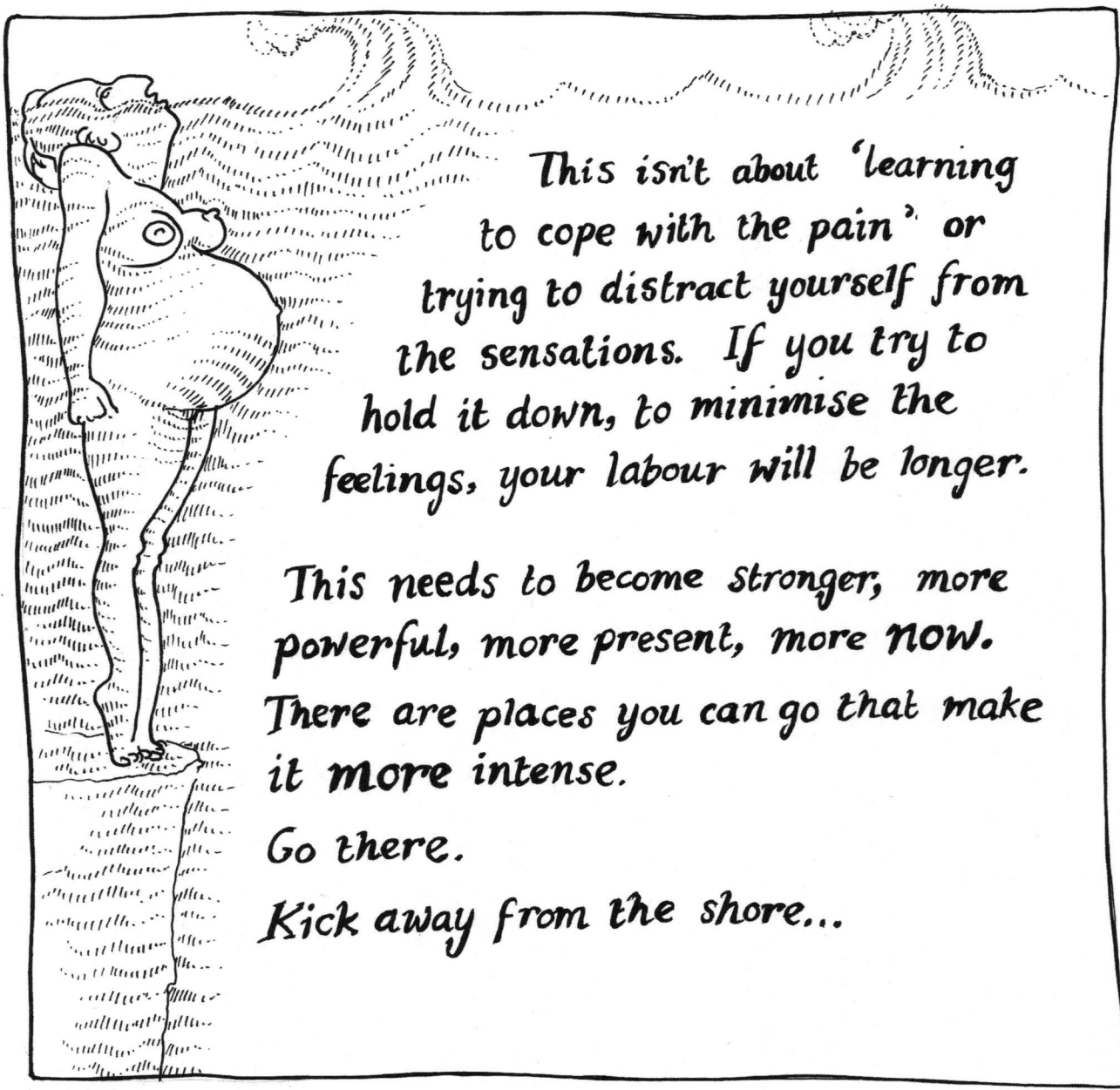

This isn't about 'learning to cope with the pain' or trying to distract yourself from the sensations. If you try to hold it down, to minimise the feelings, your labour will be longer.

This needs to become stronger, more powerful, more present, more now. There are places you can go that make it more intense.

Go there.

Kick away from the shore...

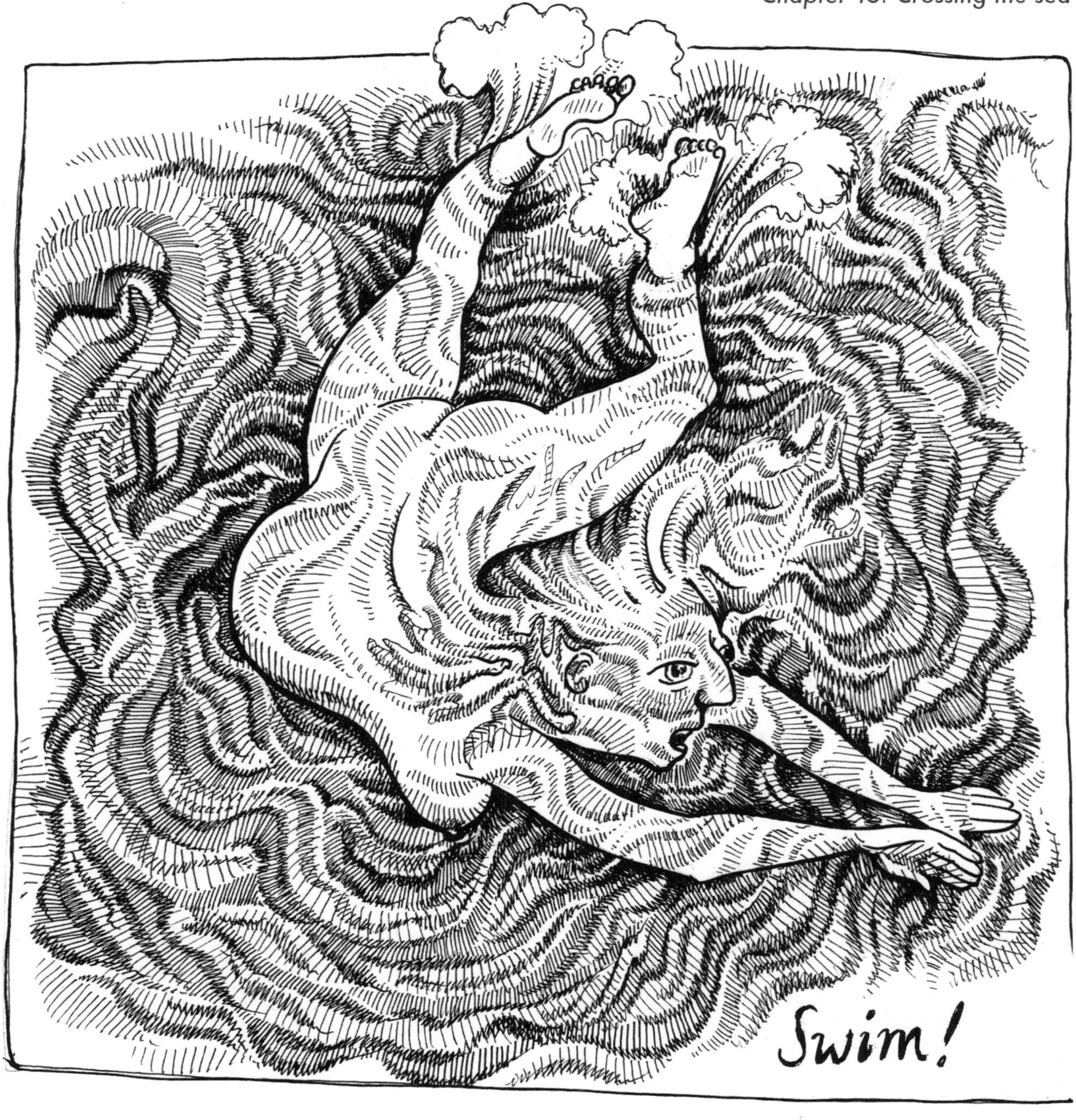
Swim!

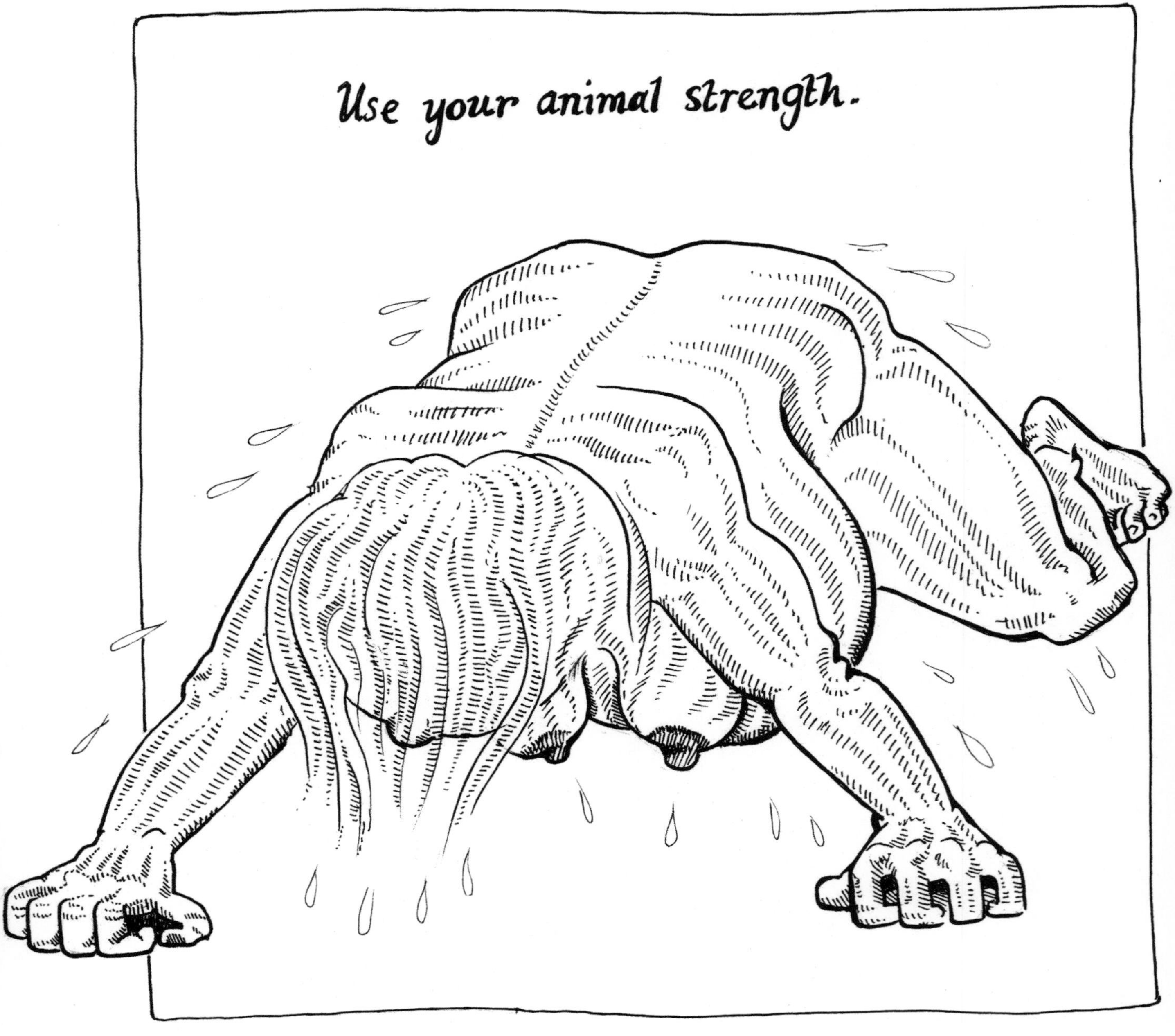
Use your animal strength.

Use the panting, sweating, shaking, biting, scratching, licking, puking, pissing, pooing, shouting, swearing beast within you.

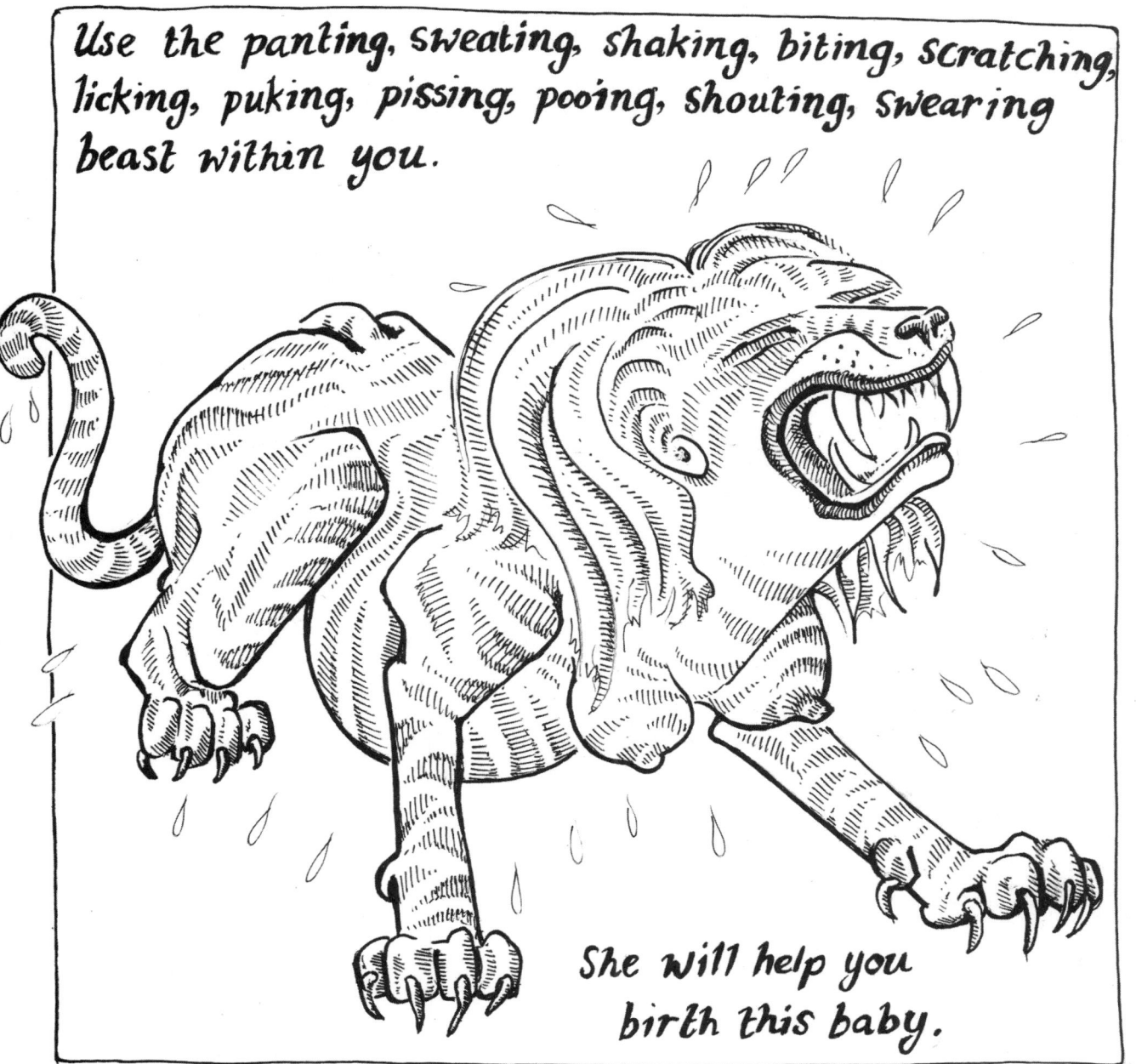

She will help you birth this baby.

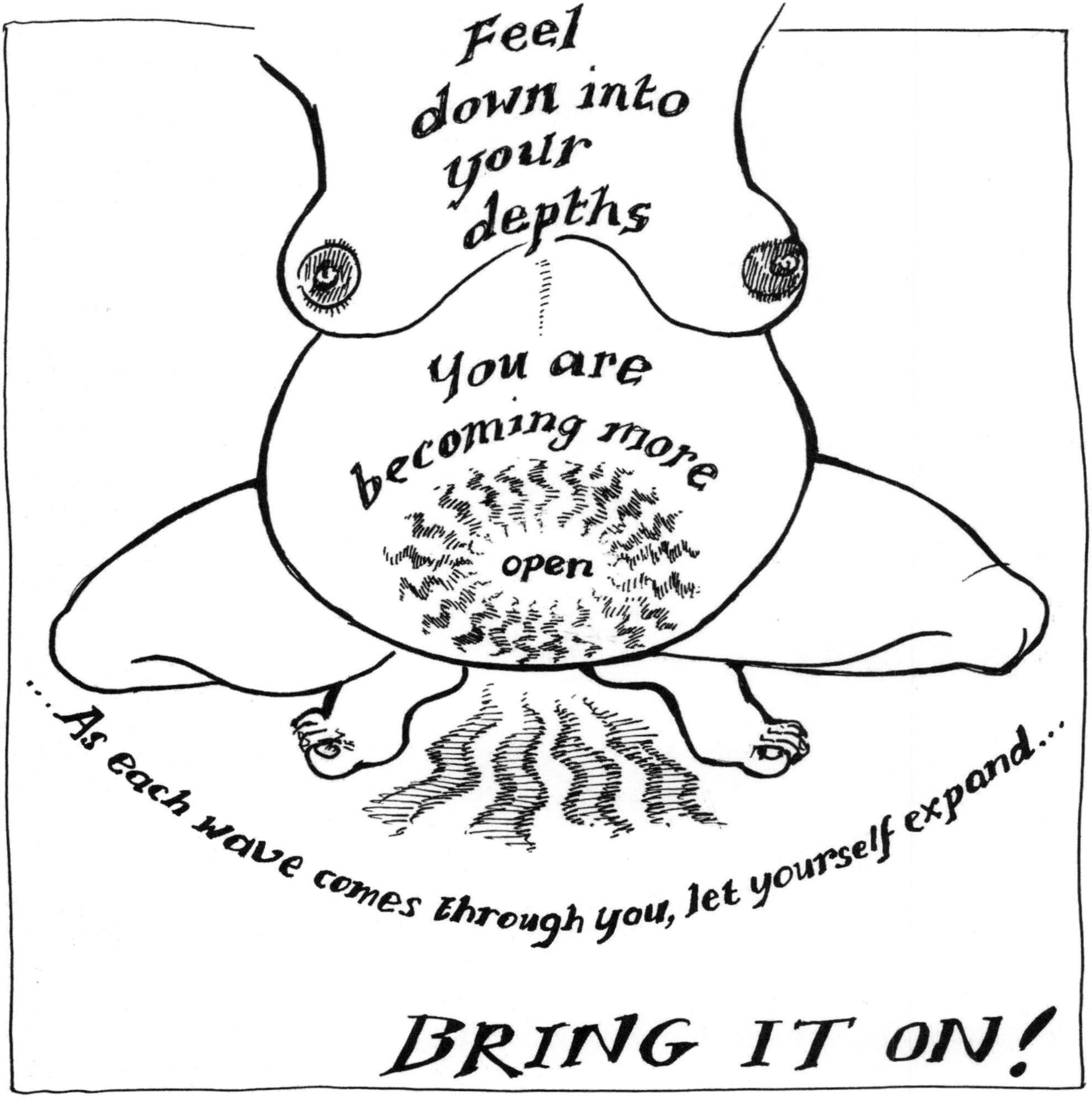
Feel down into your depths
You are becoming more open
...As each wave comes through you, let yourself expand...
BRING IT ON!

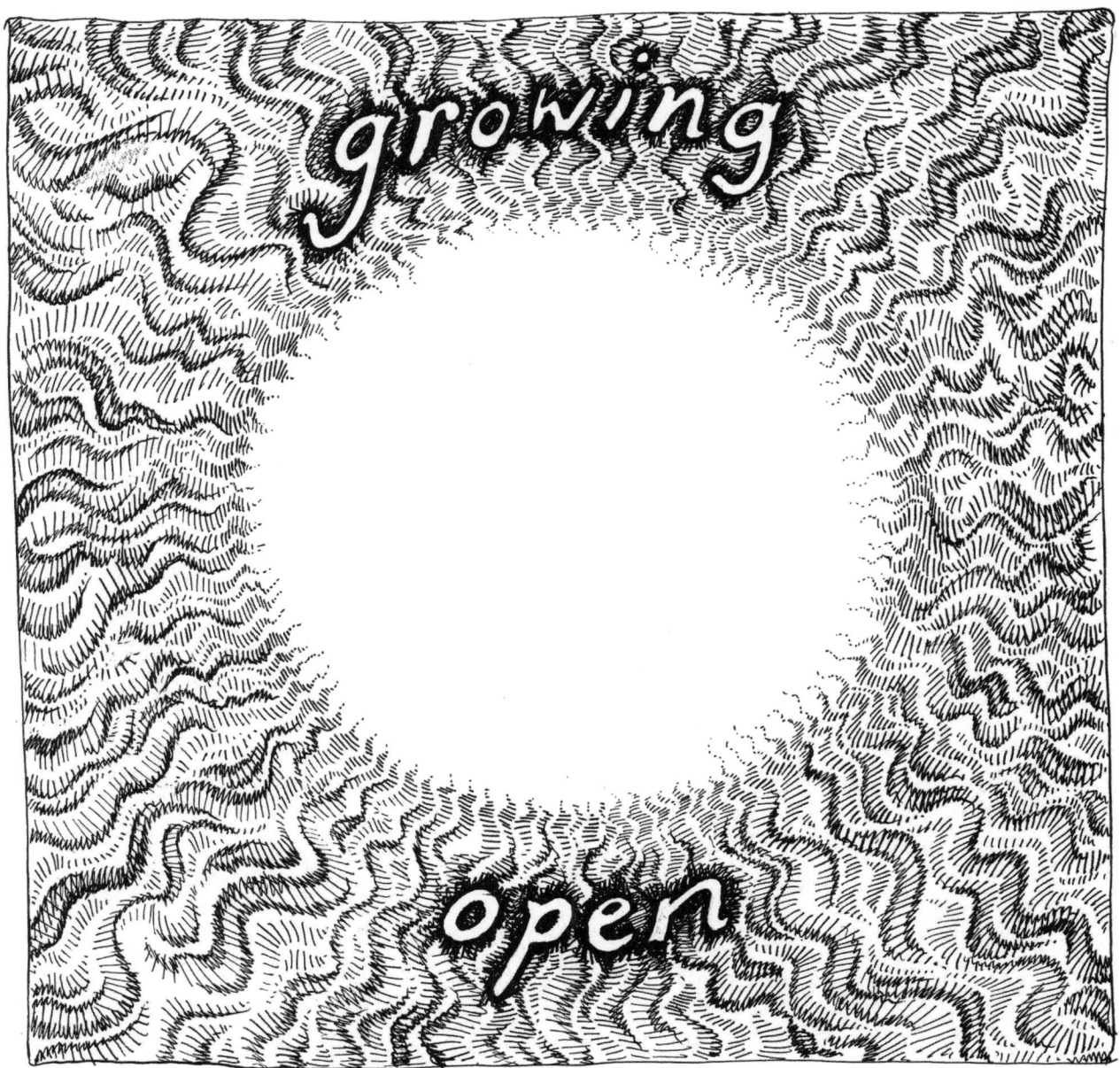

This is exactly how open you're becoming.

Remember
your baby loves you.

Close your eyes and journey in
your mind to somewhere
beautiful with your baby.

Talk to your baby.
Tell them it's time to come through.

Remember
this is the right place
to have your baby.

Even though it probably isn't
exactly how you planned
it would be.

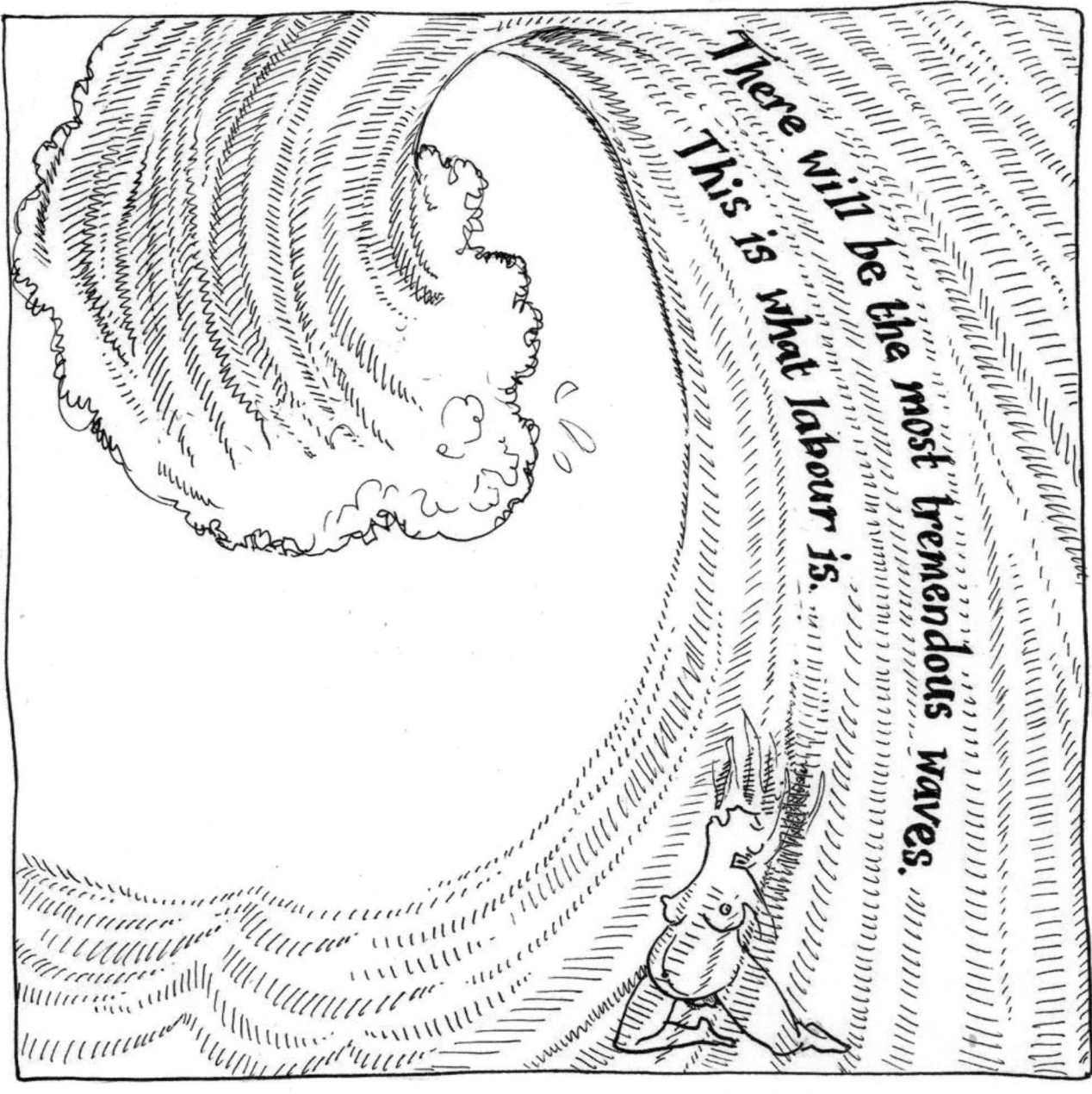

There will be the most tremendous waves. This is what labour is.

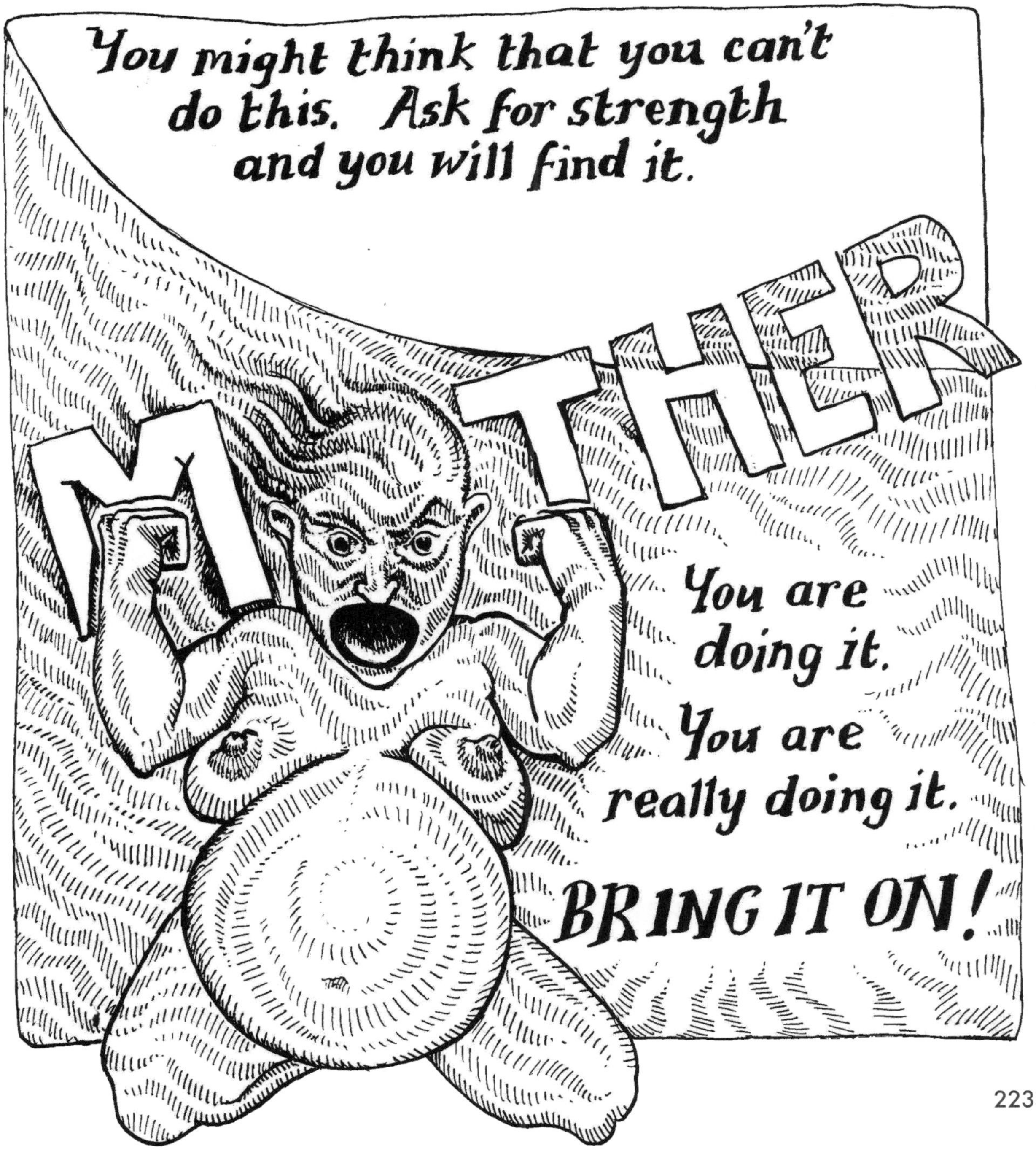
You might think that you can't
do this. Ask for strength
and you will find it.
MOTHER
You are
doing it.
You are
really doing it.
BRING IT ON!

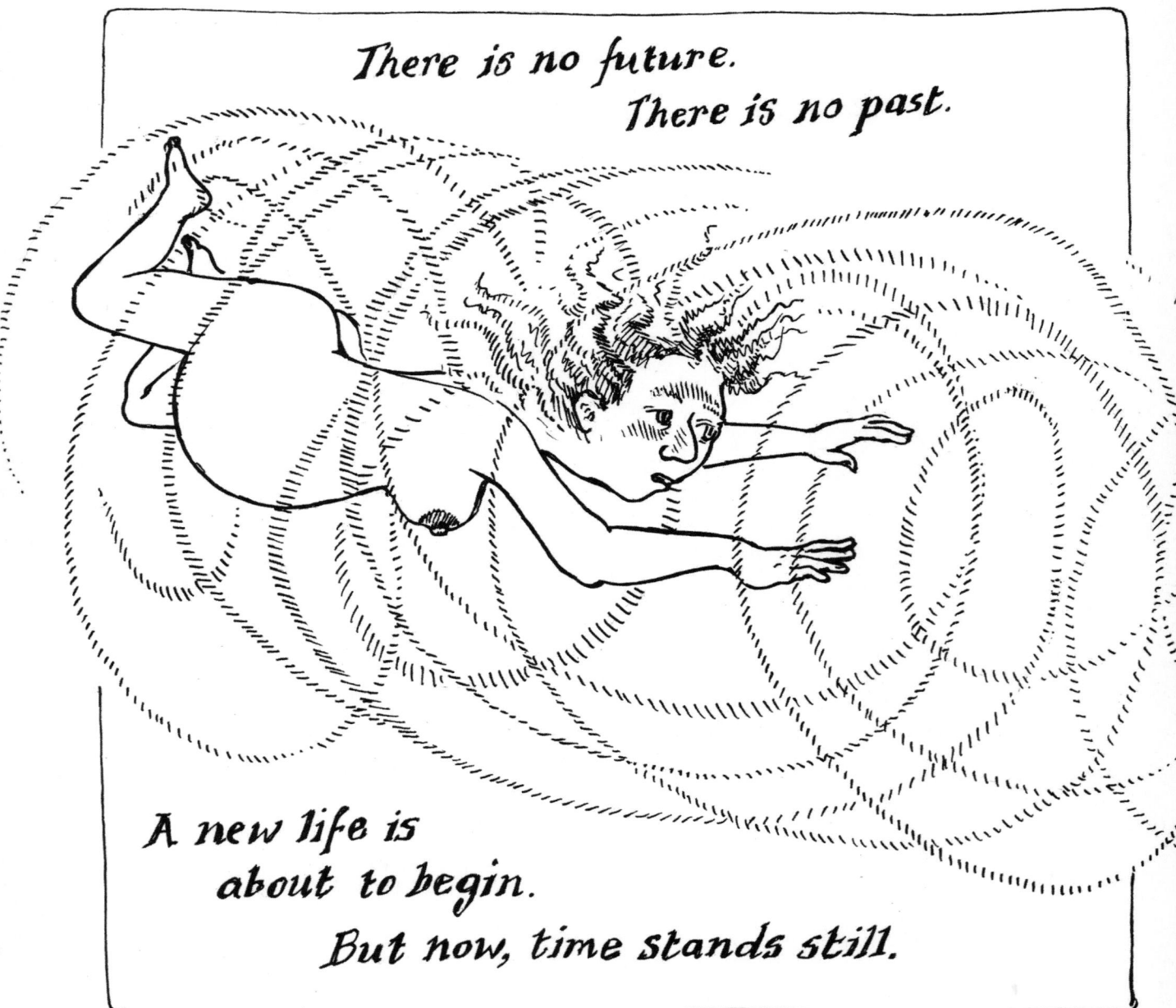

There is no future.
There is no past.

A new life is
about to begin.
But now, time stands still.

A new life.
A new narrative.
But now, you are
beyond words.

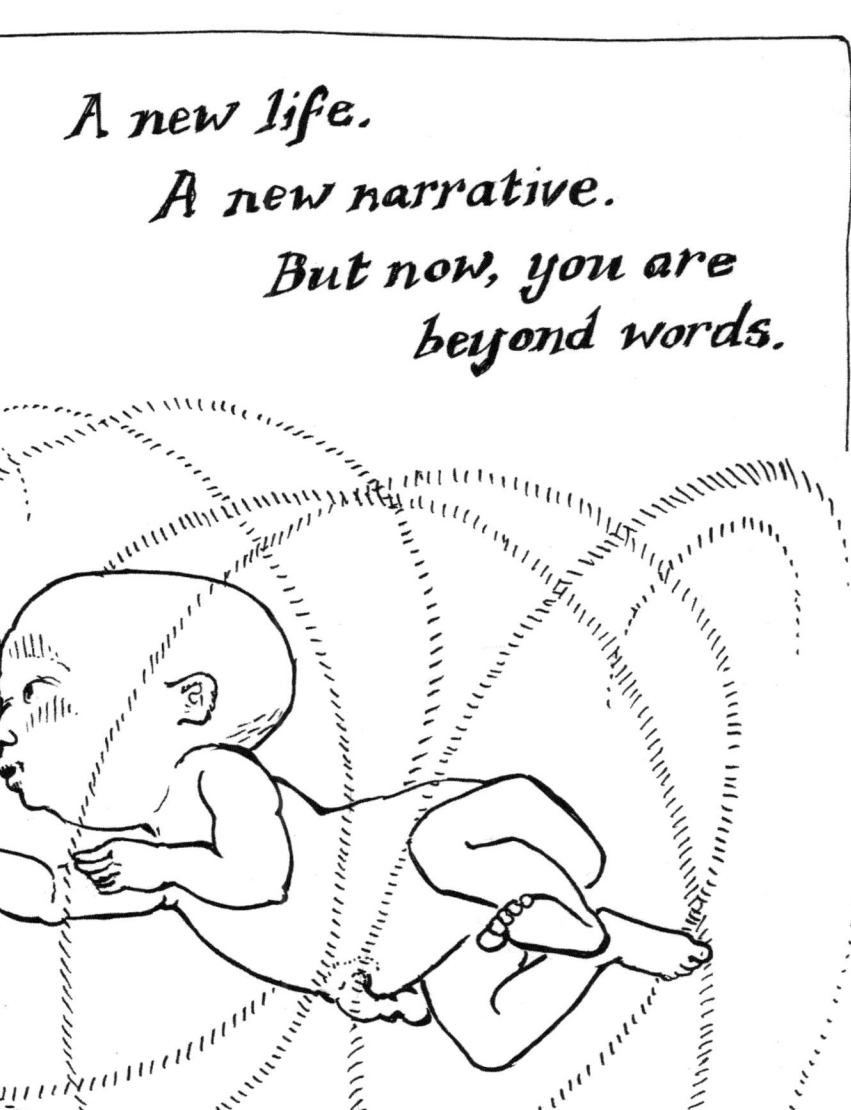

PICK YOUR OWN ADVENTURE MOMENT!

That was the most important part of the book.
It was about being in your labour; entering into the process of birth.

You now have a choice.
There are two equally valid stances that a pregnant woman
can take when preparing for labour and birth.

You can trust in yourself.

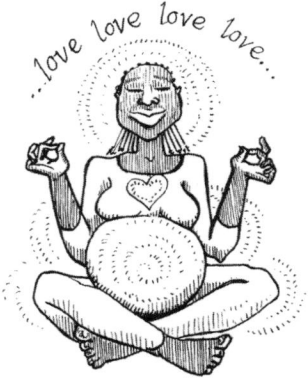

Be in the moment and let events unfold.
This approach works particularly well
if you have a known, loved, experienced
care-giver who will definitely attend
your birth.

You can stop reading now.

Cut this book down the spine at this
page and throw the second half away.
You have no need of it.

And you can learn from others.

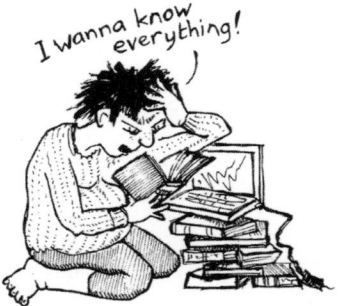

Some women prefer empowerment
through information. If you want the
details about birth, including some
gory ones, read on…

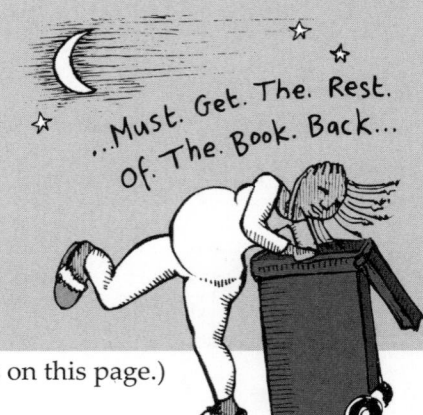

(It is possible to feel more than one of the emotions on this page.)

16 *How monkey mama does it*

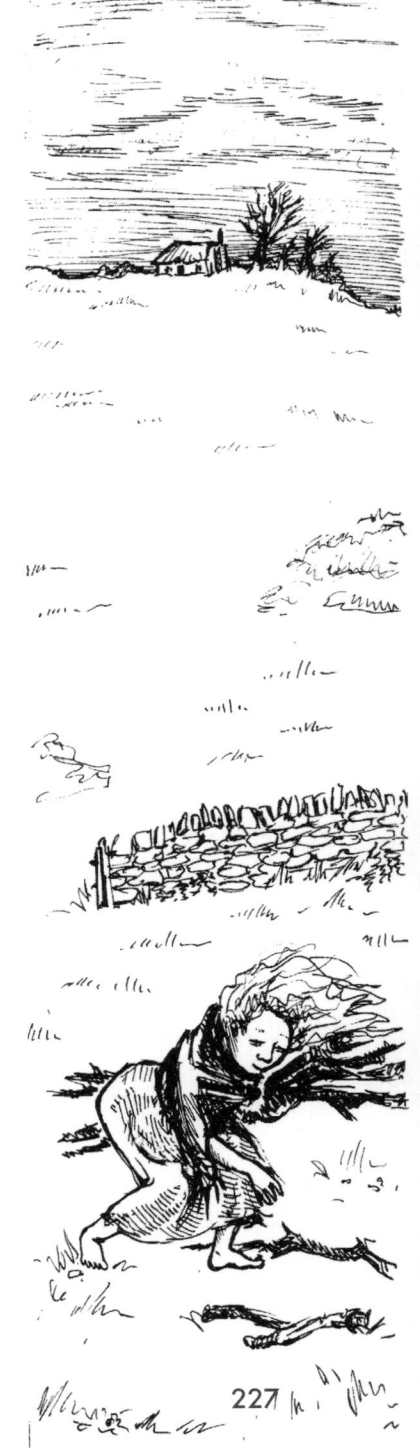

When I market-tested this chapter, some readers assumed it was about home birth. It's not. It's about birth. It's about what has happened when women have had babies since time immemorial. I gave it a historical setting because it's a primal creation myth: it's the story of a maiden, a mother and a crone. Oh, and I also wanted to be able to draw women with hairy fannies without it being a political statement.

Let us introduce the principal actors in this birth story.

Once again the **womb** is the star of the show. Hasn't she put on weight since we last saw her? Just wait. She's about to really let herself go...

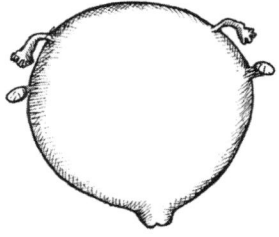

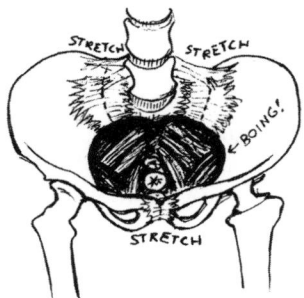

In a supporting role, the **pelvis**, and the bouncy, supple-yet-stretchy **pelvic floor**. The fun bits also play a larger part than you'd expect.

Also starring… the **baby**!

It's a rites-of-passage movie for our baby here. Rites of birth passage, to be precise. And the baby will make a surprising twist in the plot.

To make this all a lot easier, the maternal pelvis is not one solid ring of bone, but three separate pieces, linked together with extra-stretchy ligaments. And the baby's skull is not one bone but seven, that can meld and move over each other as they pass through the birth canal.

227

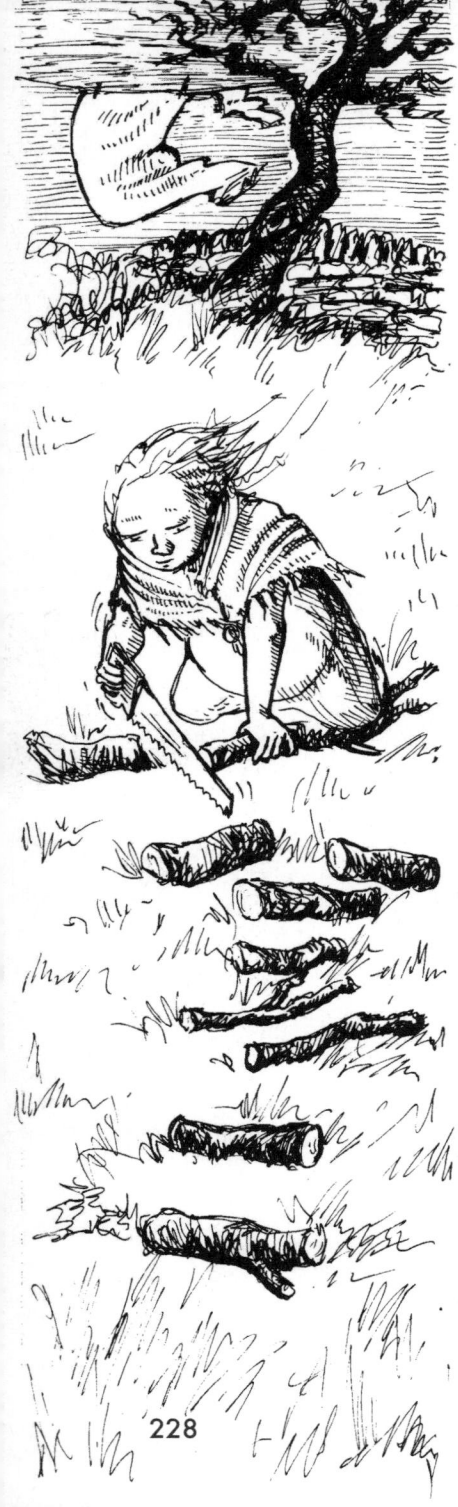

While the baby has been fattening up in the mother's belly, so has the pituitary gland, deep within her brain. Both mother and baby are about to get the hormone rush of their lives.[1]

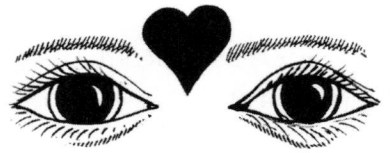

Oxytocin is the hormone of love. It makes us feel calm, connected and empathetic. It is the chemical that makes contractions happen, and its name is derived from the Greek for 'quick birth'.

Beta-endorphin is a natural opiate, which works on the same brain receptors as morphine and heroin. It is the hormone of transcendence. It is produced in response to pain.

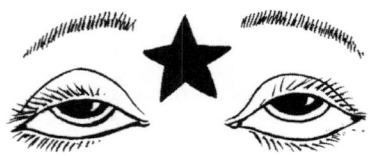

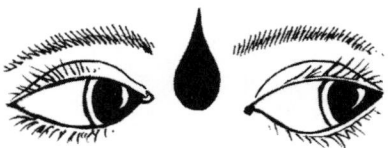

Prolactin is the hormone that makes breastmilk. As well as relaxing, loving feelings, it promotes a sense of vigilance in the new mother.

Catecholamines (adrenaline and noradrenaline) enforce a 'fight or flight' response to fear or stress. In early labour they quell contractions, diverting energy from the womb to the mother's limbs so she can run to safety. Right at the peak of birth, they perform a different function, as we shall see...

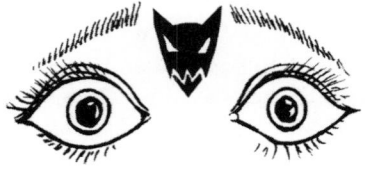

Here is monkey mum-to-be.[2] She hasn't given birth before.

Now, at the end of her pregnancy, her progesterone levels fall and her oestrogen levels surge, activating the oxytocin receptors in her womb.

The womb does some painless practice contractions, co-ordinating its movements for the effort ahead.

Prostaglandins soften the fibres in her cervix and the amniotic sac around the baby swells and weakens.

As the baby drops down within her, pressure on her cervix sends a signal up her spine to the pituitary to release more oxytocin. And these trigger some more movements in her womb – a little less painless and a little more purposeful.

The plug of jelly-like juices that have sealed the womb come away. A 'show'. Labour is near.

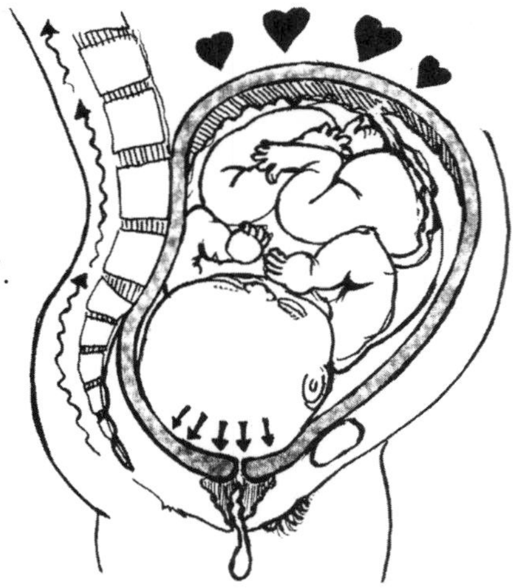

The baby has hormones too. A surge of catecholamines matures his lungs and liver in readiness.[3]

And these hormones from the baby give the mother a burst of energy. Like most animals, she needs to prepare a safe, private space for the birth.

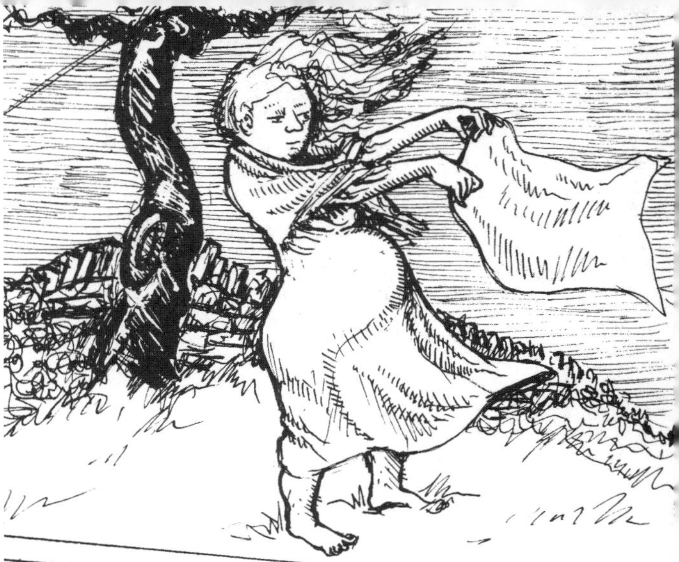

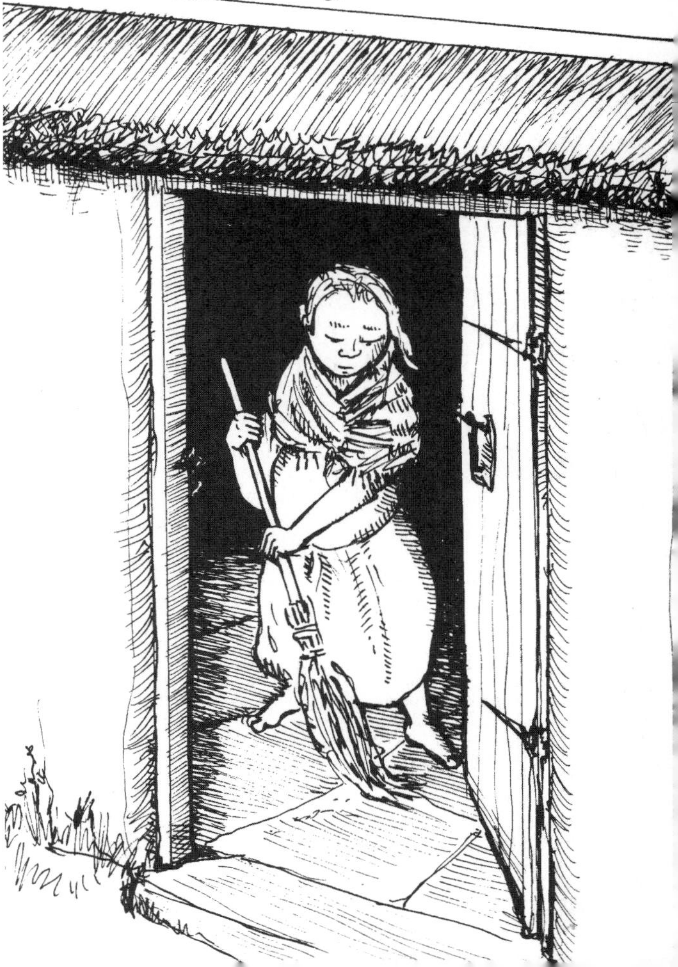

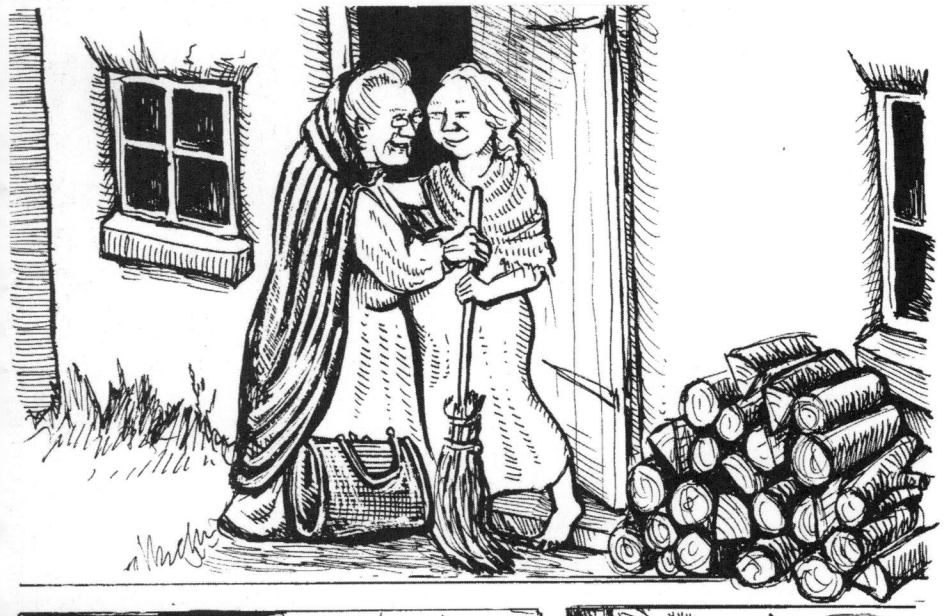

Like whales, elephants and gorillas, the human monkey seeks a birth companion. Someone she knows and trusts. A woman with a wisdom born of experience of many births. A midwife. A profession that is as old as humanity itself.[4]

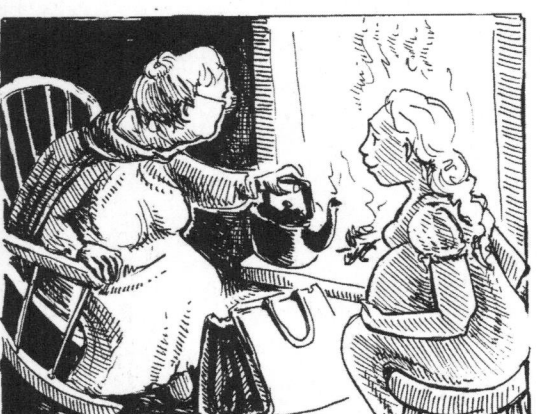

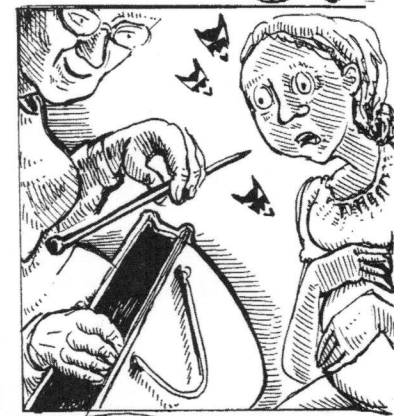

The midwife brings the tools of her trade…

…her hands, her brain and her heart.

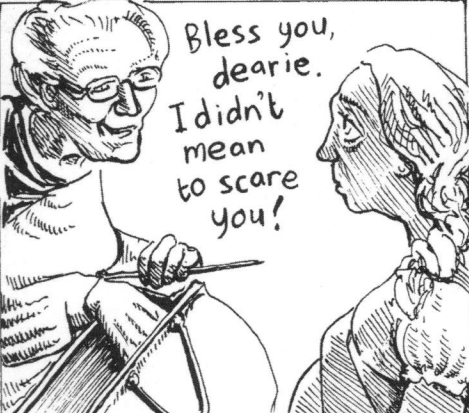

Bless you, dearie. I didn't mean to scare you!

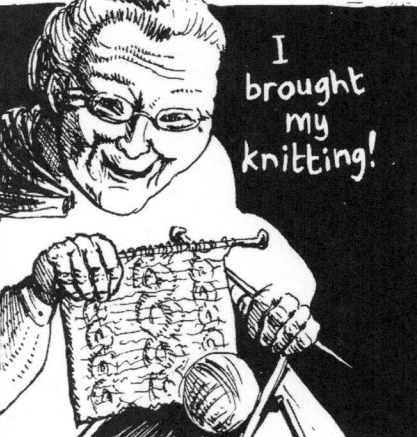

I brought my knitting!

When monkey mama feels anxious, catecholamines rush through her, and her contractions are suppressed.[5] It is the job of the midwife to seek out and soothe such stresses.

Kindness and humour can instantly dispel fear.

To enter into the state of birthing, monkey mama needs privacy. Oxytocin, a sex hormone, comes on stronger in a dark, private place. Being undisturbed by strangers is as important for giving birth as it is for making love.

In the first part of labour, the womb creates expansion (not contraction!) in the cervix, to let the baby out. As the cervix has been locked tight for nine months, holding back the weight of the baby and the waters, it takes some time to soften and retract.

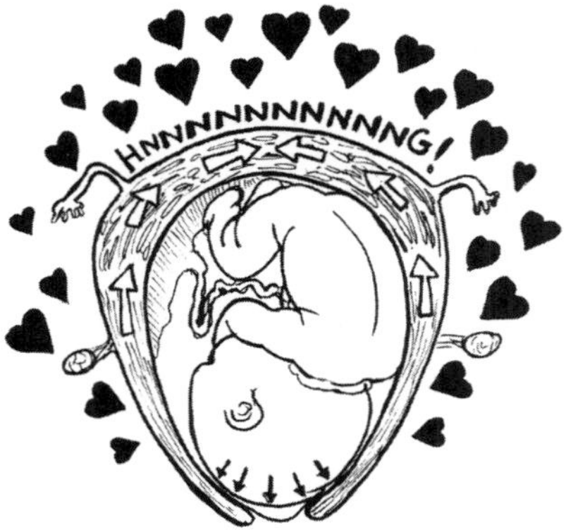
HNNNNNNNNNNNG!

With each wave, the muscle fibres in the top half of the womb thicken and pull towards each other, easing open the gates below. The bulging bag of waters presses more incessantly upon the cervix. More oxytocin is released.The waves grow stronger.

As oxytocin floods the baby's system, neurons in his brain quieten down, so he can survive with less oxygen (if need be) during the rigours of birth.[6]

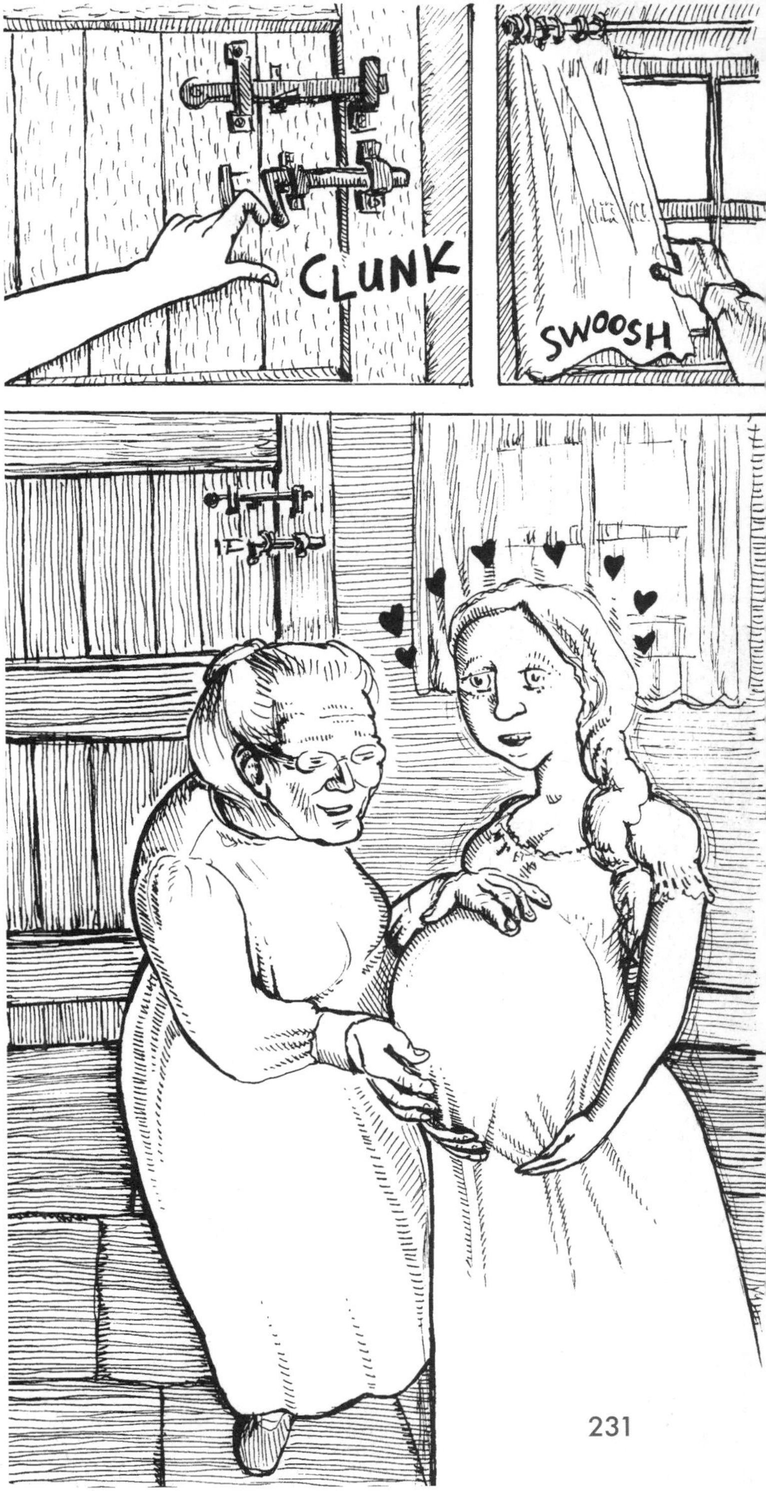
CLUNK
SWOOSH

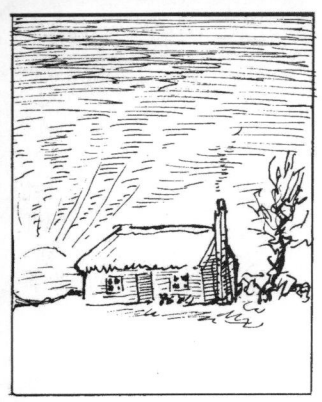
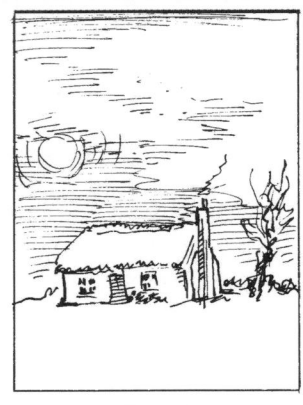
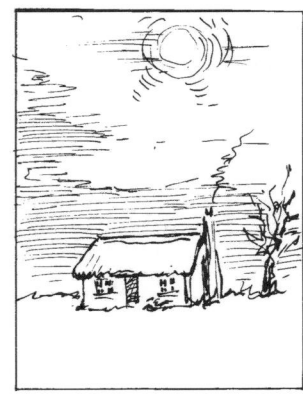

How long does this first 'stage' of labour take?

It can take any time at all. It can be stunningly quick, or timelessly, eternally slow.

Perhaps it will be this long…

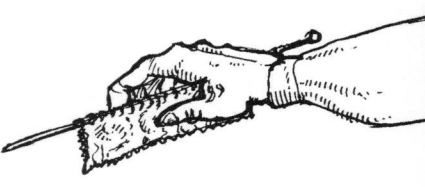

Or maybe it will be this long…

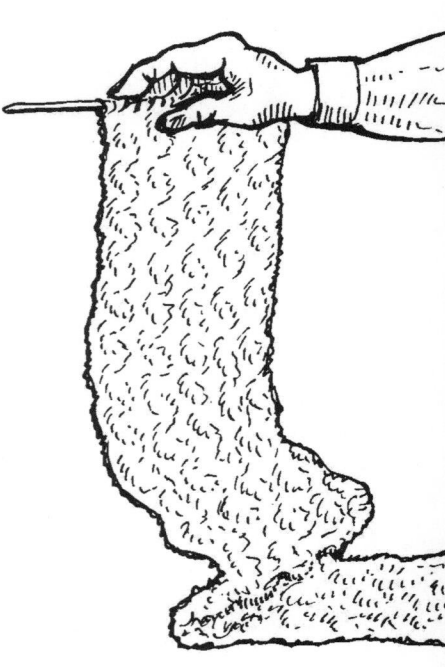

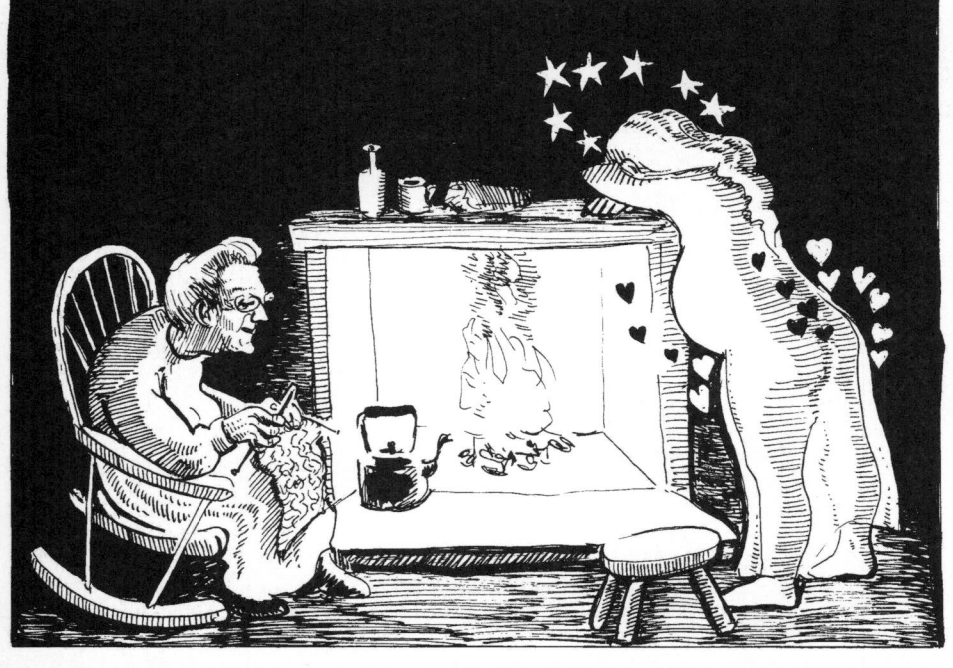

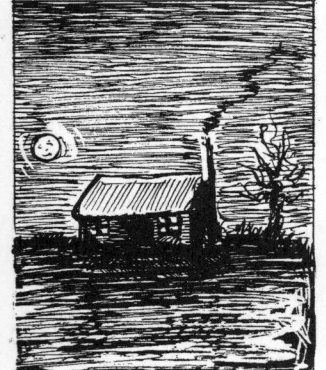
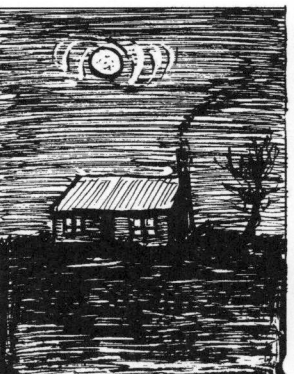

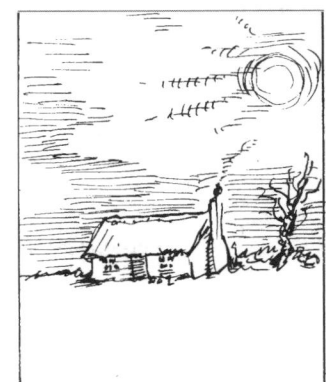
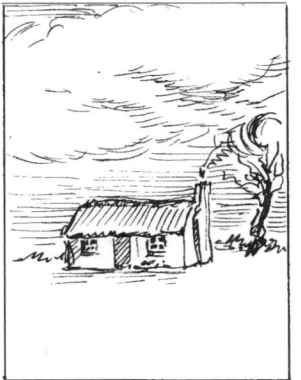
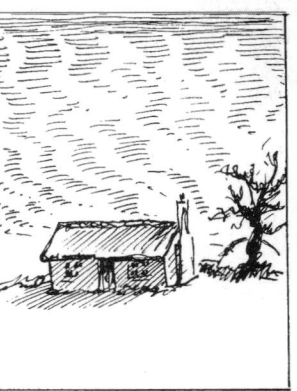

In response to the pain, monkey mama's brain sends out beta-endorphins, spacing her out so time loses its meaning. When the outer 'thinking' human brain, the neocortex, is less busy, the inner, ancient, mammalian brain can take over – sending out more hormones, and making more womb-work.

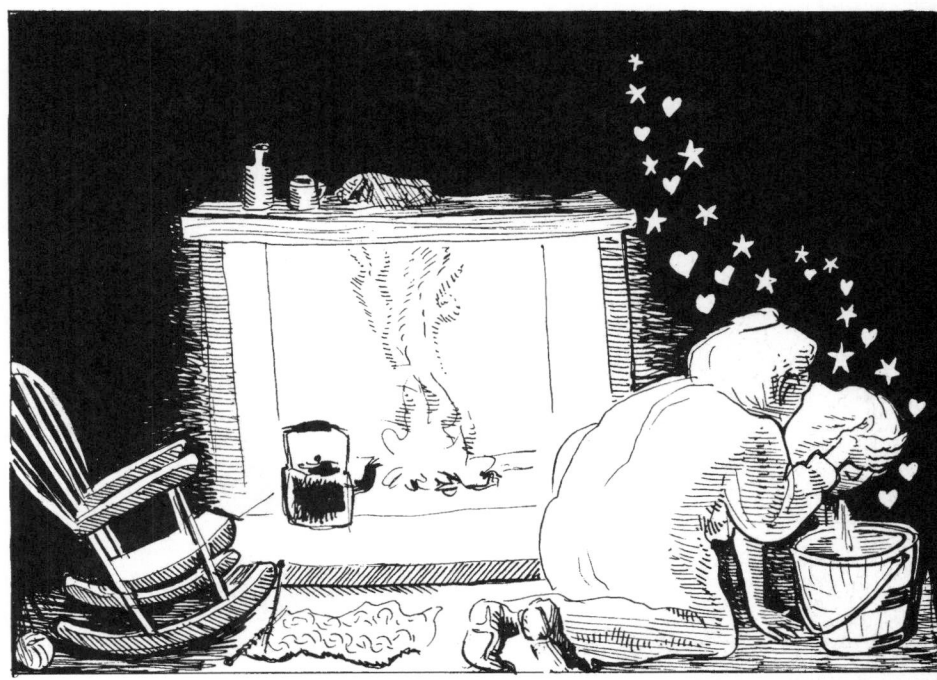

Part of the work of labour is endurance. How long can monkey mama go without sleep? How long can she go without food? She tries to eat, but her stomach repels food. Her energies are needed elsewhere.

More babies are born at full moon, when fewer predators prowl.[7]

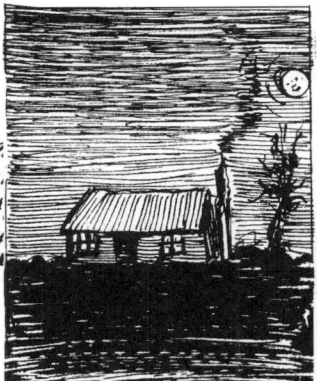
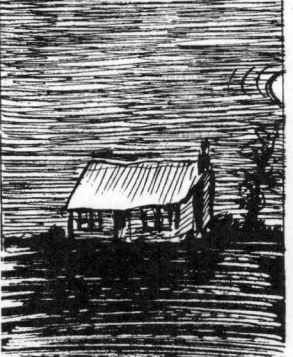
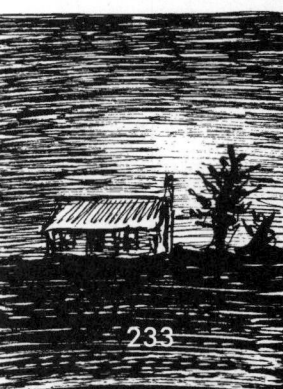

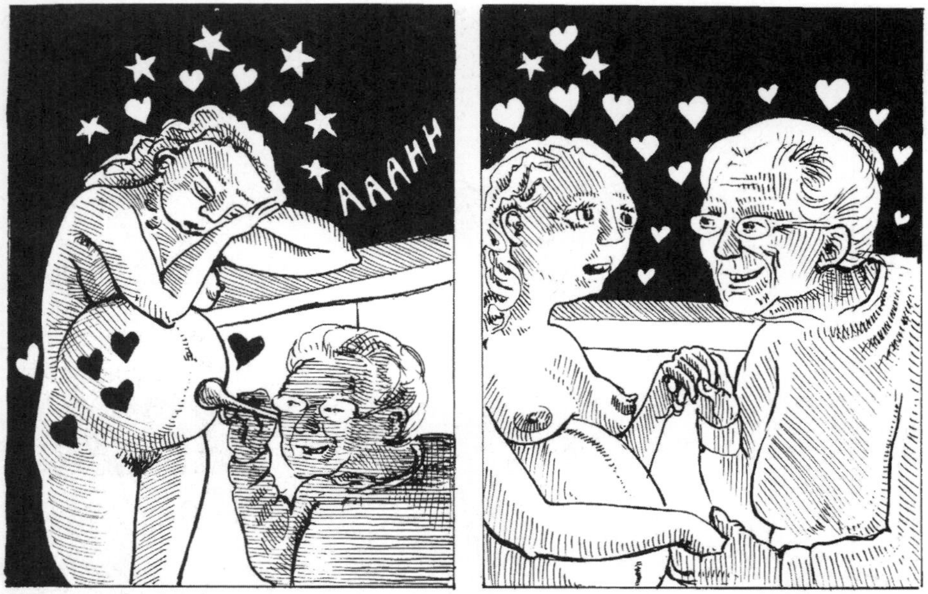
AAAHH

And what is monkey midwife doing? She *listens* to the mother and the baby. Much of what she hears is communicated without words.

She soothes, she comforts, she *understands*. The midwife produces oxytocin too. The hormone of connection, it acts upon all the people present at the birth.

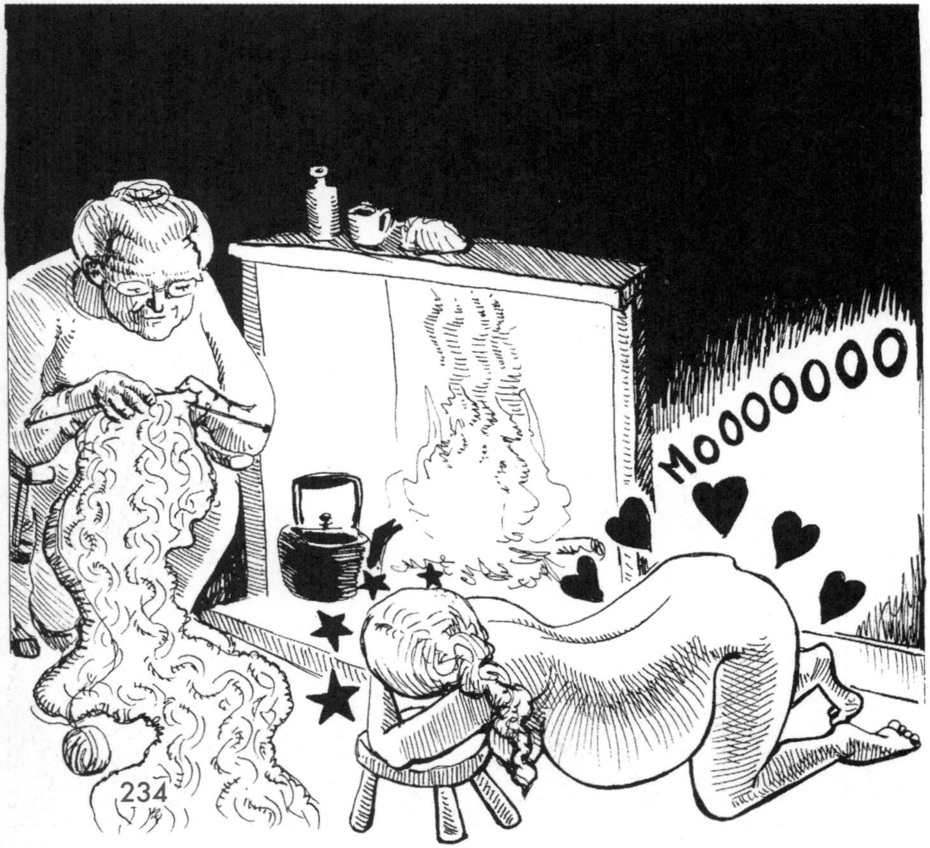
MOOOOOOO

Mainly, she knits[8]…

'Spontaneous labour in a normal woman is an event marked by a number of processes so complicated and so perfectly attuned to each other that any interference will only detract from the optimal character.

'The only thing required from the bystanders is that they show respect for this awe-inspiring process by complying with the first rule of medicine – nil nocere *[do no harm].'*

Gerrit-Jan Kloosterman,
Professor of Obstetrics, 1982

…and she *watches*.

A dark red line makes its way up monkey mama's bum-crack. From its progress, monkey midwife can see how close the birth has come.[9]

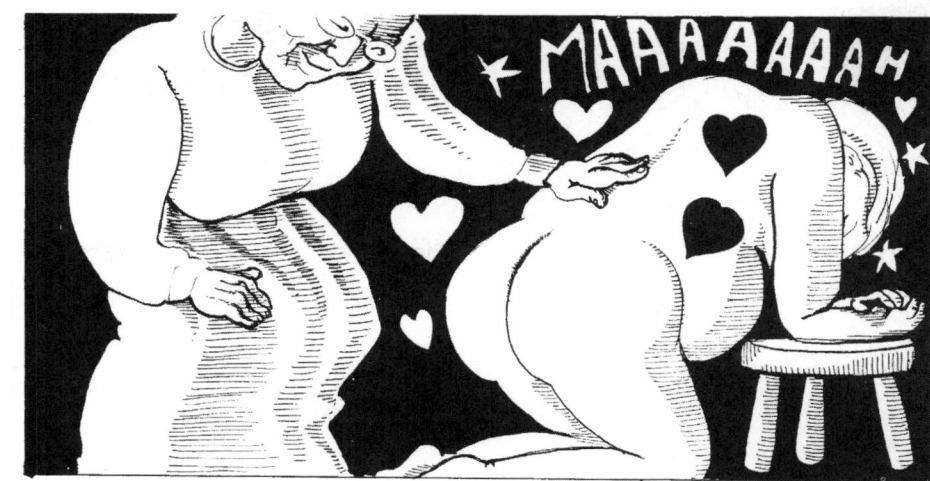

As monkey mama opens fully, great waves of passion come upon her. The baby's head has slipped from her womb, poised for the next stage, the journey through the pelvis towards birth.

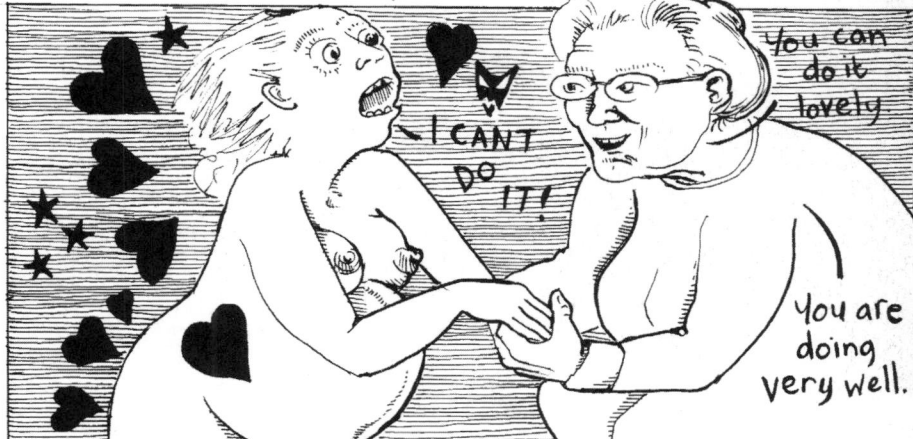

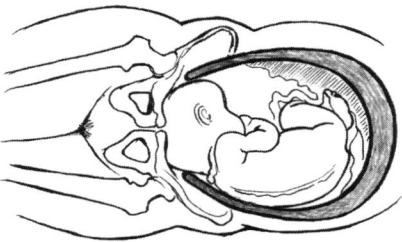

And then… nothing. Monkey mama sleeps deeply. She must 'rest and be thankful', gathering strength for the next stage.[10] It is thought that this lull gives time for the fibres of the womb to loosen up around the baby's body.

Monkey midwife isn't worried. She listens, and she watches, and she stokes the fire.

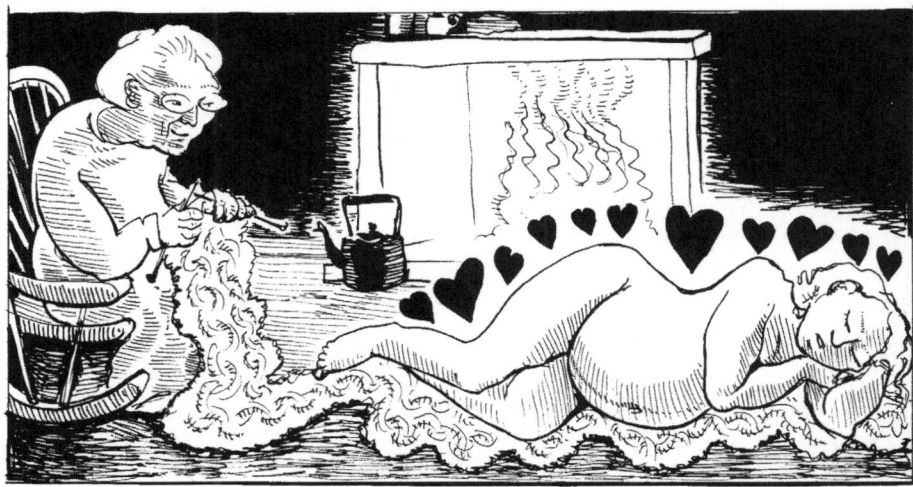

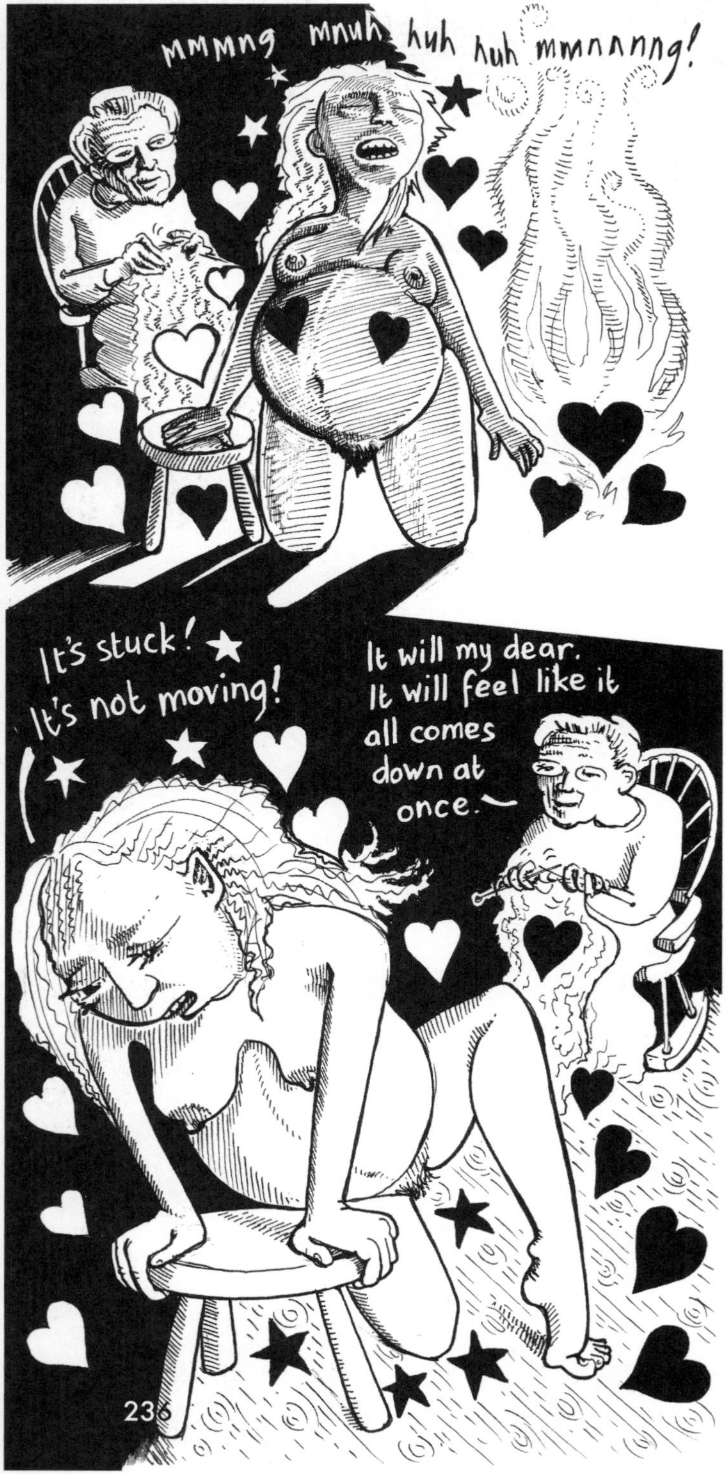
MMMng mnuh huh huh mmnnnng!
It's stuck! It's not moving!
It will my dear. It will feel like it all comes down at once.

Flames leap up. Monkey mama arises. Her womb bears down.

Instinctively, the mother shifts position, helping to shape the baby's head within her with the precision of a sculptor.[11] It takes some time.

Here's the twist in the tale. The baby comes into the pelvis sideways, and then wriggles around a quarter-turn to slip his head under the pubic bone.

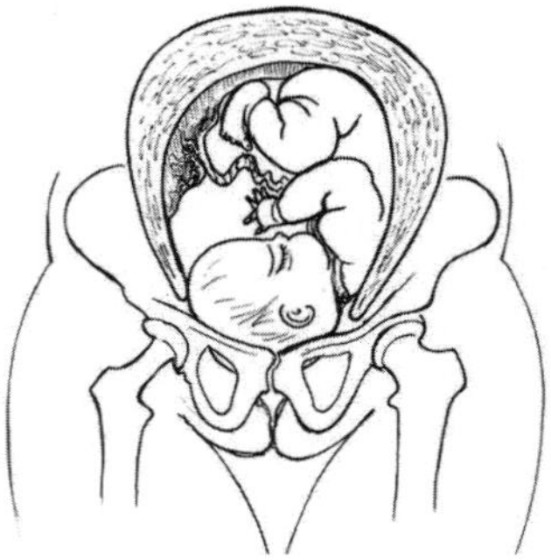

As his head slips down, then back, the tension in the pelvic floor muscles gives him resistance to bounce against and complete his rotation.

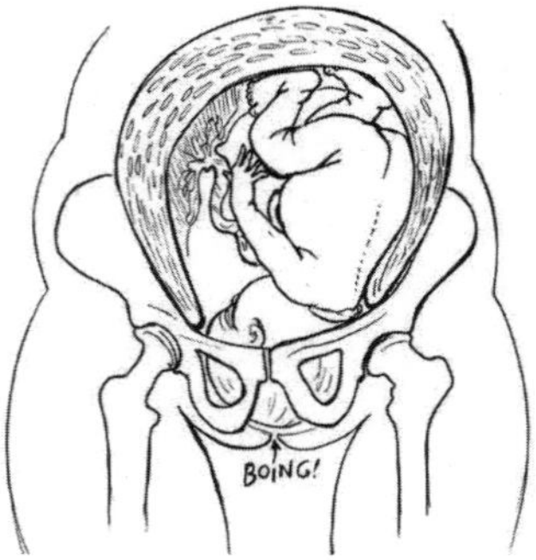
BOING!

Down, then back, a little further down, then back again, a delicate dance.

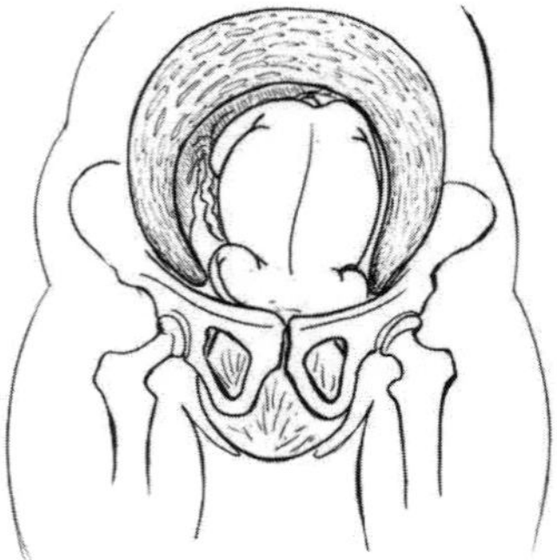

Blood rushes down inside monkey mama. Her internal clitoris swells immensely in size: the erectile tissue there engorges and expands. A hot wet cloth massaged over her vulva eases and increases it.[12]

The baby moves within her, the waters gush, the womb redoubles its efforts. Oh! The intensity!

As the head fills the birth canal, another wave of endorphins overwhelms her, this time accompanied by an immense surge of catecholamines.[13]

Monkey mama cries out in anger and fear…

Monkey midwife says nothing. A spell has been cast that must not be broken.

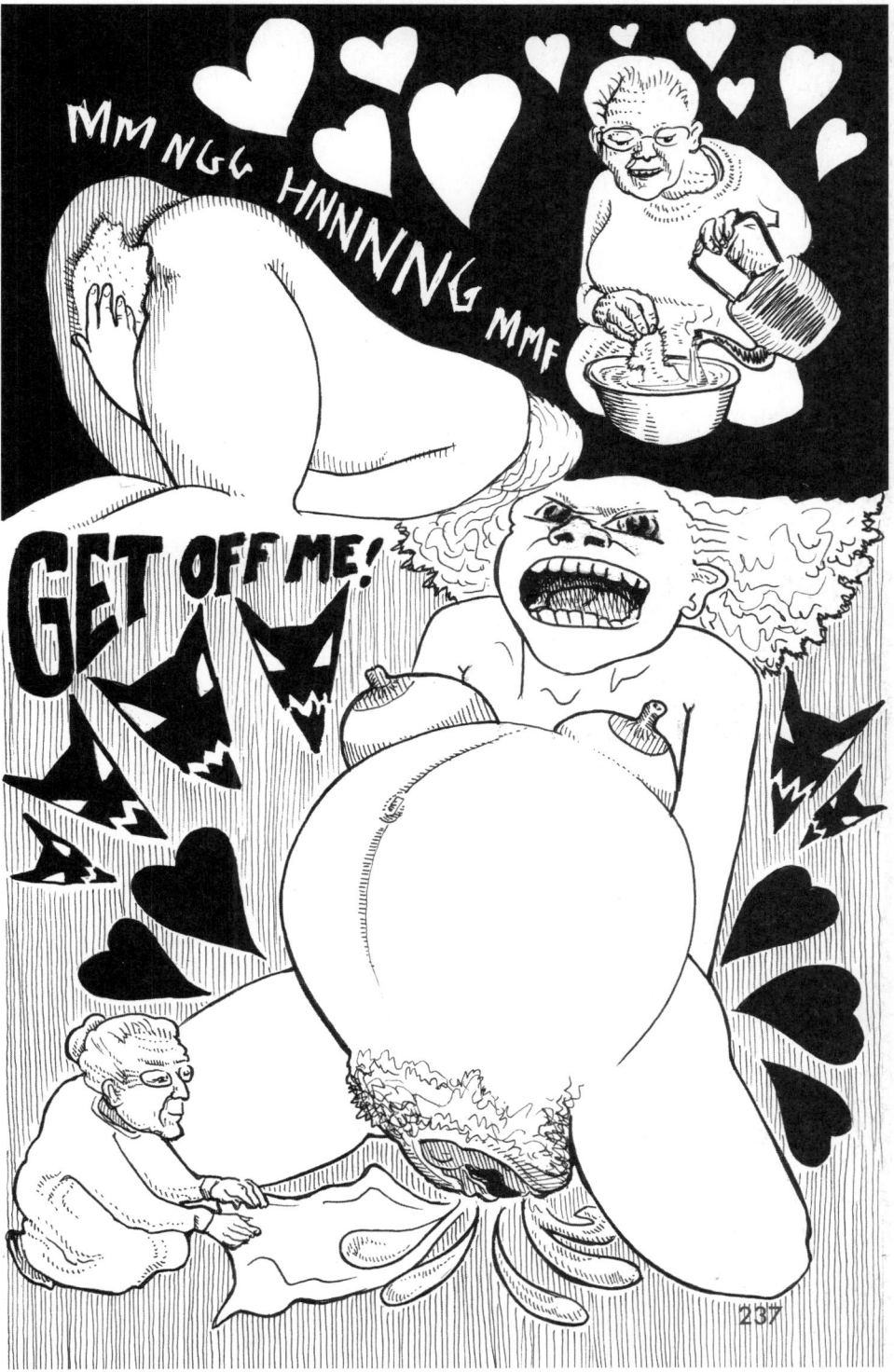

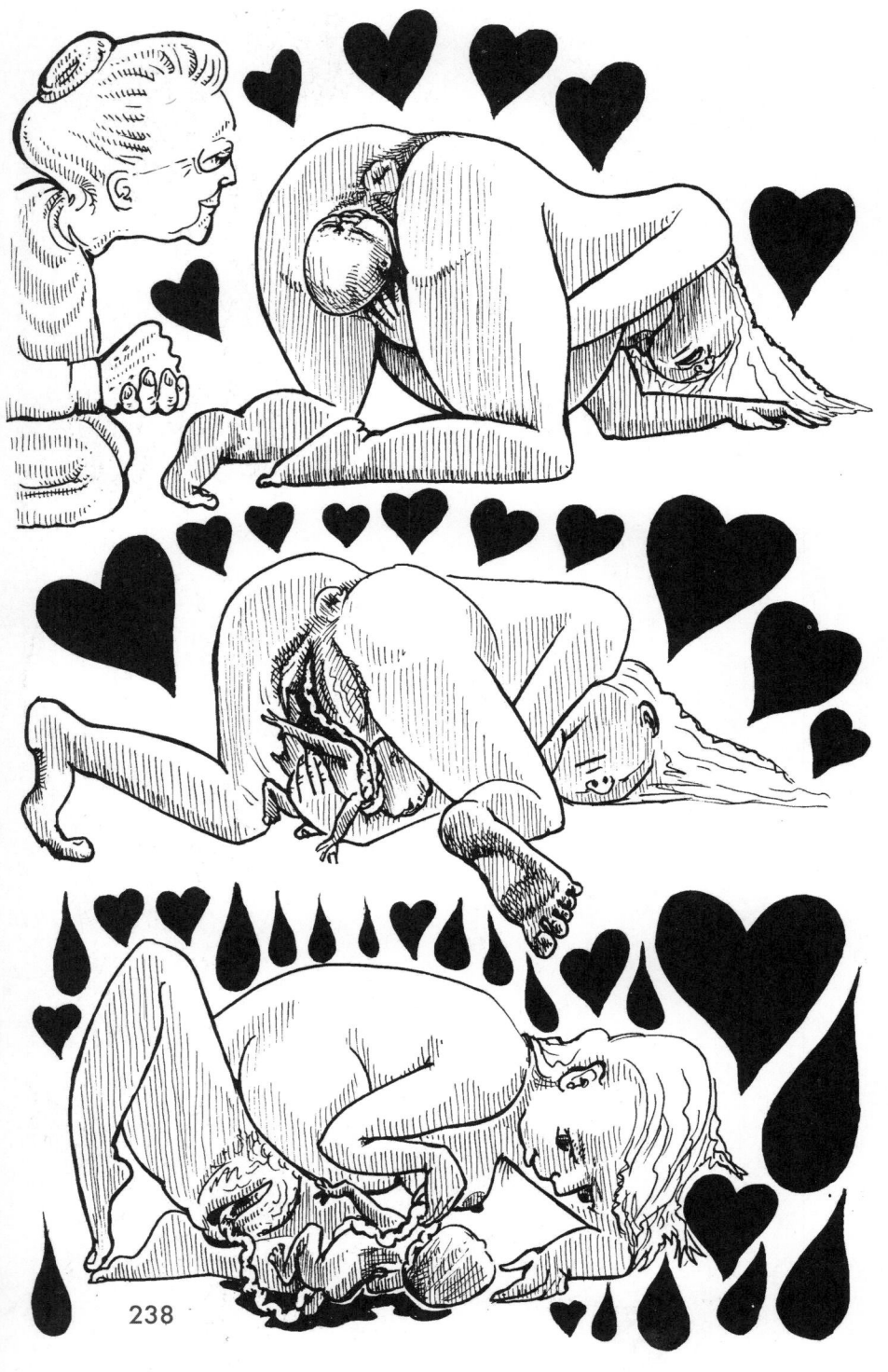

The head is out.

His eyes blink open on a new world.

The pressure of the birth canal squeezes the amniotic fluid from the baby's lungs.

The mother feels for her child.

His body wriggles round and, with the next surge, the baby tumbles free.[14]

Fresh, oxygenated blood pumps steadily from the placenta into the baby, perfusing pinkness into his limbs, and expanding the alveoli of the lungs.[15]

Monkey baby takes his first breath.

Awestruck in amazement, monkey mama touches his head, and his fingers and toes.

Monkey baby gazes back calmly. The surge of catecholamines gives clarity to his first moments.

The mother gathers her child in her arms. The cord still pulses between them. They are two people, yet they are still one.

The baby rests, soothing away the stresses of his birth. The mother shivers as the catecholamines recede. Oxytocin and prolactin flood through them both.[16] Love, and relief, and wonder.

Time stands still. This perfect moment stretches on for an eternity.

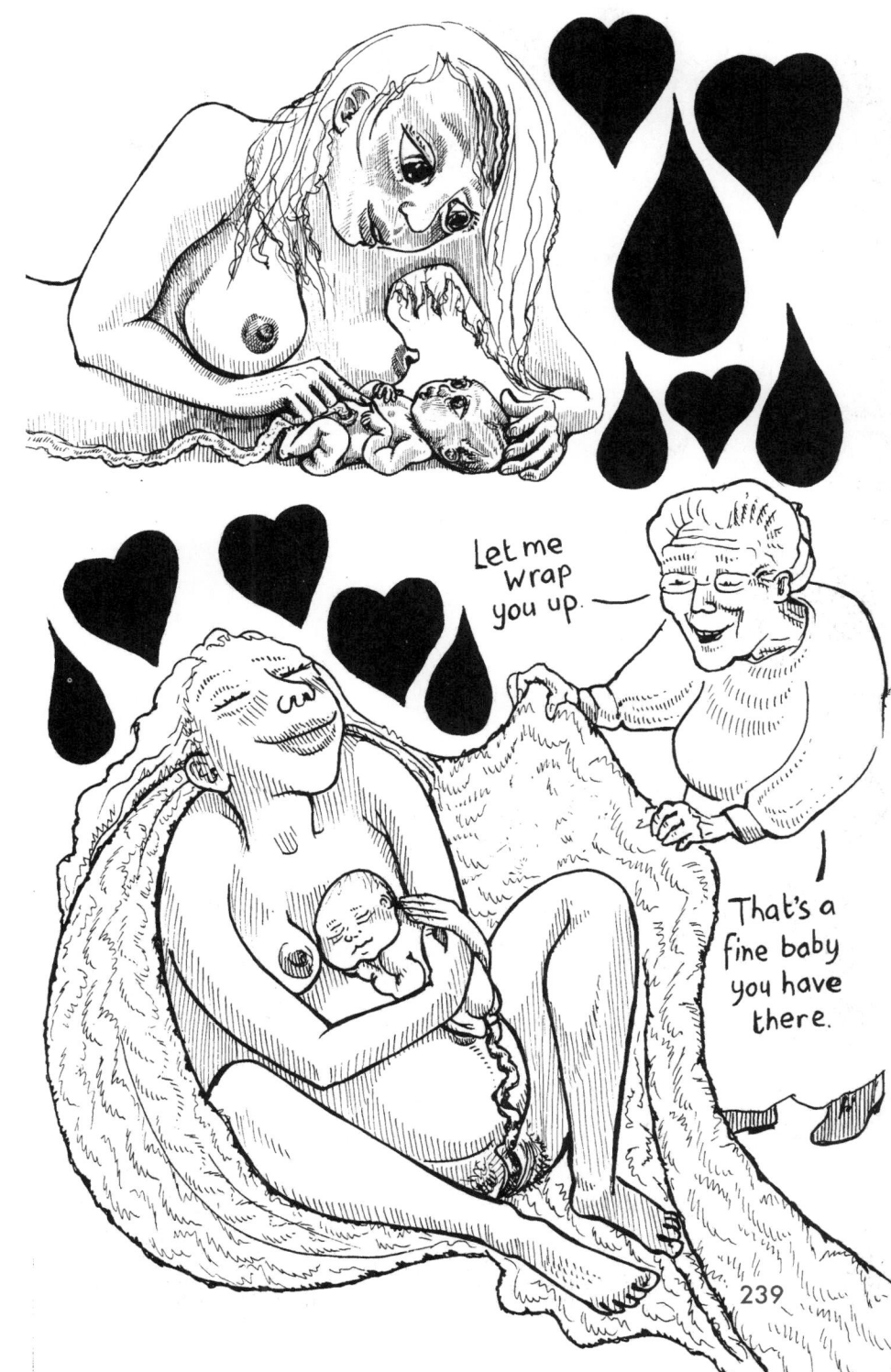

239

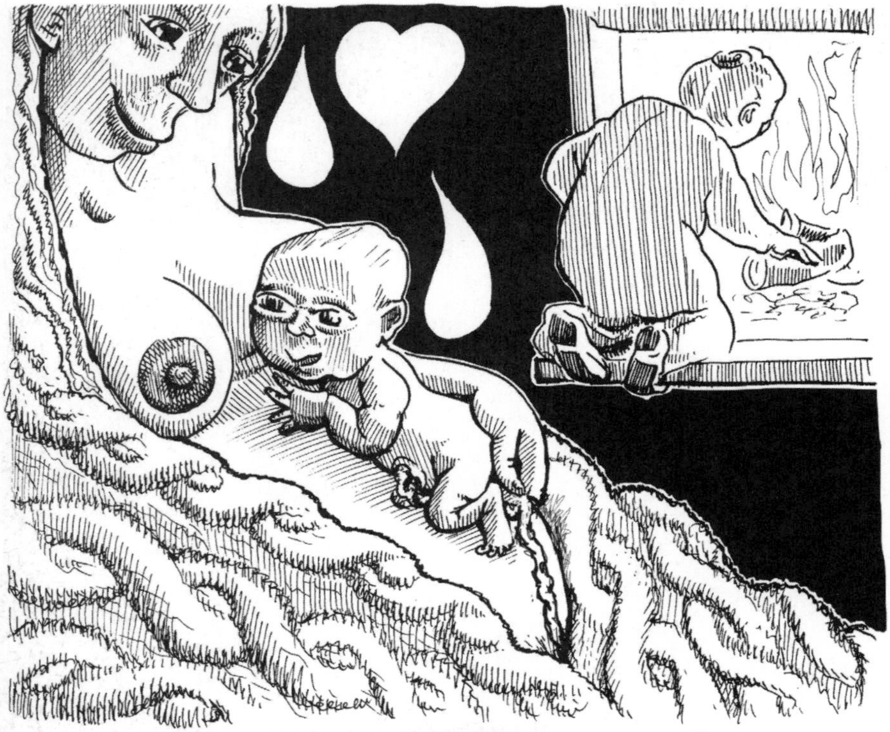

Some time later, he sucks his hands and bobs his head about. He can smell her milk, and moves towards it.[17] There it is. A dark circle on a paler background. There is a reason why this is the international symbol for a 'target'.

The birth isn't yet finished. Now the placenta must detach, and it must do so perfectly. A million tiny roots must come free of their earth in the womb.

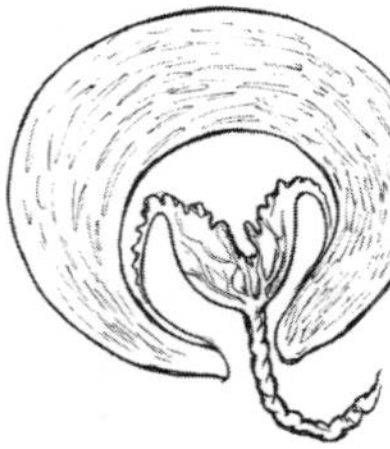

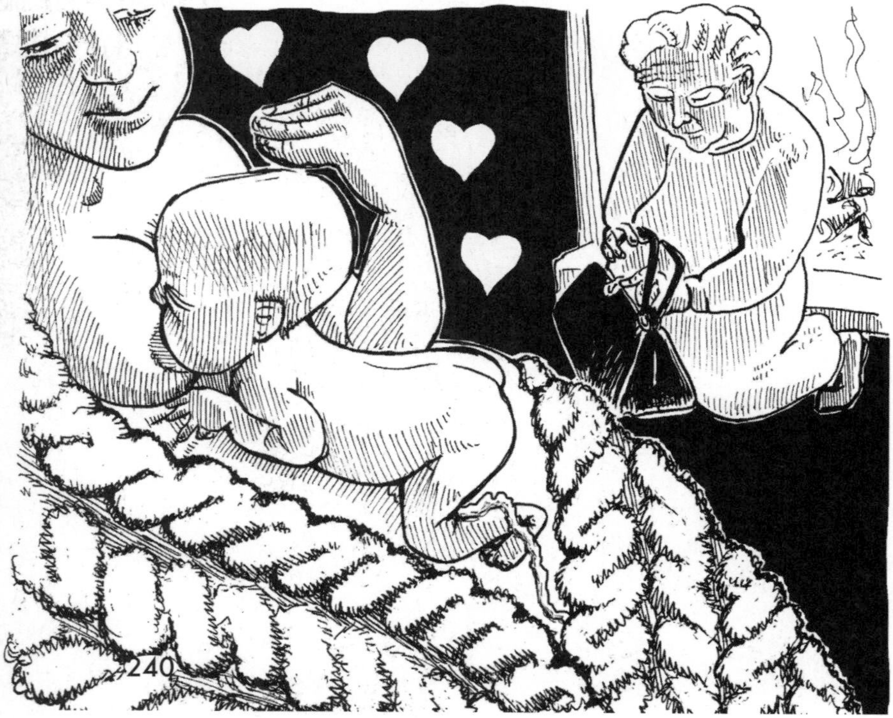

To achieve this, the womb completes its last act of procreative genius. The muscular walls contract down in a mesh of cross-ways fibres. And as they do so, they clamp down on every tiny blood vessel, forming 'living ligatures'.

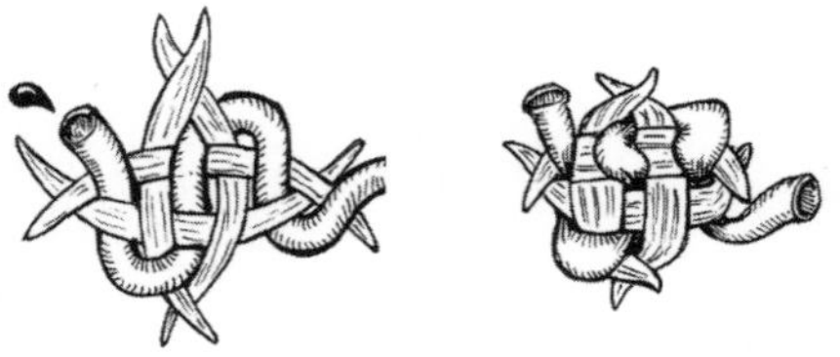

The baby helps, massaging his mother's abdomen as he steps his tiny feet.

Here comes the placenta. A soft, warm feeling, and out it slides.

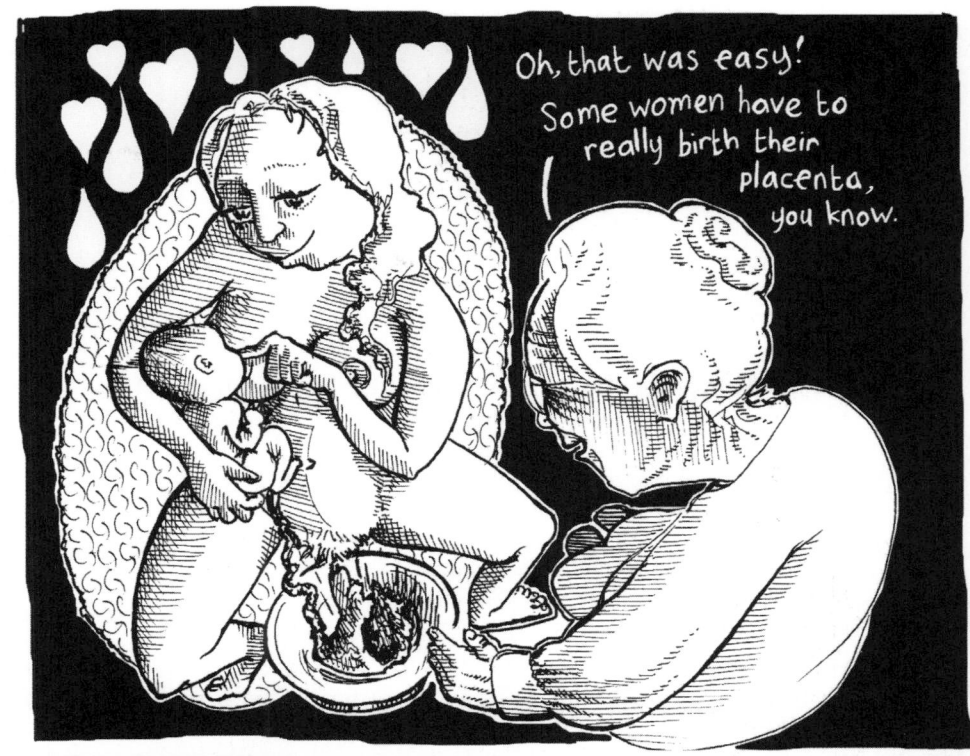

He suckles contentedly. With the first drops of milk, more endorphins pass from mother to child.

Monkey man is born.

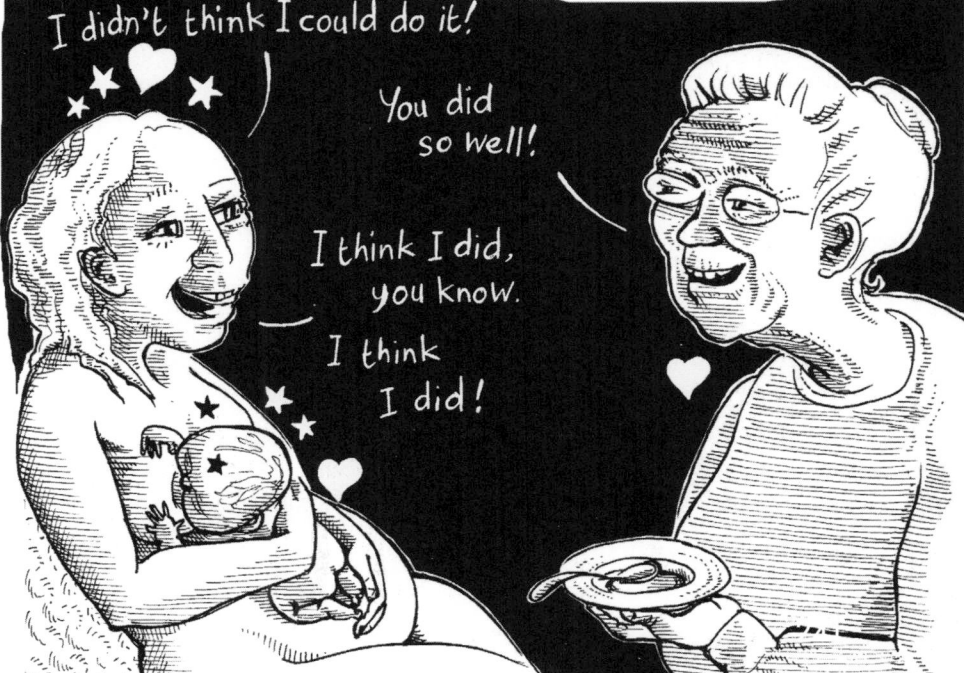

17 *Totally bananas*

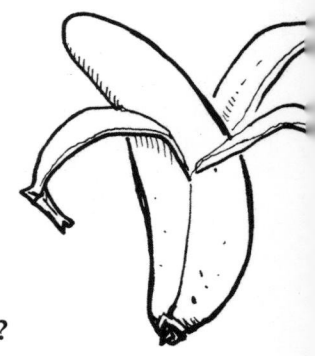

Who put men in charge of childbirth? I mean, honestly, what was that about?

First, it's a bad idea to put a subset of people in control of a physiological phenomenon that they have no direct experience of. That is not to say that men or childless women can't make very good midwives and obstetricians – they can, and do. But the last four hundred years of history have seen the implementation of some utterly bonkers ideas in obstetrics, on the untested whims of organisations of powerful men.

Secondly, on the occasions when you need a medical professional to get hands-on and help you give birth, you want that person to have very small hands.

This chapter is a whistle-stop tour of some of the rituals around childbirth that the medical profession adopted wholesale, without checking whether they were a good idea or not, together with the recent research that proves that, really, they weren't.

Because I thought that the accompanying pictures might be a little bit alarming, I have illustrated it throughout using gorillas in frilly nighties. In fact, this chapter is quite full-on.

Skip it if you want to, and turn to page 261. Or, if not, please bear in mind that some of this is history, and brilliant obstetricians and midwives are working hard to reverse these practices.

Making women lie on their backs

The reason women give birth lying on their backs with their legs in the air is so that the birth attendants can have a nice clear view of proceedings. The 'lithotomy position', as it's known, originated in France in the mid-1600s, possibly at the insistence of King Louis XIV, who had a fetish for watching women in labour.[1] In all the ethnographic evidence of birth practices all around the world and throughout history, no one else has made women birth in the stranded-beetle position. Maybe they know something that we forgot?

The largest central artery and vein in the body run down a pregnant woman's back, pumping blood to and from her lower limbs. When she lies flat, her womb compresses these, causing 'supine hypotensive syndrome' (or 'lying-down-flat low-blood-pressure problem' in non-medicalese). Less oxygenated blood running round the mother's body means less oxygen gets through to the baby.[2] Not a good idea.

This fall in blood pressure can also make a woman feel anxious and shaky. Anxiety leads to the release of stress hormones, the catecholamines, that slow labour down. Also not a good idea.

Flip back to page 188. See how the baby has to slip around a curve between the base of the spine and the pubic bone? The good news is that the spine is flexible, and that tailbone can move to accommodate the baby. Unless it has been immobilised by being lain upon. Lying or sitting leaning back on the bottom during birth reduces the space available to birth the baby by up to 30%.[3] Really, not a good idea.

When women stand, kneel or squat to give birth, then gravity helps to deliver the baby. But make them lie on their backs, and the birth canal curves upwards. This isn't going to help! These last two factors might explain why, when women birth on their backs, they are more likely to need drugs and medical instruments to assist them with their labours.[4]

Women tear or get cut more in lithotomy position.[5] Spreading the legs widely apart puts the skin around the vagina under tension, so it doesn't stretch as easily around the emerging baby.

A significant number of pregnant women suffer Pelvic Girdle Pain, and have a medical reason to keep their knees together. Lithotomy is the worst position for them to be made to give birth in.

Plus, it's humiliating! This is important! Remember, stress stops labour. Women are made to lie down and expose their genitals before fully clothed birth attendants who stand over them, directing operations. This is fundamentally disempowering. It could be particularly traumatic for a woman who has (as so many of us have) experienced sexual assault or rape.

And finally, lying women on their backs makes their labour pains worse.[6] This alone is a good enough reason to get up off the bed and walk away from it.

So, why is it that when we see births on the telly, or at the movies, or even when we imagine what birth will be like in our own heads, it's invariably with the mother lying flat on her back with her legs in stirrups? Culturally, we expect to birth like this, and we are expected to too. When interventions are needed to help birth along, as they sometimes are, when care-givers have reason to examine a woman internally, or use ventouse or forceps to help the baby out, the mother is often told to lie back with her legs apart. Because it has always been done like that. Not because it should be, now or in the future.[7]

If you are asked to assume the stranded beetle pose in labour, an appropriate response would be 'Why?' Wait for some reasoning that convincingly outweighs the disadvantages that are listed here.

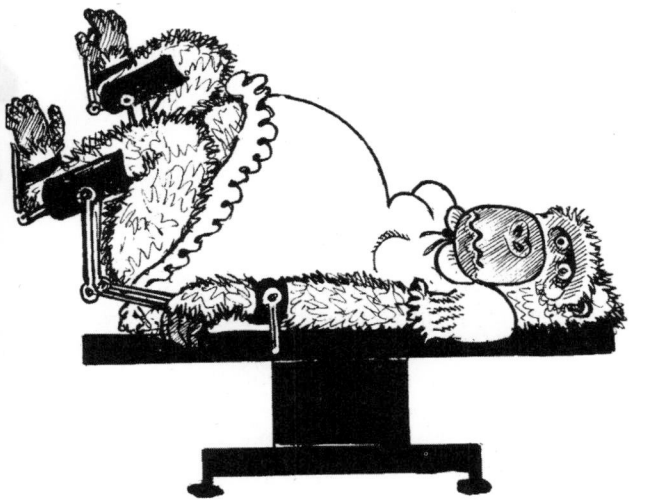

Drugging women up

Once birthing women have been made to lie in an inefficient and humiliating position that makes labour a lot more painful, they're going to want pain relief.

Um, perhaps I should qualify that last statement. I've had two children and I know what it can feel like. I figure that most women think about pain relief at some point during labour, because the sensations involved can be pretty extreme, and some of them will choose to have medication for the pain. This is good. Because the operative word in that sentence is 'choose', not 'have chosen for them'.

Chloroform was the first anaesthetic administered to labouring women, most famously to Queen Victoria for the birth of her eighth child. It had the unfortunate side-effect of killing people.

In the early 20th century, a mixture of morphine and scopolamine was developed as a safer option. These drugs were marketed as 'twilight sleep' which sounds quite pleasant. It wasn't. It rendered women temporarily insane, and did little to dull the pain. They were tied to their beds with lambswool, so the restraints left no marks on their limbs.[8] (No, I'm not making this up!) Afterwards, the amnesia induced by the drugs meant that they had no memory of anything that had happened, and were bewilderedly presented with babies they found it difficult to bond with.

Things have moved on from those horror-film zombie days. We now have ways to remove pain from the birth process that are a lot more humane.

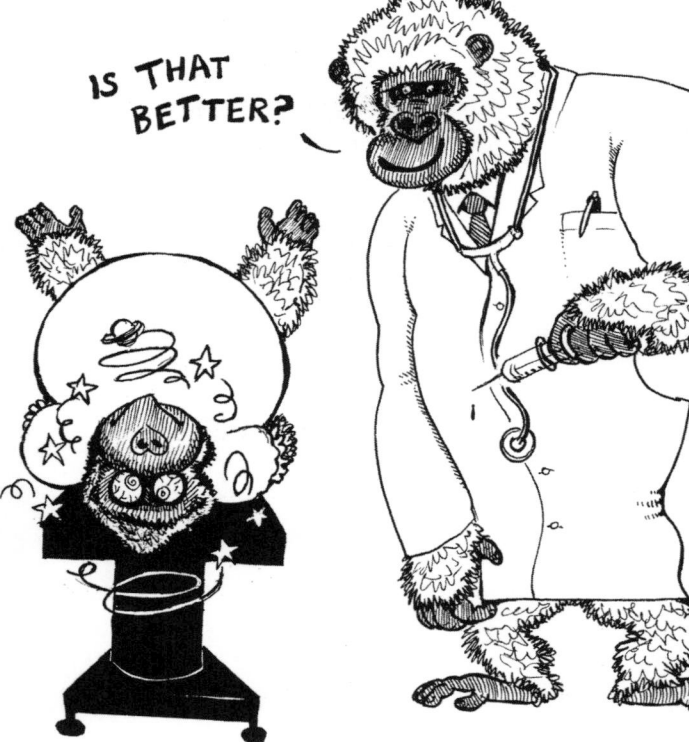

IS THAT BETTER?

Wonder drug number one!

Epidural anaesthesia is a marvellous invention. I mean that, literally, I think we should all take a moment to marvel at the fact that many modern women are offered an injection of a combination of a cocaine-derived anaesthetic and an opiate drug into the cerebrospinal fluid around the fourth lumbar vertebra. Wow.

It doesn't mean it's always a good idea.

An epidural is a surgical procedure, and, before it is carried out, the risks should be explained to the woman. The consequences of incorrect administration, the chance of an adverse reaction, the likelihood of a fall in maternal blood pressure, fever, how likely it is to work well – these are the kinds of things that tend to be discussed. But because anaesthetists never see undrugged, positive birth experiences, they rarely tell mothers what they will be missing when they choose an epidural.[9]

The brain suddenly loses the sensations of labour, so it produces less of the hormones that keep it going. Oxytocin levels drop.[10] There is no catecholamine rush to make super-efficient contractions in the final stages, and to infuse the baby with quiet alertness immediately after birth.[11] The pelvic floor goes floppy, so the baby can't bounce against it and turn in the birth canal.[12] The birth usually takes longer and the baby is more likely to need assistance.[13]

While anaesthetised women don't suffer the 'lows' of tempestuous labour pains, they also miss out on the 'highs' of the endorphin, oxytocin and prolactin rushes that accompany unmedicated birth. Does this affect how mothers and babies bond? One study found that women who had been given epidurals spent less time with their new babies in hospital,[14] and another found that mothers tended to rate their babies as more difficult to look after if they had an epidural during birth.[15] Babies are less likely to breastfeed successfully immediately after epidural anaesthesia, particularly if higher doses of opiates are used.[16] (Please note: this does *not* mean that if you choose epidural pain relief you won't be able to love or feed your baby! Keep your baby skin-to-skin lots and sniff their yummy smell, and you'll bond just fine.)

It's not just the pain that is lost with an epidural. The mother stops being the active agent in her own destiny, and is tethered to a bed. She is now a patient, dependent on others to move. An epidural is usually associated with continuous foetal monitoring, a drip in the arm, and a catheter for urination. That's a lot of tubes and wires.

Having said all that, epidurals completely remove the pain for nine out of ten women who have one. *This is empowering*. Because there is more than one good way to have a baby, I can argue this both ways. Mothers should be given swift access to effective pain relief when that's right for them. And you are allowed to change your mind about epidural anaesthesia as your birth unfolds. Not everyone has to do the natural childbirth thing. It's the 21st century. We have a choice.

Wonder drug number two!

Opiates such as pethidine, morphine and dia-morphine (heroin) are all commonly administered to labouring women. These take over the job that beta-endorphins should already be doing in a labouring woman's brain (provided that she isn't scared and stressed).

The synthetic versions have some disadvantages. They're not very good at blocking labour pain.[17] They make labour take longer,[18] so that's presumably more pain in total, not less. And they make mothers drowsy, nauseous and detached from their surroundings.[19] This isn't a great combination. Childbirth is a big day for a woman – it's the moment she gets to meet the child she has made and must raise. It would be nice if she could remember it clearly, rather than throwing-up in an opiate haze.

Babies are affected too. They are markedly less likely to feed immediately after birth,[20] and some have problems with their breathing.[21] The drugs last a lot longer in the system of a tiny baby than in an a large adult. In fact, the effects could stay with them for life. It has been proven that adult heroin addicts are more likely to have been exposed to multiple doses of opiate drugs at birth.[22] This says something very profound about how important the very first moments of life can be. (It *doesn't* mean that every woman who chooses pethidine at birth will go on to parent a junkie. It's not a straight cause-and-effect thing.)

Wonder drug number three!

What about nitrous oxide, also known as 'gas and air'? I'm not going to be down on this one. It takes the edge off things,[23] it's self-administered, and if you don't like it you can stop taking it. But I do know women who used it who felt disconnected from their birth experiences and wish they hadn't taken so much at the time.

Afterwards is a different matter. If you end up with a tear, and choose to have it stitched (yes, it is your choice!) then that's a great time to have gas and air. You have to really honk on it to get it to work.

So what's the problem?

Painkilling drugs are no longer compulsory. No one's going to strap us down with lambswool and inject us against our will.

But the problem, the 'totally bananas' thing,[24] is that there are still people working with birthing women who see it as their job to deliver them from terrible suffering, and who have a range of painkilling options that they're all too ready to offer. When a woman is in the middle of a tremendous wave of labour, she is very vulnerable; it's not a good moment to lean over her and say, 'Here's a little something for the pain.'

Hardcore painkillers can sometimes be presented as the preferred option for labouring women, and mothers who refuse them are thought to be in some way exceptional or misguided. That undermines women's abilities to try to find their own way through birth.

And since sedated, anaesthetised women are much easier to care for than rampaging, raging mothers, you have to ask why it is that some birth assistants are quite so keen to 'relieve' that pain?

Speeding things up

I made an observation back on page 38 that textbooks may state one thing, but women's bodies frequently do a whole range of other ones. This is still true 208 pages and nine months later. But! There is a way that women's bodies can be made to conform! Welcome to **Wonder drug number four: syntocinon!** This is chemically synthesised oxytocin that can be administered to birthing women. It puts doctors in charge of when and for how long women labour. There are three ways that it's commonly used, and here are two of them.

Induction of labour

We have a 'deadline' for pregnancy in the UK of 42 weeks. If women haven't gone into labour by then, standard practice* is to induce the baby, first by inserting a pessary of prostaglandins to soften

* There is more information on alternatives to induction on page 276.

the cervix, then by breaking the waters to see if labour starts, and then by giving them syntocinon through a drip.

The reasoning behind this is that the stillbirth rate rises after 40 weeks' gestation. Actually, it's highest at 35 and 36 weeks, dips down towards 40 and then climbs back up. In individual terms, we are not talking about a large increase in the likelihood of this happening. You are 99.9% likely to not have a stillbirth if you labour at 40 weeks gestation, and 99.85% likely to not have a stillbirth if you give birth at 37 or 43 weeks.[25] (Although relative risk in this context is meaningless, because when you're nine months pregnant *nothing* is more important than your baby not dying. Nothing.) What happens after 43 weeks? We don't know.

Bear in mind that we don't know why a large proportion of stillbirths happen. There is a theory that when pregnancies continue past 40 weeks the placenta stops working as efficiently; it 'ages' and endangers the life of the child. It's a theory. It hasn't been proven, and it has been disputed,[26] but some medical authorities take it as fact, regarding all post-dates pregnant women as a ticking time bomb, needing intervention to save them from their 'inability' to give birth.

There is variation in all natural processes, and it could be that some women can safely carry their babies much longer than others. But research isn't being

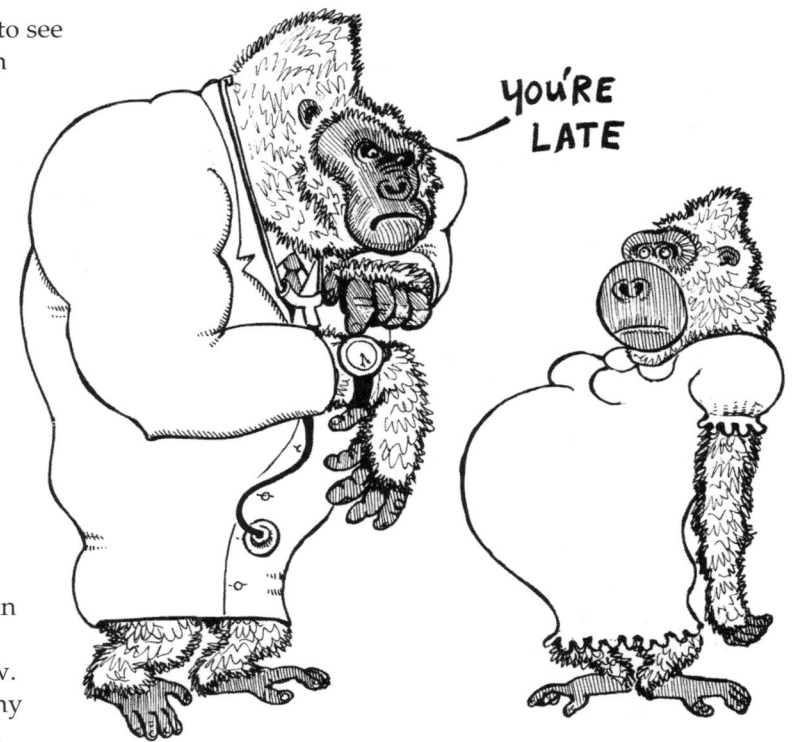

YOU'RE LATE

done into how we can tell what a healthy 'post-term' pregnancy is, because the protocol is that they all have to be induced. The doctors have the syntocinon, and they're not afraid to use it.

Partograms

In the 1950s doctors derived a chart, the partogram, to show the pattern of dilation that women are expected to conform to in labour. Upon admission, a woman's cervix is examined, and her progress charted against the graph. According to the Friedmann curve, women are in 'established' labour once their cervix is three centimetres dilated (open), and from then on the cervix dilates

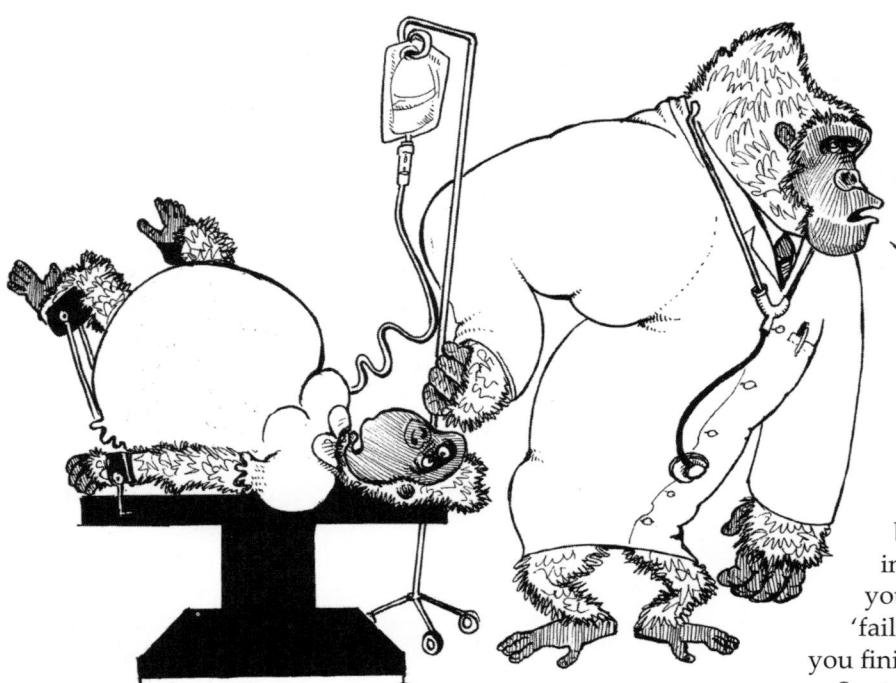

CAN WE GET THIS ONE DONE BEFORE LUNCH?

are inadequate, that's a self-fulfilling prophecy. Birth is a natural hormonal process, a bit like sex. If a doctor walked in when you were, er, pleasuring yourself, and diagnosed you with 'failure to orgasm', would that help you finish the job?

Syntocinon really is a wonder drug. It does make contractions happen, fast and hard. But it hurts.[29] And this is in a context of a process that has the potential to really hurt anyway. Why add something that really, really, really hurts into the mix?

In undrugged labour, the brain produces beta-endorphin, as part of an intricate pattern of hormonal feedback, keeping the sensations of labour approximately tied to what a woman is able to bear. Flood the system with syntocinon and the body's natural painkillers can't keep up.[30] So it's usual for women with augmented labours to have an epidural, which can make the labour longer, and then they need more syntocinon…

When women make their own oxytocin, it infuses through their brains, priming them with feelings of love. Injected synthetic oxytocin can't

at a rate of one centimetre per hour. The 'first stage' of labour (the cervix-opening part) lasts for no longer than 8.5 hours for women having their first babies (less for a subsequent child) and the 'second stage' (the pushing part) no longer than one hour.[27]

Wanna bet?

Fifty-seven per cent of low-risk, first-time mothers, who are good contenders for undrugged, straightforward births instead have their labours 'augmented' (speeded up) with syntocinon drips.[28] Just who is failing here? Should these women be diagnosed with 'failure to progress', or are we faced with an epidemic of 'failure to wait' on the part of the medical professionals concerned? When women are told by experts that their labours pass into the brain, so women miss out on that positive hormone rush.[31] We don't know if there are consequences for mothers' bonding with their babies. Nobody has studied this.

We do know that super-fast contractions aren't the best thing for the baby. The pauses between contractions are there to let fresh oxygenated blood pulse into the placenta. Overstimulate the womb, and the oxygen supply to the baby drops.[32] Yikes! Yet women are frequently given syntocinon because staff are concerned about the condition of the baby. Isn't that a little like fighting fire with gasoline?

Once a woman has a syntocinon drip, the recommendation is that the baby's heartbeat should be continuously monitored.[33] This usually means two elastic belts and leads attached to a TV screen and a drip in the hand. Tethered like this, it is difficult to move around, which makes it even more likely that she'll need an epidural for the pain. Women are asked to pick one card of medical intervention, and are then dealt the whole pack.

The administration of syntocinon for 'slow' labour is an intrinsic part of our healthcare system, but its effectiveness has only very recently been evaluated.[34] And guess what? It doesn't help! The drug doesn't improve outcomes for mothers and babies. Syntocinon augmentation doesn't improve babies' condition at birth or prevent them being admitted to neonatal intensive care. It doesn't reduce the likelihood of Caesarean birth or instrumental delivery. It does reduce the average length of labour by about two hours, but it is most effective if started early on; by the time the labour has really dragged on, it may not make

as much difference. And it increases the risk of overstimulation of the womb and has negative effects on babies' heart rates (although the study concluded that this wasn't associated with lasting ill-effects).

Given this stunning lack of any discernible positives, the recommendation from this research is that 'the decision whether to undergo this treatment is one that can reasonably be left to women to decide'. But how many women who accepted syntocinon augmentation over the past 40 years did so with informed consent? Were they asked, 'Would you like a drug that makes your labour a lot more painful, but means we can shift you out of the delivery room two hours quicker?' Or were they told 'We have concerns about your baby's condition', 'Your labour is ineffective' and 'You need this drug to save your baby from your body's inability to give birth'?

Recent attempts to redefine the Friedmann curve found that 26 hours of active labour isn't inherently problematic for a first-time mum.[35] And three centimetres' dilation might not be the right point to mark the 'start' of established labour. Researchers found that after the cervix has expanded to six centimetres, that's when things really get moving.[36] Women are not fitted with automatic garage doors that open at a predictable and steady rate. It might be more useful to expect a woman to labour moderately or intermittently for some time without much evidence of 'progress', until she hits the right mix of hormones. Then, boom! Off she goes.

It is also possible for a cervix to close back up again.[37] That's why it's important to be nice to labouring women and help them feel safe.

Should women even be given vaginal examinations to assess the dilation of the cervix? Since women's labours don't all progress at the same steady rate, then what useful information do these impart?[38] They encourage a kind of lazy mental arithmetic. The thinking goes: 'Oh, it's taken me six hours to dilate from 3cm to 4cm and I have another six centimetres to go, so that means, six times six, I'll be labouring for another 36 hours! Yikes! Gimme the drugs!' But that's not the case. This woman could spring right open in one massive mega-contraction 15 minutes later, and then be ready to push. Or, yes, she might labour for days more (there are suggestions for help with long labours on page 278). My point is that past progress is no indication of future performance.[39]

Vaginal exams are surprisingly imprecise, especially when conducted by different care-givers.[40] Women are usually expected to lie down for them (although they can be conducted in any position) and, once they're in bed on their back, many women stay there.

And they are intrusive. This is a personal issue. Some women don't mind having their cervix examined. Some are reassured by it. But for others it could trigger memories of sexual assault. Is it fair to make a potentially traumatic procedure routine in order to compare women with charts that have been discredited?

Once again, I invite women in labour to respond to a request for a vaginal examination with the question 'Why?' There are some very good reasons for doing one if the midwife is concerned about your baby (see 'prolapsed cord' below), but, if it's just

a case of checking how far your labour has come, well, that's up to you to decide. (And if you're interested in your degree of cervical dilation you can also check your cervix yourself!)

Labours should be assessed by the condition of the mother and the baby, and not subjected to an arbitrary time limit. The Cochrane Collaboration, which represents the gold standard of medical research, concluded in a recent review that *'we cannot recommend the partogram as part of standard labour management and care'*. But many hospitals still do.[41]

Breaking the waters

Some hospitals break every woman's waters as a matter of routine. Others do it when labour is taking 'too long'. The belief is that it helps the baby's head to press more insistently on the cervix, increasing the strength of the contractions and shortening the labour.

Recent research has proved this isn't true.[42] This intervention doesn't shorten labour and it doesn't improve outcomes for mothers or babies. This could be because the bulging bag of waters can help keep the cervix open, so rupturing it is unhelpful. Also, while the baby is still cushioned in its sac, it enjoys a little more freedom of movement, which it can use to wriggle around the birth canal.

Some women experience a dramatic increase in the intensity of their contractions when their waters are broken, an unfortunate side-effect of an intervention with no proven benefit. And, if the baby's head isn't down snugly in the pelvis when the waters gush out, the umbilical cord can drop down (prolapse) and become squashed, which is a real medical emergency. Prolapsed cord is very rare, but extremely serious, so it's best not to do anything that might cause it to happen.[43] The Cochrane review is clear. '*Evidence does not support routinely breaking the waters for women in normally progressing spontaneous labour or where labours have become prolonged.*'

Nil by mouth

Birthing a baby is bloody hard work. And, unsurprisingly, banning women from eating and drinking during labour does nothing to help their energy levels.

Hospitals used to to restrict food and fluids to all labouring women, on the grounds that they might need a general anaesthetic. They don't any more, because that was silly. Here's Cochrane again: '*women should be free to eat and drink in labour, or not, as they wish*'.[44]

It won't necessarily stay down anyway. Apparently, being sick helps labour to progress. Great.

Continuous foetal monitoring

This invention is a surprising addition to the 'totally bananas' list. Listening to the baby's heartbeat during labour is a very good idea. Midwives have been doing it for millennia,[45] using their ears, and funny little wooden 'Pinard' stethoscopes, or, more recently, hand-held Doppler sonic aids. Logically, it should follow that strapping heart-rate monitors to a mother's belly would be effective at preventing foetal fatality. Once cardiotocography (CTG) machines became available, hospitals rushed out to buy them. Their effectiveness was only evaluated years later, and the results were surprising.

When compared to 'intermittent auscultation' (the listening that midwives have been doing for centuries), CTG monitoring doesn't prevent neonatal deaths. It doesn't improve babies' Apgar scores at birth (a measure of wellbeing), doesn't alter the number of babies who need hospital treatment after birth, doesn't prevent babies from experiencing oxygen deprivation, and doesn't change the incidence of babies with cerebral palsy. The only aspect of babies' health that improved when their mothers were strapped to monitors is that they were less likely to have a seizure after birth, but seizures are rare in any case, and we don't yet know if they carry any long-term ill effects.[46]

The risks to the mother were substantially increased. Forceps or ventouse were used to extract the baby more often, and far more babies were born by Caesarean. The figures show that 667 women have to be given CTG monitoring to prevent one baby suffering neonatal seizures, of whom between 15 and 61 will have an unnecessary Caesarean as a result.[47] That's avoidable major surgery, which endangers mothers' lives,[48] their mental health,[49] their future fertility,[50] and makes serious complications in subsequent pregnancies and labours more likely.[51]

The problem is that CTG monitors throw up false positives. Take the ominous sign of 'multiple late decclerations and decreased variability'. It can be an indication that the baby has cerebral palsy. In 0.2% of cases. For the other 99.8% of babies showing this pattern, it doesn't.[52] But once the medical staff have spotted the trace, they feel compelled to act. Let me remind you

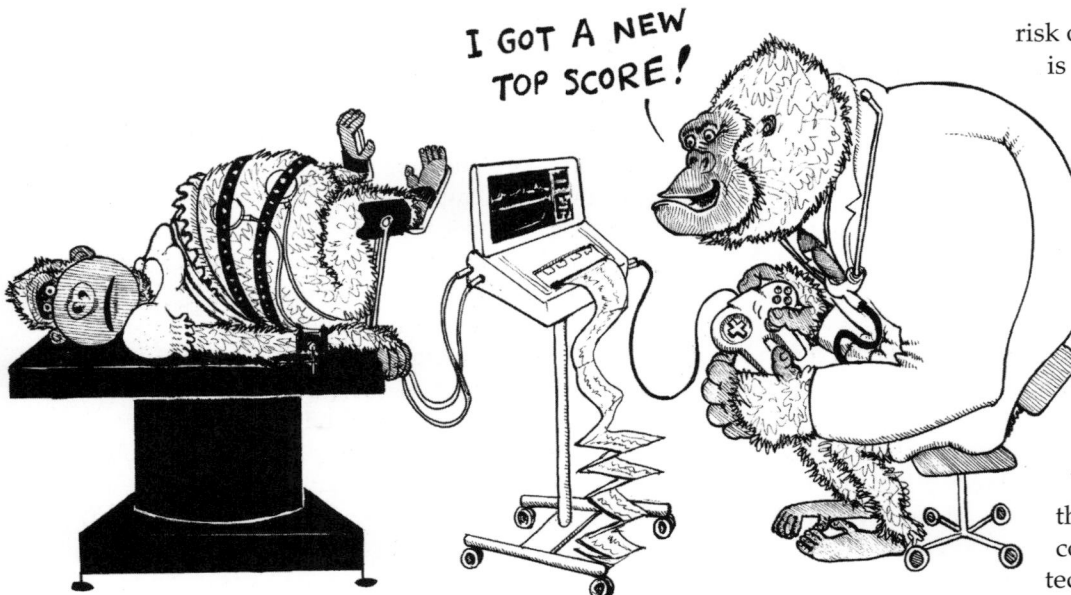

I GOT A NEW TOP SCORE!

that intermittent monitoring is *just as effective* at identifying babies in trouble and preventing them from developing cerebral palsy as a result of their birth.

Strap a mother to a monitor, and that TV screen becomes the focus of all the activity in the room. The midwife looks at the monitor. The midwife looks at the trace. The worst example of this is where labouring women are left alone attached to monitors which then relay information to a central bank of screens. What? Are we on *Star Trek* or something? Take the TV screen away, and the care-providers return to providing care to the mother and listening to the baby directly.

I meant it with the *Star Trek* analogy. We tend to think that every problem in human life can be solved with the application of the correct technology. In birth, it can't. Although we are lucky to live in an age and a nation where the

risk of death during birth is very slight, we can't remove it altogether, and to pretend otherwise does grieving mothers a disservice. Maybe that's a hard thing for medical staff to cope with. Maybe that's why they like CTG, because it gives them an illusion of control. In reality, the technology can promote a false sense of security, as professionals have admitted themselves[53] – it's not a good substitute for monitoring women directly.

Hospitals also like to create physical records of the heart rates of babies in labour in the belief that it protects them against future legal claims of medical negligence. In fact, every time an aberrant trace shows up on a CTG monitor, the actions of care-providers present are then infused with a sense of panic. They know that, once that record is there, they could be sued if they don't intervene. So hospitals become more vulnerable to litigation, and mothers become more vulnerable to interventions.

The scientific review that evaluated CTG's effectiveness found the same results across all groups of women. But this has been translated into national guidelines that state that continuous monitoring should not be used on low-risk women (the 'straightforward' ones), but still recommend it for women in the high-risk ('we-found-something-to-fuss-about') group. Why exactly is this? The report itself points out that it's strange.[54] Is it because we paid for all this technological equipment, so now we have to ensure that someone uses it?

Surely the risks of unnecessary surgery are higher for women with diabetes, or obesity, or heart disease? Surely they have greater reason to need mobility in labour without heavy belts and leads tethering them to one spot? Obviously, high-risk women need careful monitoring, but the science doesn't show that this is better achieved by attaching them to TV screens (where the temptation then is to leave them alone) than by paying a midwife to pay them proper attention.

There has been one randomised controlled trial of continuous versus intermittent monitoring for women attempting to have a vaginal birth after previous Caesarean surgery (VBAC). It found that CTG monitoring didn't improve the outcomes for babies, but it did increase the rate of repeat Caesareans for mothers.[55] So women trying for a VBAC are being strapped to equipment that purely serves the function of increasing the likelihood of the very event – a Caesarean – that they're specifically trying to avoid.

Bananas.

Hydrophobia

Not all innovations in childbirth are unhelpful. There is a marvellous new aid for labouring women that gets excellent results.

A paddling pool.

(Well, it's a bit deeper than that, with some design modifications for hygiene and stability, but that's essentially what it is.)

Labouring in warm water is lovely. No longer 'heavily pregnant', women become weightless,[56] mobile, and upright[57] are more relaxed,[58] and have lower blood pressure.[59] They are more likely to have uninterrrupted care from one midwife, yet other staff seem more willing to grant them privacy[60] – perhaps we all have social inhibitions about barging in on somebody in the bath? All these factors contribute to making the first stage of labour shorter in water.[61]

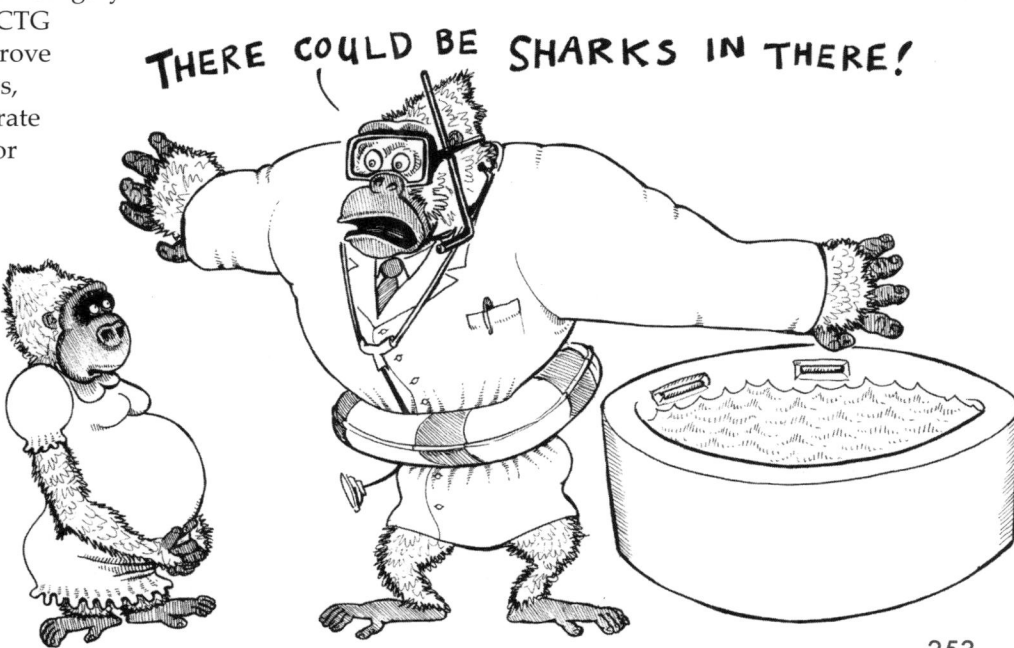

THERE COULD BE SHARKS IN THERE!

A birth pool doesn't completely remove the pain of labour, but it does become much easier to bear – women feel more in control[62] and are less likely to resort to epidural anaesthesia.[63]

Giving birth in water is lovely. A healthy baby won't take her first breath until she is brought up to the surface,[64] and when she does, she rarely cries.[65] It's a gentle way to come into the world. (Oxygen-deprived, distressed babies should not be born underwater in case they don't do this. That's why it's important for a midwife to keep checking the baby's heartbeat.)

You would think that such an innovation would be widely adopted? Think again.

'*I have always considered underwater birth a bad joke, useless and a fad, which was so idiotic it would go away. It hasn't! It should!*' That's the editor of respected scientific journal *Pediatrics* writing in a professional capacity.[66]

It would appear that empowering women to hit a peak of good birth hormones while floating in a dimly lit pool[67] is a scenario that's way outside some doctors' comfort zone.[68] It's very difficult to do things to a slippery, moving, water-birthing woman. Maybe that's a problem for the doctors? Maybe less so for the mothers?

Perhaps as a result of this, access to birth pools is limited. In some hospitals, high-risk women face a blanket ban. Partly this is because they are required to have continuous monitoring (and they can't invent a waterproof CTG device? Yeah, right!). Also, in an emergency, how do we get the mother out of the pool quickly? (I don't know, but since we're capable of putting astronauts into orbit I feel that a technological solution to this problem is not beyond the wit of humankind.)

Women are discouraged from getting into the pool until they are more than five centimetres dilated, on the (probably erroneous) belief that it will slow their labour down.[69] Instead they are encouraged to stay at home and cope with early labour pains, maybe by relaxing in a warm bath…

Could this technology be offered to more women? Are current restrictions on its use valid? Will research be done into this area? Not if some doctors get their way. (These doctors are in America. We're in Britain. Don't worry, we are a lot more holistic in our attitudes to birth over here. I just put these quotes in because I was so gobsmacked by their arrogance!) '*There are no proven clinical benefits*,'[70] they write, and '*underwater birth should not be performed except within the context of an appropriate clinical trial.*'[71] Unlike every single other innovation in this chapter, none of which was tested first.

Telling women when to push

This is another aspect of birth that we're familiar with because we've seen it on the telly. Inevitably, when a woman gives birth, she has a cheerleader positioned strategically between her thighs, telling her to 'PUSH-PUSH-PUSH-PUSH-PUSH-PUSH!!!'

Women in the second stage of labour are routinely told to take a deep breath, tuck their chins down, not make any noise and continuously strain to push their babies out, all the way from the beginning of a contraction to the end. 'Just a little bit more, now – PUSH!' This is called the 'Valsalva manoeuvre', or 'directed pushing', and it's common practice in maternity hospitals around the world.

Several hundred years after doctors[72] adopted this practice wholesale, scientific research was conducted into it. And would you believe it – it's not a very good idea.

Once that cervix has opened up, and the baby has dropped down,[73] women are going to push anyway. The urge is undeniable. Strangely, out of all the creatures in the animal kingdom, humans are not uniquely designed to be unable to give birth without someone telling them how to do it.

Instructing non-anaesthetised women to override the indications their bodies are giving them as to when to push, how much to push and what noise to make does not get the baby out faster.[74] (Although, since the desired aim is to birth the baby swiftly, one study[75] has found that getting women into upright postures and leaving them to it helps them give birth *45 minutes faster* than lying them on their backs and telling them what to do.) Moreover, the research indicates that directed pushing can be dangerous. When women hold their breath, instead of breathing freely throughout the second stage of labour, it reduces the oxygen that is available for the baby.[76]

Straining like this is more likely to make the mother exhausted,[77] because she's not matching her efforts to the cues her womb is giving her about when her pushes will work best. More forceps and ventouse deliveries are the result.[78]

Directed pushing makes it more likely that the perineum will tear[79] – an outcome that we would rather avoid. And it can damage pelvic floor muscles,[80] which could lead to a risk of incontinence.

And it's stressful.[81] Shouting at a woman to maximise her efforts gives her the impression that this is an emergency, and her baby is at risk from the natural processes of her own body. What's actually endangering the baby is the drop in the oxygen supply that results from the unnatural instructions being yelled in her ear.

Apparently, directed pushing is sometimes accompanied by a doctor inserting fingers into a woman's vagina with the instruction 'Push my fingers out.' What the...? Why? In case she has forgotten where her baby is coming out? Have you ever heard of anything more patronising?

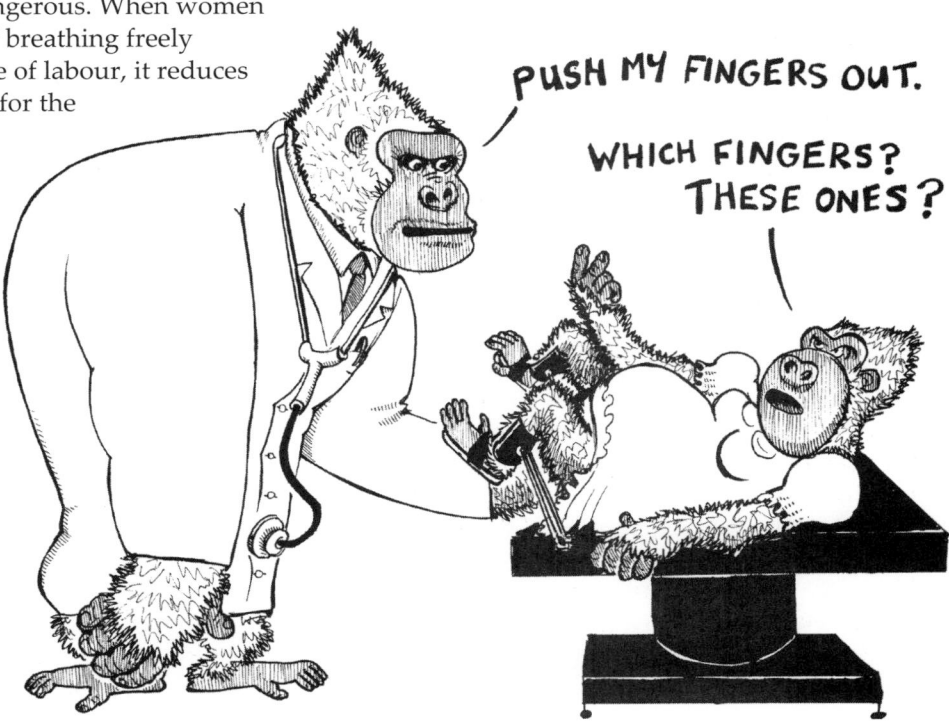

255

There are no benefits in telling women when to push. The scientific evidence on this is very clear,[82] yet it seems that old habits die hard in some maternity rooms.

This then begs the question, are there any benefits in telling women not to push? In current obstetric practice, before a woman is 'allowed' to progress from the first stage of labour to the second, her cervix is checked to make sure it's fully dilated. If it isn't completely open, she is told not to push yet, in case the cervix becomes swollen from the pressure of the baby's head (which really wouldn't help). But surely that's only likely if she's being shouted at to strain? If we allow women to follow their own pushing urges, rather than imposing external ones, what's the danger?

This is a question that needs more research to answer,[83] partly because we don't come from a medical tradition of trusting women and empowering them to listen to their own bodies.

Ubiquitous use of instruments

In 1920, American obstetrician Joseph Bolivar DeLee published a hugely influential paper: 'The Prophylactic Forceps Operation'.[84]

I think it's fair to say that Dr DeLee wasn't a fan of natural childbirth – he likened it to the woman being impaled on a pitchfork and the baby having its head crushed in a door. Instead, DeLee detailed exactly how to drug a woman into 'twilight sleep' and what to do to her next (that she would still be able to feel but be unable to remember afterwards):

1. Cut a large 'episiotomy' (an incision at the vaginal entrance).
2. Pull the baby out with forceps.
3. Sew her back up so that 'virginal conditions are restored'.

Dr DeLee also stated that tokophobia – fear of childbirth – was on the increase among women. I can't imagine why.

An epidemic of forceps births resulted. Here in the UK, they were used in more than 50% of births in the 1930s.[85] Some hospitals performed episiotomies on virtually every labouring woman[86] until the 1990s – the Association for Improvements in the Maternity Services even has a record of a woman being given an episiotomy after the birth, because the midwife was afraid she would be reprimanded for failing to do one![87] Unsurprisingly, these interventions were subsequently proved unhelpful. It's never a good idea to pull a newborn baby about by the head.[88] And routinely cutting women's genitals to prevent them from being damaged is logically nonsensical.[89] These procedures are no longer routine, and are being relegated back to the 'emergency' drawer, where they belong.

Phew!

Clamping the cord

At the moment of birth, the baby, having just squeezed through quite a (marvellously stretchy) narrow gap, has left about a third of its blood behind in the placenta.[90] It takes a while for that blood to pulse back into the baby, where it expands the alveoli of the lungs, increases the efficiency of the liver,[91] and helps the heart and lungs to adapt to the new phenomenon of 'breathing air'.[92] This blood is full of red blood cells,[93] essential for efficiently transporting oxygen around the body, and it represents a store of extra iron that lasts the baby for months,[94] possibly years.[95] In these first moments after birth, a billion stem cells flood into the baby, with a magical ability to heal any trauma.[96]

This then, would be the wrong moment to clamp and cut the cord. But that is precisely what hospitals have been doing for the last 30 years.

As usual, it has been up to proponents of natural birth to prove that the 'new', physiological, 'we-did-it-like-this-for-millennia-before-hospitals-came-along' method is superior to the 'normal' untested established procedures that the medical profession unquestioningly adopted. So we now refer to waiting a little while before clamping the cord as 'delayed cord clamping'. This is silly. We should call the other type 'premature cord clamping'. Still, that's the terminology, and we're stuck with it.

Delayed cord clamping carries overwhelming benefits for the baby, so official guidelines[97] have now been changed. They now state that medical staff should wait a few minutes before cutting the cord… unless the baby requires resuscitation.

Whoa! Let's have a look at that last proviso again. A baby is born who is having trouble breathing. While that baby is still attached to the mother after birth, it receives a supply of oxygenated blood. When doctors clamp and cut the umbilical cord, they sever the baby's lifeline. And that's official best practice!

Totally bananas.

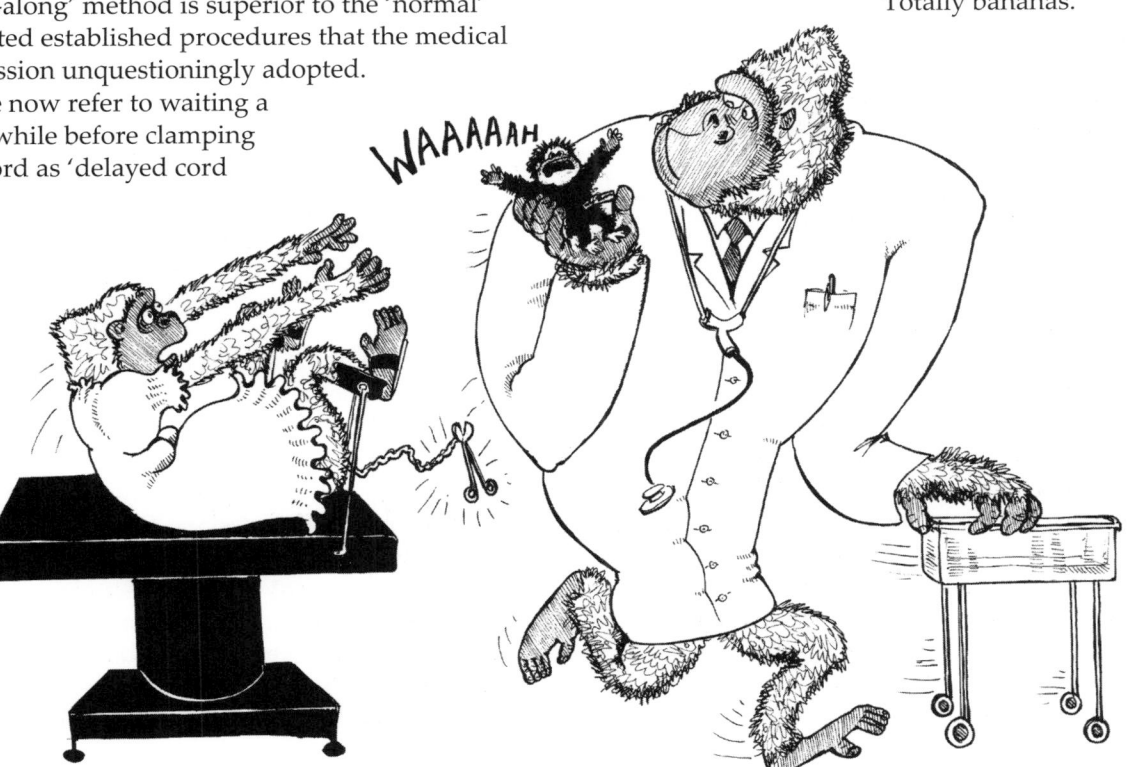

WAAAAAH

It's unconventional for a medical team to work on a baby while its still attached to the mother, but since it's in the baby's best interests, conventions should change. We can empower women by educating them to be part of the resuscitation process. A newborn baby knows its mother – her touch and her voice play a vital role in helping it transition into this crazy thing called life.[98]

Cord wrapped around baby's neck at birth? Don't clamp and cut it. It's possible to deliver a baby with the cord tight round the neck[99] – you saw a picture of it back on page 238. If a baby has suffered from a slightly reduced blood supply during birth it needs that extra postnatal placental perfusion.[100]

Premature baby? Don't clamp and cut the cord. Preemies have left a whopping 50% of their blood behind in the placenta. A delay in clamping of just 45 seconds reduces the risk of complications, including life-threatening necrotising enterocolitis.[101] Waiting until the cord stops pulsing would be optimum. LifeStart mobile resuscitation trolleys have been invented, but now we need our cash-strapped NHS to fund them.

Don't clamp and cut the cord.

Whisking the baby away

There has been some interesting anthropological research into the significance of the very first moments of a new baby's life. It found that in more peaceful societies, the mother and baby were left together undisturbed. But other cultures conducted a ritual separation of the mother and baby shortly after birth, and these people were more warlike.[102]

What does that say about our society, where for many years it was standard hospital practice

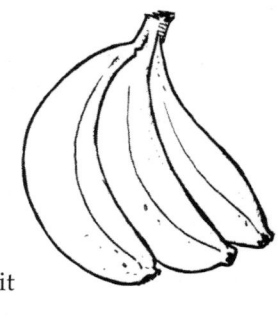

to smack the baby on the bum, stick a suction tube up its nose, tag it, weigh it, measure it, put eyedrops in its eyes and injections in its thighs, scrub off the vernix, bundle it up, wheel it off to the nursery and feed it formula milk?

It doesn't have to be like this. Scientists have done studies into the alternative – what we did for millennia before hospitals came along.[103]

Take the baby immediately after birth and move her to the mother's belly. The mother can do this herself if she doesn't have a drip in her arm. (Drips are quite disabling. They are great for ill people, but not very well designed for active birthers. I wonder if they could find a way to get IV fluids into a woman that doesn't knock out the use of one of her limbs?) Pat the baby dry with a towel so she doesn't get cold, and wait.

At first, nothing much happens. There is a pause of at least fifteen minutes, while the mother thinks, 'OMG! I've had a baby!' and the baby thinks, 'OMG! I'm breathing air!' Then the baby makes sucking movements with her mouth and starts bobbing her head around, like she's looking for something. After about half an hour, she'll probably put her hands to her mouth. Then, partly guided by smell, and partly by sight, the baby starts to crawl about, kneading the mother's tummy with her tiny arms and legs. She does little push-ups with her arms. Sometimes she'll change direction as she shuffles about. It's all very cute.

At about the one-hour mark, she'll find the nipple and spontaneously start to feed.

This is pretty incredible. Everyone will tell you that 'some mothers can't breastfeed' and 'breastfeeding is terribly difficult'. I have written a whole book to help mothers and babies learn to breastfeed in our nipple-phobic society. But babies are born knowing how to breastfeed! They can do it perfectly – we just have to let them show us how.

It has been estimated that 22% of neonatal deaths could be prevented if all babies were breastfed in the first hour of life.[104]

There are a couple of ways to derail a baby's instinctive feeding behaviours. You can give the mother pethidine in labour. About half of babies born to mothers who have had artificial opiate pain relief don't find the breast unaided, and, of those that make it, some try to suckle incorrectly.

Or, after 20 minutes of skin-to-skin contact, you can take the baby off the mother, weigh her, measure her, jab her, etc., then plonk her back on. Just as she's starting to work out where she is and what she's meant to do, a series of bewildering and disorienting things happen to her. These babies can still root around and find the breast, but around half of them self-attach poorly, in a way that could hurt the mother's nipples.

Of course, mums and babies still have days, weeks or months to get breastfeeding to work for them. It's just a bit bananas that hospital procedures don't make it easy from the start.

Syntometrine-tastic!

While the mother is enjoying a moment of blissful connectedness with her baby, buoyed up by a profound sense of relief that she's not in active labour, the midwives start doing some serious fretting.

Medical staff have to be alert to the possibility that women will haemorrhage after birth if the placenta doesn't detach correctly. They are standing by with that wonder drug syntocinon (commercial oxytocin), sometimes mixed with a little ergometrine… Syntometrine!

They are very keen to give this drug to mothers. That way they can stop worrying, get the womb to clamp down hard, pull the placenta out by the cord, bundle the parents out of the delivery room and get on with the next birth. This is called 'active management of the third stage of labour', and it's so common that some midwives have never seen it done any other way.

The alternative is to wait. The oxytocin rush that the mother and baby get from each other's company is the natural version of the same drug. In time, she can birth her own placenta – no one has to pull it out.

Which technique is better? The science on this presents a mixed picture. The most recent Cochrane review[105] of the subject found that active management results in less immediate blood loss, and that's why it's still standard hospital procedure. But there are concerns about this research. It didn't properly separate mothers who are at higher or lower risk of haemorrhage. The definition of haemorrhage could also be too strict[106] – given that pregnant women have an extra 1,250ml of blood in their body, perhaps blood loss of a little more than 500ml at birth shouldn't be judged as a problem?

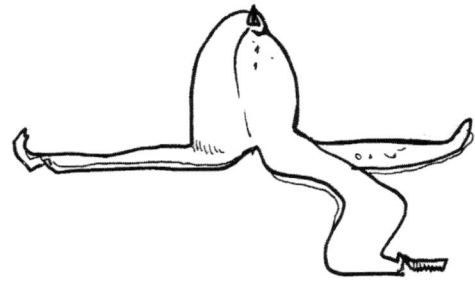

Two recent studies have found that active management increases the chance of haemorrhage for low-risk women.[107] One of these gives some interestingly strict criteria to help optimise natural birth of the placenta:

- The mother feels safe, secure, trusted and respected.
- The midwife is confident and calm.
- The setting optimises natural hormone release, with warmth, privacy and subdued lighting.
- The baby is kept on the mother directly after the birth and does all its cute wriggling and suckling. The pair are undisturbed.
- The midwife doesn't fiddle about with the cord or the mother's belly.
- The mothers have no medical complications for their pregnancies and labours, and are not given epidurals, syntocinon drips, forceps or ventouse deliveries.

Women birthing their placentas under these circumstances are seven times *less likely* to haemorrhage if they are not given oxytocic drugs.[108]

Epidurals and syntocinon drips increase a woman's risk of haemorrhage, and medical staff wouldn't be so keen to use these interventions if they didn't also have syntometrine to finish the job. Birth is a complicated mix of very finely tuned interdependent processes. Mess with one, and you interfere with all the others.

So for some women, active management remains the best option. If this is you, you may have to remind your care-givers that waiting three minutes before giving you the drugs and clamping the cord ('delayed cord clamping') is proven to have absolutely no effect on your risk of haemorrhage, and means the baby gets 90% of the placental blood that they need.[109]

But when the birth has been straightforward, hasn't been messed about with and wasn't insanely long, then why assume that a woman needs a dose of drugs to get the placenta out? The side-effects of severe womb cramps and feeling sick can interfere with her enjoyment of her first moments with her baby, and that is a special time that she can't get back again.

Natural oxytocin helps a mother to love her baby. Prolactin helps her to make milk. Synthetic syntocinon interferes with these vital hormones. We should be absolutely sure that they're necessary before we use drugs on a woman at birth.

NEXT!

SPLOP

18 Risky business

I guess that, by now, you're expecting me to be a fan of home birth. You probably assume that I think that all women should give birth in huts, with broomsticks, and open fires, and large amounts of Arran knitwear. Actually, I don't. I think that hospitals are amazing, life-saving establishments. If I were to be knocked down by a bus tomorrow, I would like to be taken by ambulance to the nearest hospital with an A&E department and an intensive care unit. I would not like to be brought home to die of hideous injuries on my sofa.

The debate about how to empower women to give birth safely and with satisfaction is too complicated to be reduced to a simplistic 'home birth = good/hospital birth = bad' equation, or vice versa. There will always be some mothers who are better off giving birth in hospital, and some who will be fine at home. I just want both hospital births and home births to be the best they can be.

Let's have a look at the basic requirements of a labouring woman.

- She needs to feel safe.
- She needs a space that she feels comfortable in, can move around in, and can make her own.
- She needs warmth and darkness or dim lighting, plus some music would be nice.
- She needs the company of an experienced, trained care-provider she knows and likes, who stays with her throughout the birth.
- But, other than her chosen companion(s), she also needs privacy.
- She needs to feel respected, trusted, and in control. (The paradox is that this is so she can fully lose control and place her trust in others.)

And:

- Some women also need access to an operating theatre, an anaesthetist, a surgeon and a team of nursing staff. Hospitals are very good at providing this, and that's something to be profoundly grateful for.
- Women can choose to have painkilling drugs, and it's good that these are available.
- There can also be times when oxytocic drugs are useful to help birth a baby.

When hospitals fail to fulfil the first six basic requirements, they make it more likely that women will need the last three.

Note: when I talk about 'hospital' in this chapter, I'm referring to large obstetric units with operating theatres attached – the places that high-risk women are encouraged to attend. There are also midwife-led units and freestanding birth centres. These are excellent, but their services tend to be targeted towards women deemed to be low-risk.

Safety first

A lot of the discussion about home birth versus hospital centres on risk. Women are invited to ponder how incredibly dangerous it is to give birth without the safety-net of easy access to major surgery. 'But what,' they are asked, 'would you do if Things Went Wrong?'

This question implies that hospitals are able to eliminate all risk from childbirth, which they can't; that women's bodies are inherently dangerous, which they aren't; and that dwelling on the worst-case scenario is the most appropriate way for pregnant women to make decisions, when it isn't.[1]

For the vast majority of mothers in our affluent, well-nourished society, things are not going to 'go wrong'. In birth, it's more useful to plan how things are going to go right,* because a woman's confidence and faith in her ability to give birth could be the deciding factor in making it easier.

It's hard to assess exactly what the relative risks are of home versus hospital birth for women with no obvious complications. Like so many innovations in maternity care, the move to hospital birth took place without being scientifically assessed for effectiveness.[2] In the 1950s and '60s, home birth for low-risk women was widely practised and well supported. In 1970 everything changed and everyone went to hospital. No randomised controlled trials were made to justify the move, and now the opportunity to do such research has been missed. Would you let a researcher tell you where to give birth to your baby? I wouldn't either.

Instead, we can evaluate the likelihood of life-threatening events occurring in low-risk women and, from them, calculate the likelihood of a baby dying at home that would be saved by a hospital birth. We are not talking about large amounts of risk. For any given set of parents, the chances of one of them being killed in a road traffic accident before their child reaches school age is significantly higher, and fear of a car crash doesn't stop people walking the streets.[3]

But risk works the other way too. The same paper points out that hospitals' failure to provide optimum conditions for natural labour (those first six points on the list) can be problematic for birthing women. And there are superbugs in hospitals, not in the home.

Another way to study the subject is to trawl perinatal mortality records and work backwards to see where babies were born. These studies need to be careful, though, to differentiate between women who have been screened for potential problems and are birthing in the presence of a qualified midwife (low-risk), and desperate mothers who give birth unexpectedly, unassisted and in complete denial about the fact that they were pregnant at all (extremely high-risk).[4]

From time to time, a piece of research hits the headlines which presents home birth as more dangerous than hospital birth.[5] And at other times large, well-conducted studies are released that show that there's no difference,[6] but these ones don't attract the same media interest. 'Nothing particularly unsafe' doesn't sell newspapers.

Anyway, the question isn't 'Is a woman safer in hospital?', it's 'Does she feel safe?' And that depends on the woman. For people who are familiar and comfortable with them, a hospital could feel like home-from-home. But for others it's

---

* Using the words 'wrong' and 'right' in relation to birth is problematic. Sure, some babies need help to be born, but no woman's body is ever 'wrong'.

a place that is indelibly associated with previous serious physical trauma or bereavement. There will always be women who don't feel safe in hospital.

Personal space

Hospitals are a centralised repository of expensive equipment and medical expertise. They are under pressure to ensure the best use of resources. And they are underfunded. This means that there isn't enough space for a woman in early labour to go there and settle, and let her labour build.

When women turn up 'too early' they are often told that they aren't in 'established labour' yet, and sent home again. This damages their faith in their ability to labour 'properly', and denies them their instinctive urge to find a safe place of birth in early labour. The acceptable time for a woman to go to hospital is when she's having massive contractions, and is trying not to give birth into the footwell of the car. Why are we subjecting labouring women to these crazy car rides – and the general public to speeding vehicles that have to run red lights?

There's also a strange double standard at work here (thanks, Midwife Thinking blog for pointing this one out). The message is that labour is very dangerous, so all women must go to hospital, but women are then sent away to labour *with no medical supervision at all*. So which is it? Are women's bodies dangerous or are they not?

Aesthetics

The traditional hospital delivery room is a large, brightly lit space with a bed in the middle of it, with weird stirrups attached for a woman's legs, and a range of technological equipment prominently on view. Everything about this set-up says 'lithotomy position'. It takes no account of a birthing woman's need for privacy, ambient lighting, or freedom of movement.

Architects and hospital planners are just starting to experiment with redesigning delivery rooms, getting rid of the bed, dimming the lights and introducing softly padded spaces, birth balls, ropes to swing from, CD players and ambient scenes of nature. There is a place for a woman to unpack her bags, to take ownership of the room. Medical equipment is hidden in cupboards, because it does nothing for a woman's confidence in labour to be staring at a neonatal resuscitation unit.

This is a decided improvement. There is some evidence[7] that changing the decor like this helps women give birth more easily with fewer interventions; they feel more positive afterwards and find it easier to breastfeed. No risks have been detected for mother or baby.

Continuous care

There is an overwhelming consensus of scientific opinion that, when women are continuously supported in labour by a known midwife, every aspect of birth works better.[8] They are less likely to be induced, to need epidurals or assisted births, their labours are shorter and their babies are less likely to need resuscitation. Oh, and they enjoy the experience more.

Hospital staff work in shifts. Sure, you can have continuity of care there, as long as you manage to squeeze your baby out before the end of the working day. As for having met your midwife beforehand? You'll be lucky.

There have been some pioneering attempts to make continuous care in midwifery a reality.

It's called 'caseloading', and one example was the Albany practice which ran in Peckham, south London from 1997 to 2009.

Pregnant women were assigned the attention of a personal midwife, with a guarantee that they'd know the person who attended their birth. Their midwife visited them at home for their antenatal checks, getting to know their individual circumstances and learning their hopes and fears about the birth. Continuity of care throughout the pregnancy meant that health problems were more likely to be spotted, and social problems such as domestic violence or substance abuse could be addressed.

When a woman went into labour, her midwife visited her at home. At that point, they would mutually decide whether to go to hospital together, because there was good reason to, or to stay at home, because they could.

After the birth, the visits continued, with 28 days of on-call support. Eighty per cent of Albany mums were breastfeeding at one month, which was the highest rate in the country by far.[9] When midwives are committed to continuity of care in labour, they have to be available round-the-clock for their clients. This leads to rather unusual working patterns. But because this carries obvious benefits for mothers, the job is more satisfying, and there is no shortage of midwives willing to work like this.

Oops. I just mentioned the phrase 'shortage of midwifes'. Forget about continuity of care; with the present state of funding for midwifery, we're lucky to get adequate care. In 2010 a survey of NHS midwives found that 56% considered that they did not have enough time to do their job properly. The following year, that figure was 66%.[10] The UK birth rate is rising, NHS funding has been slashed by £20 billion,[11] a shortfall of midwifery posts has persisted, and political promises to solve the crisis have been broken.[12]

It makes no financial sense to underfund maternity services. When women don't get access to high-quality care, the effect can be devastating. Parents sue, and the sums involved are huge: 15% of the UK maternity budget now goes on compensation payouts.[13] Surely it would be cheaper to provide a proper service in the first place?

I'm sorry, I don't want to scare you, but this is information that I thought you should know.

Privacy

This is difficult to achieve in hospitals. I suppose women could lock themselves in the toilets,[14] but some delivery rooms don't even have these ensuite.[15]

Respect, trust and control

Hospitals are not set up to enable their clients to exert control over their choices. In many cases, this is entirely appropriate. There is no point in offering a menu of treatment options to someone in a coma. In hospitals, staff are empowered to make the decisions, administer the drugs and employ the surgical techniques that have been proven to be the most effective. Protocols are developed in accordance with what is considered the most appropriate intervention in any given circumstance, and applied wherever possible.

Birth is different. It's one of the most important occasions in a woman's life. It's vital that her preferences are considered and her decisions are respected. Women who want natural childbirth can find themselves constricted by hospital policies that dictate technological interventions. Women requesting epidurals or Caesarean births have to fight for these too.

Control, in hospital, ultimately resides with doctors and policymakers. It's a hierarchical system, where midwives with decades of experience are expected to defer to junior doctors, fresh out of medical school. (This isn't in any hospital patient's interests. All the staff who attend to a person, from healthcare assistants upwards, could have vital information about their condition, and should be able to contribute to decisions about their care.)

In obstetrics, the specialists, the experts, the ones with the most power, tend to be doctors who know how to apply life-saving technologies to birthing women.[16] The equally appropriate application of absolutely nothing to a birthing woman, to allow her to birth her baby herself, doesn't carry the same kudos or confer the same status. There are doctors working in obstetrics who have never seen natural births, and who have no faith in the process. They simply do not trust women to give birth unaided.

It's also hard for medical practitioners who have been positioning women on their backs, rigging them up to monitors, speeding up labours and clamping cords to accept that their actions may have been harming the women and babies in their care. It's easy to get defensive in such situations. The result has been hostile and at times vindictive and misogynistic criticism of proponents of natural childbirth.

Don't believe me? Let's have a look at some of the witch-hunts that have been conducted in recent years.

Make false accusations

Dr Wendy Savage was the first female consultant obstetrician at the London Hospital Medical College. She was (and still is) a vocal supporter of women's rights to choose how they give birth. In 1985 she was suspended from her post on trumped-up charges of professional incompetence. The following year, after a full judicial enquiry, her name was cleared completely.

The *British Medical Journal* commented that: *'The medical profession still behaves on occasions like an Edwardian gentleman's club, concerned to close ranks against anyone with nonconformist tendencies.'*[17]

Trawl the data

The Albany practice of caseloading midwives was shut down in 2009. It had an excellent safety record, despite working with some of the most deprived women in the country. The perinatal mortality rate was 4.9 babies per 1,000, considerably better than the national average of 7.9 per 1,000, and way better than the 11.4 per 1,000 that is normal for that area of south London. The Albany's Caesarean rate was 14.4%, compared to 24.1% at King's College Hospital nearby.[18]

The Albany midwives didn't just attend low-risk middle-class mums: they took everyone, including high-risk cases. They supported women's choices to birth breech babies vaginally, and to naturally birth twins, options that are not generally available on the NHS.[19]

King's College Hospital, which employed the Albany midwives, was not happy. It commissioned an enquiry into 31 months of the Albany's statistics (a weird time-frame, which included two particularly poorly babies) and claimed that babies born at the Albany were more likely than the average to be disabled. Since the Albany's stillbirth rate was so very low, this could mean that babies that would otherwise have died at birth were surviving, albeit with some problems.[20]

Or it could be an excuse to shut the unit down. Which King's College Hospital did.

Lay criminal charges

Since it's impossible to eliminate risk from birth, powerful opponents of natural childbirth have an easy weapon at their disposal. Wait until there is a stillbirth at home (as there will be, eventually, just as there will be in hospitals), and make the rogue practitioner criminally responsible for the death.

Home birth is illegal in Hungary. Obstetrician Ágnes Geréb became so disgusted by the treatment of labouring women in Hungarian hospitals that she retrained and began practising as an independent midwife in women's own homes. In 2009 she was charged with manslaughter over the death of a baby. Ágnes Geréb was held in a maximum security prison and taken to court shackled in leg irons.[21] At the time of writing, she was still under house arrest.

The lack of trust and respect that women experience in delivery rooms is mirrored by a lack or trust and respect for people who campaign for choices in birth. The president of the American College of Obstetricians and Gynecologists has likened home birth to child abuse – the organisation gave out bumper stickers at its annual conference that said: 'Home Delivery is For Pizza'.[22]

Actually, I don't have a problem with that bumper sticker. I think it's useful to remind women that they can order a tasty, hot snack of pizza at any time. Perfect for an instant meal… after they have given birth at home.

Those requirements again

Let's look back over those needs of labouring women again, and see how they can be met by home birth.

- Feeling safe? It depends on where you live, but generally, yes, because home is where you feel… at home. (This checklist presupposes that a woman has a home, by the way. Not everyone does.)
- Comfortable? Check. Nice lighting? Check. Free to move around? Definitely.
- Warm? Probably. It is a special occasion, so even women living in fuel poverty could turn the heating up for the birth of their child.
- Company of a trusted midwife? Hopefully. It would be better if we had more caseload midwifery. We address this in the next chapter.
- Privacy? This is far easier to achieve in the home birth setting, but its importance can still be underestimated. There is a fashion in home-birth circles to have all the kids, the dog and the hamster gathered around to watch the big show. This might not add up to optimum conditions for physiological birth. It's important for everyone present to remember that if, by their presence, they are not contributing something positive, they should leave. That even includes the father/other-mother if they aren't able to be supportive. Oh, and you know all those lovely 'natural birth' videos you can watch online? They are very instructive, and I have to thank those women for sharing such intimate moments with us, but none of them is actually a natural birth. Why? Because there's someone standing there with a blinking video camera! This is one day in a woman's life that she's never going to forget

(unless she chooses the pethidine). Get the camera out after the baby is born.

- Trust, control and respect are much easier to achieve in the home setting, although they can still be undermined by abusive partners, controlling parents or bullying, unsympathetic midwives.

What about the last three requirements on the list? Giving birth at home doesn't mean forgoing all access to surgery, epidurals or syntocinon. We have ambulances. When women transfer to hospital, that doesn't mean they have 'failed'

at giving birth at home, it means they have succeeded in taking advantage of what hospitals can offer, because there is a genuine need.

But it does guarantee that these won't be used when they're not needed. A woman's risk of medical interventions is increased by birthing in hospital, and the longer she is there, the more potentially unnecessary stuff is done to her.[23]

The choice of the best setting for birth is a trade-off between the optimum conditions for different scenarios. There's no one right answer, and there's more than one good way to give birth.

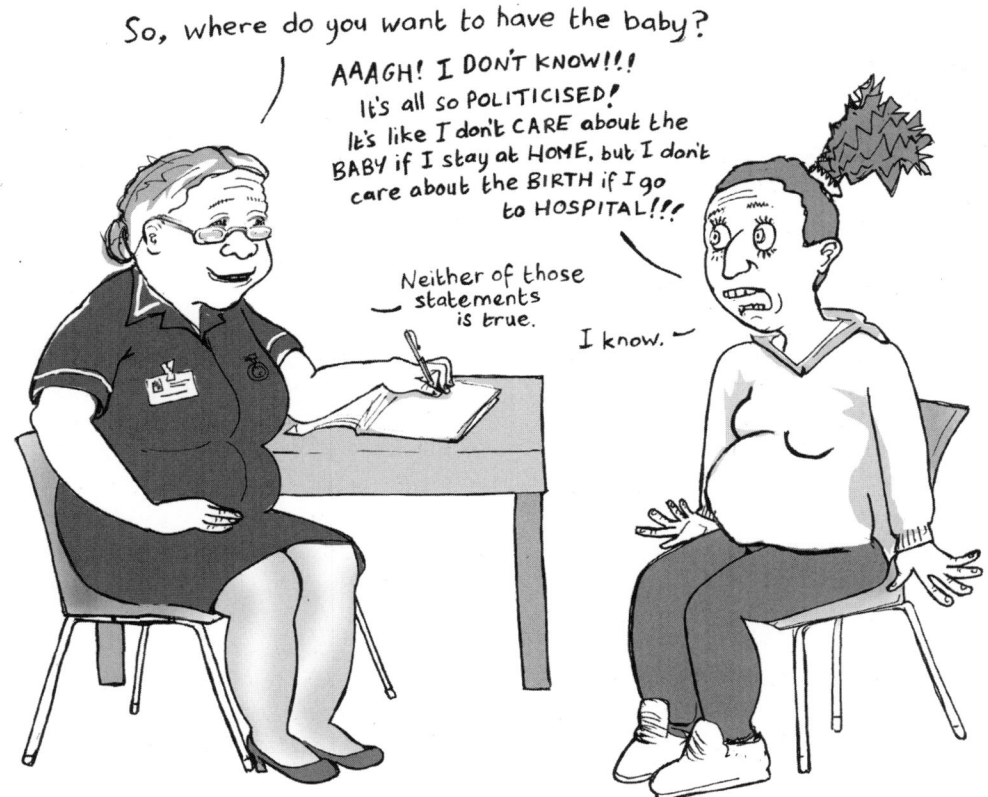

A word on the NHS

The title of this chapter is risky business, and when we discuss risk with pregnant women, at the back of our minds we're thinking about death. There's one death in particular I'd like to discuss.

The death of the National Health Service.

The Secretary of State no longer has a duty to provide people with a national health service, free at the point of use. That died with the Health and Social Care Act of 2011. The NHS in England is now just a brand, formed of healthcare companies that compete to make a profit at the expense of the public purse.[24]

The bits of the old system that it's possible to make money out of – providing drugs and surgery – have stayed with the NHS. And the aspects of medical care that are devoted to keeping us healthy, such as anti-smoking campaigns and help with obesity, have been hived off to a new body called Public Health England, and are paid for by local councils. There is no longer a legal duty to keep these services free, and in time we may start to be charged for them. This division of health services makes sense from a capitalist viewpoint. Since the hospitals are making money out of people being sick, it's not in their interests to promote healthy living campaigns that keep people well.

Antenatal education and health visitor support after the birth come under the public health part of the system, while midwifery services stay with the NHS. Can you see a potential there for fragmentation of care around pregnancy and childbirth?

We are seeing a conscious move away from the old UK system (woman's risk of dying in childbirth: 12 per 100,000) to the US system (woman's risk of dying in childbirth: 21 per 100,000).[25] Competing private providers don't just cause fragmentation of care, they don't just result in a two-tier system where the rich have better access to health than the poor, and they don't just represent a massive siphoning of public funds into the pockets of private shareholders. It's worse than that. Under the new system, the insurance companies are in charge.

We already have a system where hospitals have to be sued for negligence if something goes wrong during a birth. This is stupid. France and New Zealand have no-fault compensation schemes for medical injury. Why can't we? Litigation is unjust. We're the fifth richest country in the world.[26] We should be able to guarantee all disabled children a decent quality of life. They shouldn't have to take recourse to legal action to guarantee that.

The legal process pits the participants in a birth against each other. It puts medical staff in a position where they can't speak openly about events in case they say something that could be used against them. The lawyers are the real winners from the current

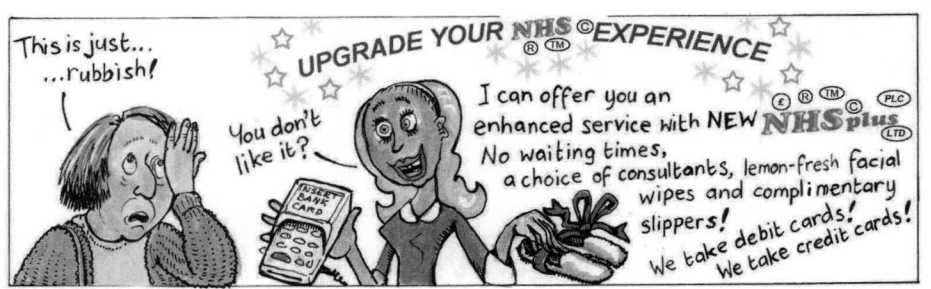

system, and they have a vested interest in making each case take as long as possible. Grieving parents don't need blame, they need closure and they need truth.[27]

And, by definition, 'negligence' means 'not doing something when you should have done something'. Natural birth works best when care providers are content to do precisely nothing, and only use interventions when clearly indicated. So a litigious culture works against natural birth. Medical staff feel compelled to do something, just for the sake of doing something, to prove that they weren't failing to do something. And once they've started meddling, and disturbed the finely tuned interdependent processes involved in the birth, then they have to meddle some more to put things right.

Once hospitals are run for profit, the choices and freedoms of women are curtailed. Patient throughput becomes more important than patient satisfaction. Fear of litigation becomes an overriding factor, because a successful lawsuit blows a hole in a hospital's finances. The protocols that determine negligent practice become increasingly strict. Insurance companies aren't run by underwriters with a sound knowledge of the principles of natural birth. They tend to think that obstetrics is like all other fields of medicine: a problem that can be solved with surgery, drugs and technology. Crazy rules result, like a requirement for all women to undergo CTG monitoring, even though it's ineffective at preventing the outcomes that hospitals could be sued for, and actually makes litigation more likely.

Insurance companies very nearly killed British independent midwifery.[28]

For many years, women unhappy with NHS maternity care have been free to employ an independent midwife. It's not cheap, but it's worth the money, and it saves the NHS £13 million a year.[29]

Independent midwives weren't able to obtain liability insurance. Their clients accepted this. They knew if they sued their midwife she'd lose her home and be declared bankrupt. They took a leap of faith and decided to trust in someone who trusted in them. All parties in the arrangement were consenting adults. You would think that would be fair enough. Then, in 2013, the government introduced regulations that made it illegal to practise without insurance, but provided no assistance for independent midwives to obtain it. A national outcry, a lot of money and hard work went into finding a solution, and insurance coverage was eventually obtained. But it remains to be seen if the process will place restrictions on independent midwives' practice – if, in effect, they will now no longer be truly independent.

Now that NHS facilities have become a front for companies such as Richard Branson's Virgin Care,[30] the £13 million that independent midwives save the NHS is money that isn't going to multinational healthcare corporations that have the ear of government ministers.[31]

Just a thought.

Right. That's enough with the doom and the gloom and the conspiracy theories. You're pregnant. You don't need to read scary stuff. Don't worry. This book is about to get a lot more positive.

19 *Birth rights*

Aim for the birth you want. I'm not about to dictate what that should be, because I'm not you and I don't know your circumstances. The good news is that you're not alone.

Where is monkey midwife these days? She's still doing what she has been doing for millennia, caring for women as they birth their babies with enthusiasm, with reverence, and with love. (Plus, nowadays, she also gets to fill out reams of paperwork.)

Birth rights are human rights, and the really good news is that they have recently been enshrined in European law. After Ágnes Geréb was arrested, one of her clients, Anna Ternovsky, took the Hungarian government to court. She was pregnant, and outraged that her freedom to give birth safely at home had been curtailed. The European Court of Human Rights saw the justice of her case and agreed that all women have the right to choose how and where they give birth.

That's not just about home birth. It's about all birth.

We have come a very long way from the 1970s, when hospitals used to print on a woman's maternity notes 'when she enters hospital it can be assumed that she assents to any necessary procedures'. These days, your consent should be sought for all aspects of your maternity care. This means you don't have to say 'yes' to everything. You can say 'no'. The case of Ternovsky vs Hungary states that you have the right to choose the circumstances in which you give birth.[1] That ruling is legally binding anywhere in the European Union.

Now to make it a reality.

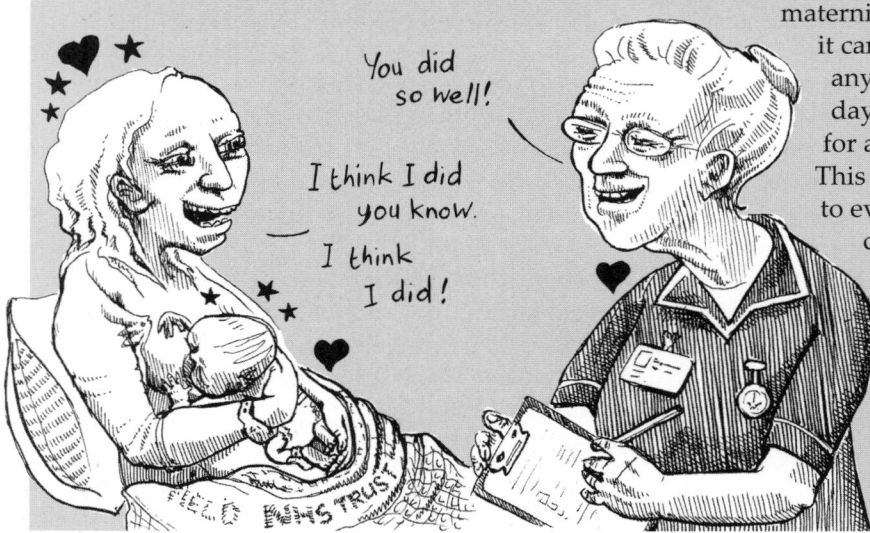

You did so well!

I think I did you know.

I think I did!

Who can help?

Midwives can help. They have been plotting together in their covens since time immemorial, sharing their knowledge of woman-centred care. In the last 30 years they have made huge progress at creating space for natural birth, both at home and in hospitals. We now have midwifery-led units within large hospitals and freestanding birth centres in small towns where midwives set the protocols, creating some imaginative, creative and beautiful birth environments.

Researchers can help. There has been some marvellous scientific enquiry into the processes of birth and the relative benefits and drawbacks of various interventions – academic enquiry that asks the right questions, and conducts sensitive, qualitative evaluations. I've tried to list a lot of it in the notes if you're minded to read further.

Activists can help. Lawyers at birthrights.org.uk are pushing for your legal right to choose. The Association for Improvements in the Maternity Services (AIMS) and the NCT are both excellent organisations. They are there for all mothers, not just those who want natural birth.

And you can help yourself. You can demand to be included in decision-making. You are being offered medical intervention: it could be something that saves your baby's life, or it might be something that just saves the midwife some time. So ask follow-up questions and decide how you feel about what's being proposed.

It is good that protocols for care exist, where they are evidence-based (which not all of them are), because overall they do reduce risk and improve outcomes. But you can still choose to be the exception to the rule. You can investigate the risks involved, make an informed decision, sign a legal disclaimer if that's appropriate, and then do what the hell you like. Birthing women are the real agents for change here. Anyone who is employed by a hospital has to abide by its policies and procedures or they're at risk of disciplinary action. So an NHS midwife can't suggest that you do something out of the ordinary. But mothers-to-be aren't tied by the same constraints. They are free to challenge the status quo, and, when enough of them do, the medical profession will adapt to accommodate their needs.

It's your birth. Pick your own adventure.

How to fight for the birth you want

Write a birth plan. Medical notes are an absurdly technical and reductionist way to record something as magical and spiritual as birth. The only point where a woman's lived experience of the process enters the record is in the little box at the end marked 'mother's reaction to baby'. You can counter this by writing a document that includes how you feel, why you feel it, and what you're aiming for.

Consider several eventualities when you write your plan, because, whatever you decide about the

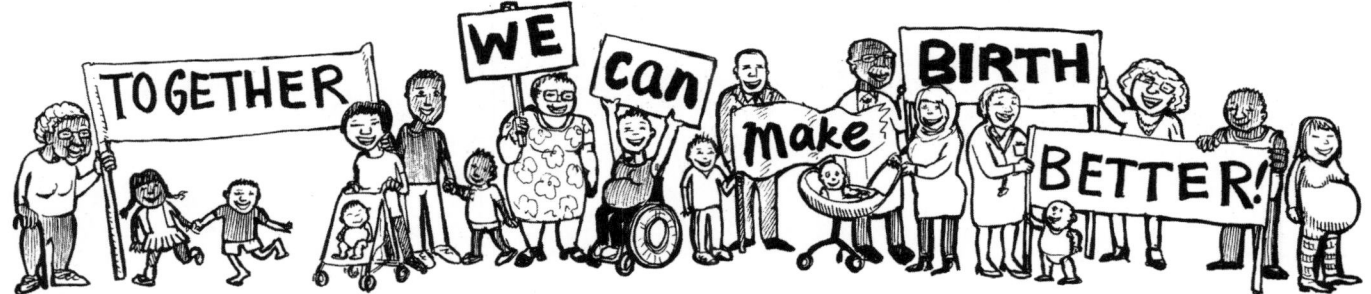

birth, your baby might have other ideas. (Welcome to motherhood! Kids are good at confounding your expectations.) In fact, every single point on your birth plan might go straight out of the window when you birth your baby, and as long as you know why this happened, were consulted and consented, that is absolutely fine.

Giving birth is not a fashion statement. A home birth with incense and candles isn't empowered if a woman is only doing it like that because her freaky, controlling, hippy stepdad is dicating her choices. A healing, empowered and transformative birth can be a planned repeat Caesarean.

So be pragmatic, and be prepared to react to changing circumstances. The research on the benefits and risks of various procedures that has been cited in this book is based on average outcomes for large numbers of women. But you are not an average, you are an individual, and your birth is unique. So even if, overall, there's no benefit in doing a procedure for everyone, there may still be occasions where it will be a good idea. Rule nothing out, but still, aim for what you want. You have to listen, but also be prepared to speak out.

Midwife Mary Cronk pioneered access to home birth in the 1980s, when women's choices in childbirth were rarely respected. She wrote this advice about negotiating with medical personnel:

I am sure that many others will explain your absolute right to refuse any procedure for any or no reason. The law, and good practice, is quite clear. A sensible

person will listen carefully to any explanations to why a procedure is proposed, and then, should she choose not to have X,Y or Z, she just says no or no thank you. The 'allowing' is done by YOU. An asssertive approach is worth cultivating. You may care to commit the following phrases to memory and practise them frequently in front of a mirror.

1. **'Thank you so much Midwife Sinister/ Mr Hi-an-my-tee, for your advice. We will consider this carefully and let you know our decision.'** *Sweet smile! This one is most useful in the antenatal stage, though it can be used in labour. It can just take a minute to consider what you either want to know, or what you decide.*
2. **'Would you like to reconsider what you have just said!'** *Fierce glare. This is useful and, for example, applies to the misuse of the word 'allow'.*
3. **'I do not believe you can have heard what I have just said. Shall I repeat myself?'**
4. **'I am afraid I will have to regard any further discussion as harassment.'** *This is used if the person does not respect your decision or persists in pressing the subject.*
5. **'What is your NMC or GMC pin number?'** *This is used if 4 is ineffective. If the person asks why you want their pin number, inform them that this is something they might like to consider.*
6. **'STOP THIS AT ONCE!'** *This to be used* in extremis. *I am delighted to tell you that this was* used *against me by a woman to whom I had taught*

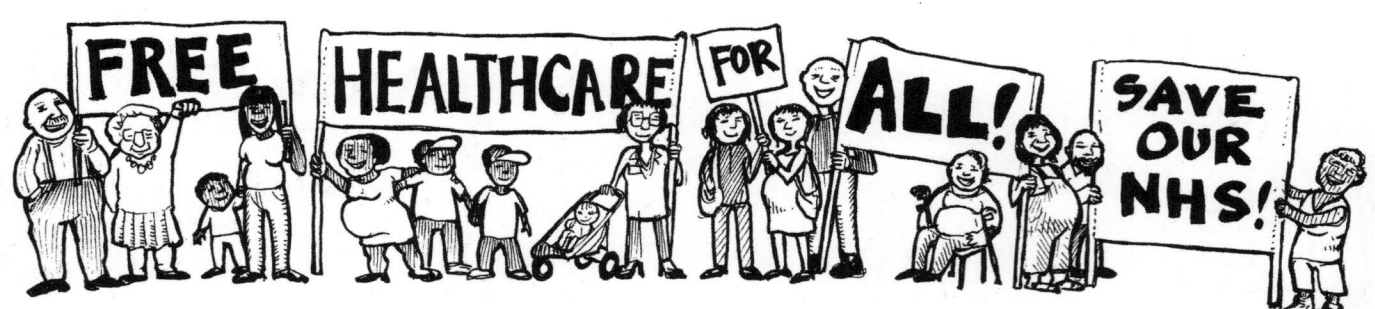

it. I was doing a difficult vaginal examination and was being too persistent. I stopped at once and learnt a lesson.

Do not argue; learn the phrases and keep them or similar for use if necessary. I am informed that it is usually only necessary to be assertive once or twice to have a much more respectful attitude from the people who are actually your professional servants.

Good luck and regards,
Mary

You may not be used to being assertive in your conversations with authority figures. Here are a few more phrases that you could keep handy:

- *What are the benefits of this procedure?*
- *What are the risks?*
- *What are the benefits of waiting and not doing this, and what are the risks?*
- *I'd like a second opinon.*
- *I'm not happy and I'd like to change care-provider.*

In an emergency, use this one:

- *I do not give my consent to this procedure,* and then get out your phone, because this is one occasion where filming a birth is a good idea.

You can find some more ideas for specific assertive phrases to use in particular situations on page 277.

How to not-fight for the birth you want

This may seem extraordinary, after the massive pep-talk I've just given you, but women can make informed and empowered decisions *not to fight.* Birth is about surrendering to mighty forces, that open up your body and your mind. The process happens best if you can disengage your rational mind and relax into being in the moment. So having to fight your corner against hostile staff is probably counterproductive.

There may come a time when you decide to go along with what's being suggested, purely for the sake of an easy life. That's OK! You're allowed to! I am really not here to tell you what to do. This is about trusting *you* to decide.

Here are some more strategies to help you overcome the paradox of aiming to surrender while remaining in control.

Request continuity of care

From your first interactions with maternity services, state that you want care from a named midwife. That way, you'll be able to have in-depth discussions with your birth attendant ahead of time. At the moment the NHS doesn't prioritise caseloading in its staffing arrangements, but since this aspect of midwifery has been consistently proven to increase safety and satisfaction in birth,

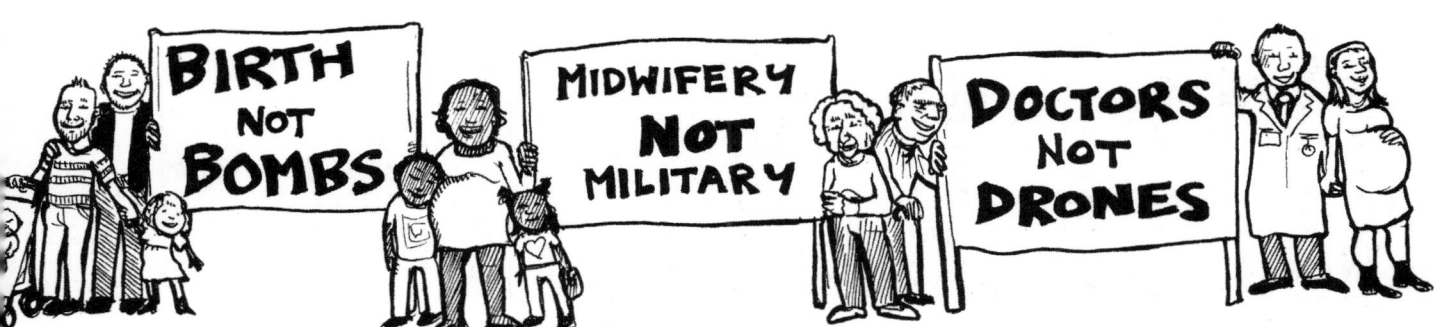

it should.[2] (And it's cheaper![3]) If you are able to choose just one circumstance around the birth of your child, this is the one to go for.[4]

There is currently a national push for continuity of care in midwifery. The campaign is called A Midwife for Me and My Baby (M4M). Lend it your support.

Get clearance ahead of time

If you want to aim for something unconventional, research your options thoroughly. AIMS can help with whatever it is that you're aiming for (and I'll say it again: this isn't just about women wanting natural birth.)

Then, take your plans first to your midwife, and then to the Supervisor of Midwives. She's an experienced, senior figure, whose role is to advocate for both midwives and patients. Many Supervisors of Midwives are happy to negotiate a deviation from standard birth protocols. If yours isn't, you can then ask to see another one. There are so many good birth workers in the NHS that you should be able to find someone to support you.

It isn't unrealistic to aim for natural birth. (If you want to! You don't have to!) If vaginal birth is an option for your baby, it works best when the hormones that govern it are allowed to unfold. Of course, not all births are straightforward,

assistance is sometimes necessary, and there could be reasons why this is more likely to happen to you, but that doesn't mean that you can't aim for an intervention-free outcome. Negotiating for natural birth in a high-risk pregnancy can involve scary discussions about 'what if' scenarios, but none of those worst-case predictions is inevitably going to happen to you. Stay calm, and carefully consider all your options.

Learn hypnobirthing

Hypnobirthing is a simple technique for deep relaxation during birth. You learn it ahead of time, with your birth partner, and then, as your labour unfolds, he or she can gently guide you into a meditative frame of mind.

This helps optimise those good birth hormones, can shorten the labour[5] and may make the sensations much easier to bear. Some women hypnobirth completely without pain, although that's not a guaranteed outcome. Hypnobirthing helps you feel calm and positive during the birth, whatever happens. My sister hypnobirthed her way to an emergency Caesarean, and it made a difficult situation a whole lot easier. Everyone can benefit from being able to go to a happy place in their mind, and it's a shame that these techniques aren't taught in state-funded antenatal classes.

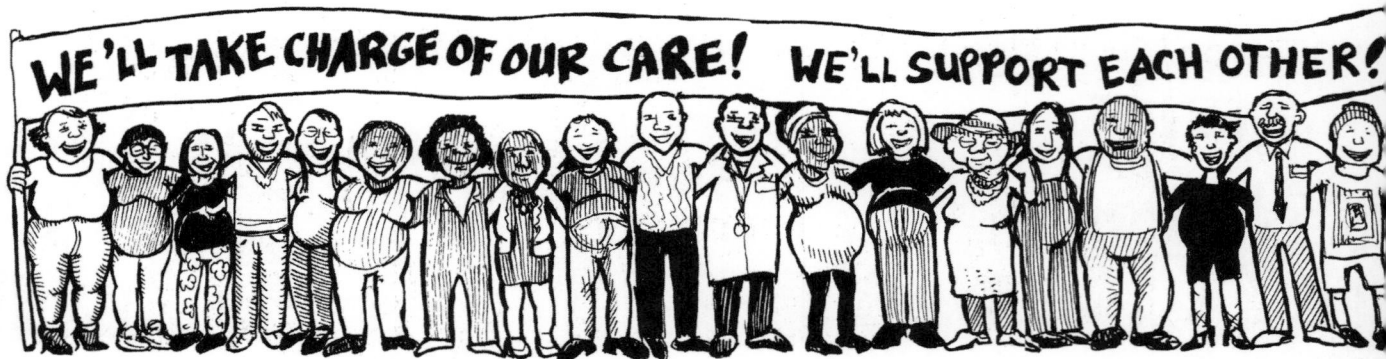

Employ an independent midwife

They're still here! And they're still amazing! You can employ someone who believes in birth, believes in you, and is completely free to help you birth your baby (or babies) in the way that you prefer.

Free from hospital protocols, that is, not 'completely free' in the financial sense. Independent midwives aren't cheap, but they charge about a sixth of the cost of the average wedding. And really, which is actually going to be the happiest day of your life?

Independent midwives are trained to the same standard as NHS midwives, are registered with the same professional body and are subject to the same system of supervision in professional practice. They often also undertake additional training in skills such as helping women to safely birth breech babies or multiples.

Your independent midwife does all your antenatal and postnatal visits as part of the care package. You can still access NHS services such as blood tests, scans and appointments with specialist consultants, where appropriate. When it comes to the birth itself, she will carry the same drugs and resuscitation equipment as NHS midwives at a home birth. If you transfer from home to hospital, she will come too and in some circumstances may still be able to be the one to catch the baby.

Find your nearest qualified practitioner from independentmidwives.org.uk.

What doulas do

Or you could hire a doula. (A what? A trained birth companion. The name comes from the Greek for 'handmaiden'.)

A doula is someone who is knowledgeable about birth, who is guaranteed to be there with you, and whose only role is to support you, in whatever way you want her to. Because your doula isn't a friend or a member of your family, she doesn't bring any emotional baggage to the place of birth. And, because she isn't employed by the hospital, she isn't concerned with getting you to behave in a certain way. She's just there for you.

Doulas have been proven to help women give birth more easily, and more quickly, to babies that are healthier.[6] And, they make a real difference to the way parents feel afterwards. They don't feel abandoned, confused or over-ridden, because they had an advocate there when they needed it.

Some doulas also offer postnatal services. You get all that birth support, then she'll pop round, do the laundry, and cook you breakfast. Bonus!

Doula? Just do it.

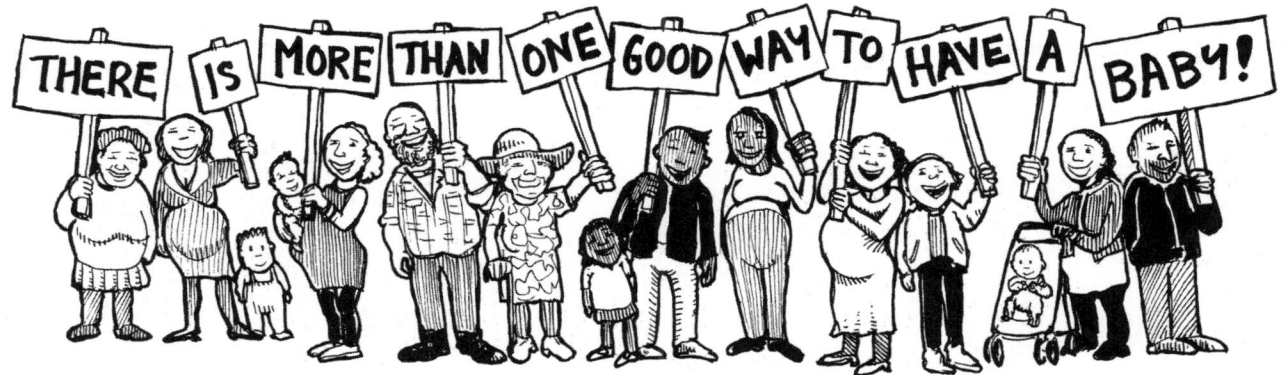

THERE IS MORE THAN ONE GOOD WAY TO HAVE A BABY!

20 *More than one good way to have a baby*

This section is about alternatives in birth. We can't cover every potential obstetric eventuality in a cartoon book – that's what your midwife is for – but here are some options for different common scenarios. You don't have to read any of this if it's not relevant to you. Sometimes too much information can be hard to handle.

Alternatives to induction

Induction of labour, first with a prostaglandin pessary and then with a syntocinon drip (see pages 246–9), is the standard protocol for all pregnancies that last more than 42 weeks, or for anyone past 34 weeks whose waters have broken. It may also be suggested if the baby seems big.

For a 'large' baby

It may be helpful to know that research has shown that assessments of the size of a baby in the womb are incredibly imprecise.[1] Artificial induction of labour for large babies has been proven to not improve outcomes for mother or baby.[2] And care-givers stressing about your baby being 'too big' is more likely to have an adverse affect on the outcome than the size of the baby itself![3]

For premature rupture of membranes

Once your waters have broken the baby is no longer sealed off, so germs could travel up from your vagina and cause an infection. (Vaginal examinations make this more likely, even with sterile gloves, as they push germs up from the vaginal entrance to the cervix.[4]) Standard protocol is to induce the birth if labour doesn't start on its own within a set amount of time. Women may also be dosed up with antibiotics to prevent an infection.

Neither of these interventions helps babies. Randomised controlled trials of 'induction' versus 'waiting' have found that the infection rates for babies are no different.[5] Preventative antibiotics are not proven to protect babies either.[6] Women are at slightly increased risk of getting an infection after the birth if they wait; but 50 women would have to be induced to prevent one infection, which is treatable, and induction carries its own risks, of instrumental and Caesarean delivery.

The studies found that more babies from the 'waiting' group were taken to the special care nursery, but that was because it was hospital policy, not because there was anything wrong with them. (There is no benefit to depriving babies of skin-to-skin contact and early breastfeeding experience 'just in case' they get ill. That's making it more likely that they will!)

When women's waters break very early in their pregnancies, they are encouraged to wait for weeks or months before giving birth, because the benefits for the baby are clear. There are cases where the amniotic sac has healed, and the leak stopped. More waters are produced all the time, so the baby doesn't 'dry out'.

Ninety-five per cent of women whose waters break at term will go into labour spontaneously within 24 hours. Watchful waiting for women who don't could involve carefully monitoring the baby's movements, eating large amounts of anti-bacterial garlic and echinacea and being alert to any sign of infection such as fever or smelly discharge.

For post-dates pregnancy

Firstly, check your due date is accurate – see page 39. Try the suggestions on pages 199–200 to enhance your body's ability to go into labour. You can ask for foetal monitoring rather than induction, which checks the condition of the baby and measures the levels of amniotic fluid.

Wait or don't: it's up to you. Any increased risk of stillbirth is worth taking seriously, no matter how remote. And the latest review of the subject has found that inducing babies that are more than two weks 'overdue' does reduce the incidence of stillbirth, and doesn't lead to more emergency Caesareans (a reassuring finding for women who opt for induction). But it also found that the chances of a bad outcome from waiting are so slight that 'a woman experiencing a prolonged pregnancy is the appropriate person to judge' what she wants to do.[7]

Some handy phrases

In the spirit of Mary Cronk's advice on pages 272–3, here are some more phrases you may want to use to ensure you have your baby *your* way.

If you want natural childbirth:

- *Don't offer me pain relief. If I need it, I'll ask for it.*

To discourage your midwife from yelling 'push!':

- *If you tell me what to do, it stops me listening to my body.*

And then, if they don't get the message, try:

- *Please be quiet.*

If you choose to refuse CTG monitoring

- *I don't need that. I need the personal attention of a midwife.*
- *The Cochrane review found no benefit for continuous monitoring for high-risk groups.* (This might carry more weight if you download the Cochrane review and print it out to show them.[8] Please be aware that the evidence on the ineffectiveness of CTG isn't widely known in hospitals, and some care-providers feel dependent on this technology in their working practice.)

If you are told that a shortage of available midwives means you have to go into hospital:

- *Well, you have a staffing problem, because I'm booked for a home birth.*

If that doesn't work, try:

- *Excuse me? Can I take your name and position, please.*

And then say:

- *We have no medical reason to attend hospital, and no intention of coming in. If you fail to send a midwife out to us as arranged, then you will be legally liable for any consequences.*

This has always worked, so far.

Ideas for long labours

Long labours really are a pain. You can feel very small, and scared, and helpless in the face of something that seems ineffective and interminable. (I did). Sometimes the body needs help to get those contractions going and move that baby down.

Here are some things to try.

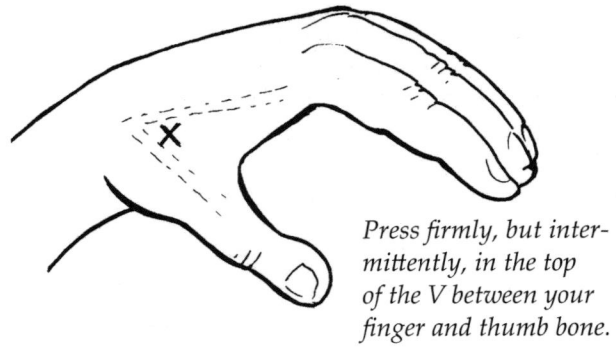

Press firmly, but intermittently, in the top of the V between your finger and thumb bone.

For a long first stage (the dilating part)

- Renegotiate arbitrary time limits. Being threatened with surgery after a set amount of time is counterproductive. Ignore the future and concentrate on the now.
- Dim the lights, turn up the music, lock the door and remind yourself that this is the right place to have your baby.
- Have sex. This can be incredibly effective, as lovemaking enhances oxytocin release. (It has to be consensual sex!) If your partner is male, the prostaglandins in his semen will also help. Don't have a partner? Try D.I.Y. (This is one labour 'intervention' that is never going to be evaluated by randomised controlled trial.)
- Or try nipple stimulation. You, or someone you love, can caress and nuzzle away. Privacy is preferred for this option too.
- Press and hold the shiatsu points illustrated on this page.
- Put clary sage essential oil in the room burner, inhale it neat from a hanky or massage it diluted into your belly and back.
- Doze for a while. Just a few snatches of sleep can revive you. Try lying on your left side or sleeping sitting up, slumped forward over something soft.
- Alternate this with staying mobile, walking, dancing and singing.

Press on the inside of your leg, behind the bone, four fingers width up from your ankle. Mark the spot with a blob of pen so it's easy to find again. (This also helps with period pain. Don't use any of these shiatsu points in pregnancy.)

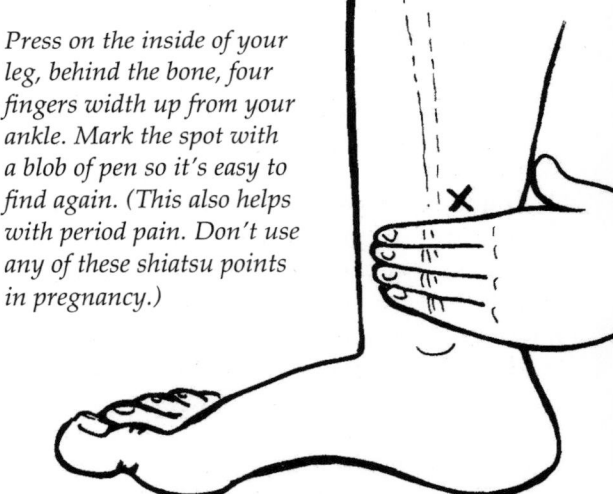

This spot on the outside edge of your little toe nail is easiest to press with a pen lid or fingernail.

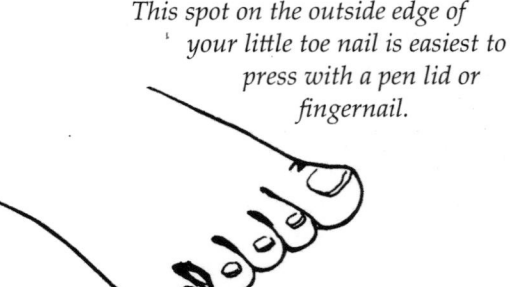

- Eat, drink, be sick, drink and eat some more.
- If you're not in a birth pool, get in one.[9]
- If you're in a birthing pool, get out and go for a walk.
- Take caulophyllum homeopathic remedy.
- Consider emotional factors. Skilled birth companions are able to help women work through their unacknowledged mental barriers to birth.
- Get rid of anyone fearful who is present: consciously reframe anything unhelpful they may have said.
- Take courage. Find your inner strength. It's in there somewhere! It really is!

For a long second stage (the pushing part)

- Arbitrary time limits are unhelpful here too. Assessment of labour should be by the condition of the mother and the baby, not by the clock.
- Some women have to really work to get their babies out. Stay mobile. Change postion every few contractions. You could try any of the poses here and on pages 281–3, and then improvise some more. Let your body tell you what works well.
- Some midwives are skilled at techniques to manipulate the pelvis to make more room.
- Keep using those shiatsu points and clary sage essential oil.
- A cup of hot, sweet tea can revive you when you are flagging.
- Emotional factors can stall labour here too.
- Use the beast within you. She will help you birth this baby.
- But don't panic. Some babies take their time.

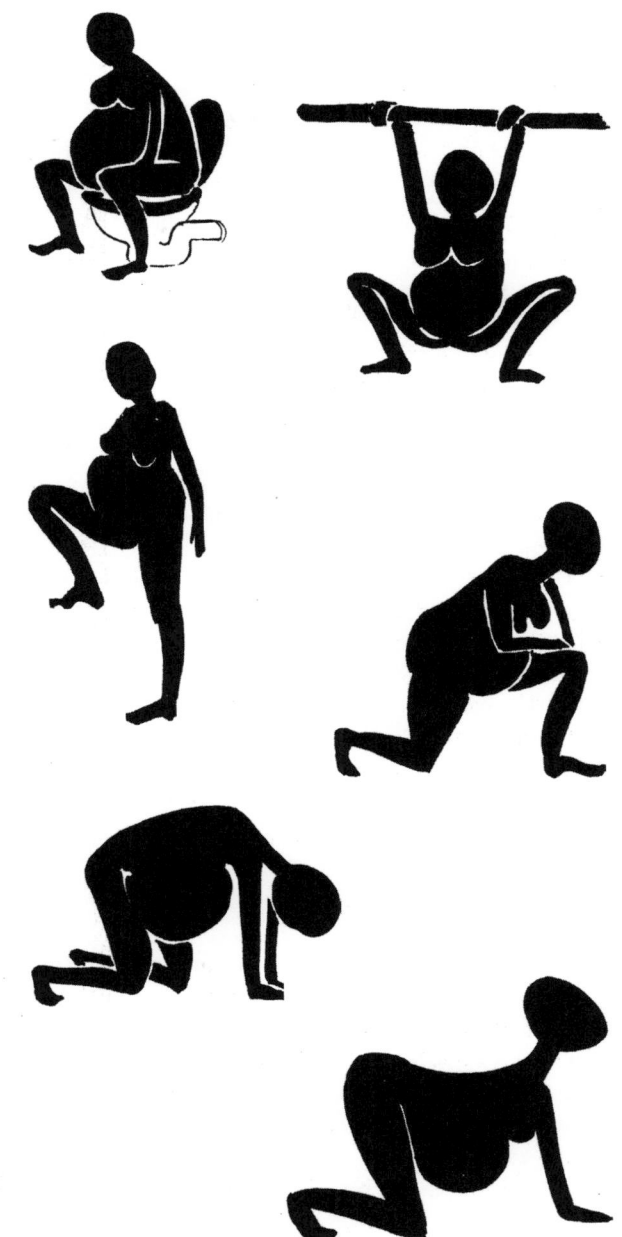

Sudden labours!

What's the alternative to very slow labours? Insanely fast labours!

If your baby is coming RIGHT NOW like a steam train:

- Phone for an ambulance if there are no qualified care providers present.
- Remind yourself that it's OK. It's over-whelming, but it's amazing.
- Massage your clitoris to help engorge the tissues around the vagina.
- Ignore any instructions to 'PUSH', instead breathe the baby out.
- If your baby arrives before medical help does, rub him dry with a towel or a T-shirt or something, snuggle him on your bare belly or chest and cover him with a fresh dry item of clothing or blanket.
- He should start to breathe spontaneously. If he doesn't, blow on his face, rub his hands and feet, talk to him and tell him to get his act together. If he still doesn't get the message, give a soft puff of air from your mouth sealed over his nose and lips.[10]
- Sit tight, and wait for the emergency services.

More than one good way…

Not every birth is straightforward. The point of this book is to inspire you to help your birth go well, but no one can guarantee that it will. There is such a thing as obstructed labour: hours of fast, hard contractions, with 100% effort but very little result. Our midwives should be expert at helping women work with the sensations of normal labour, so they can intuit when the pains are too great and something is wrong.

There is no shame attached to choosing anaes-thesia, augmentation or assisted delivery when your body has done all it can do.

There is more than one good way to have a baby.

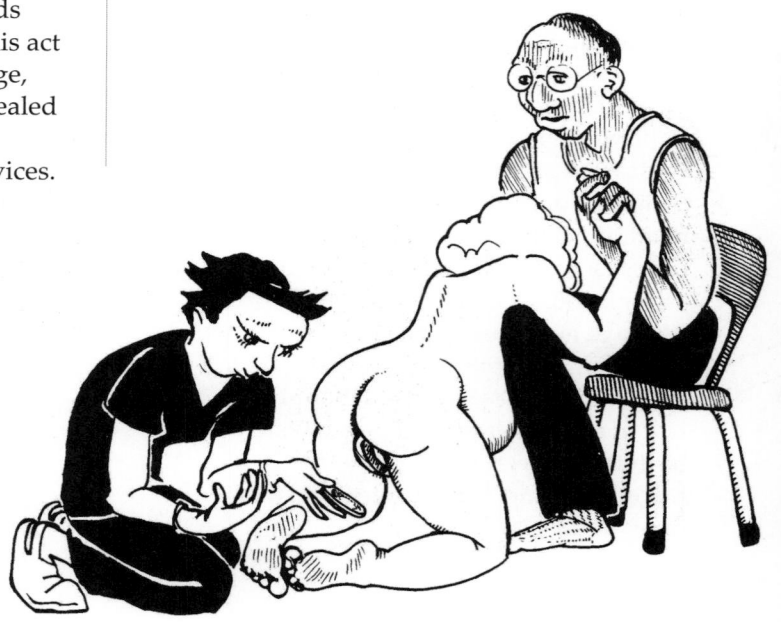

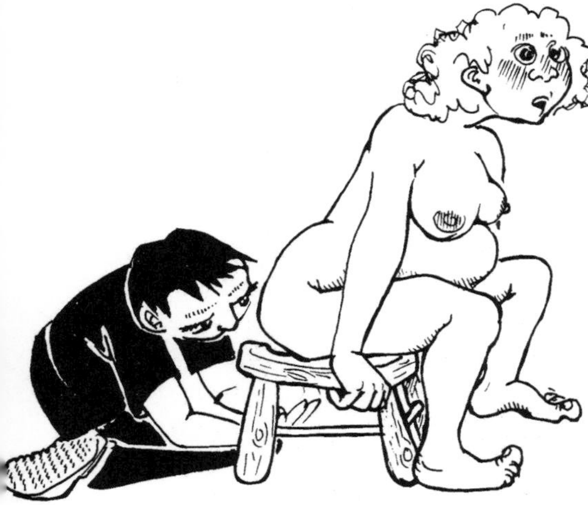

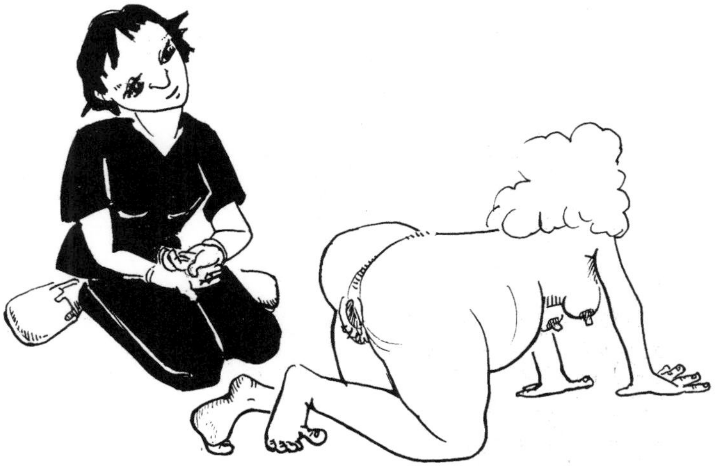

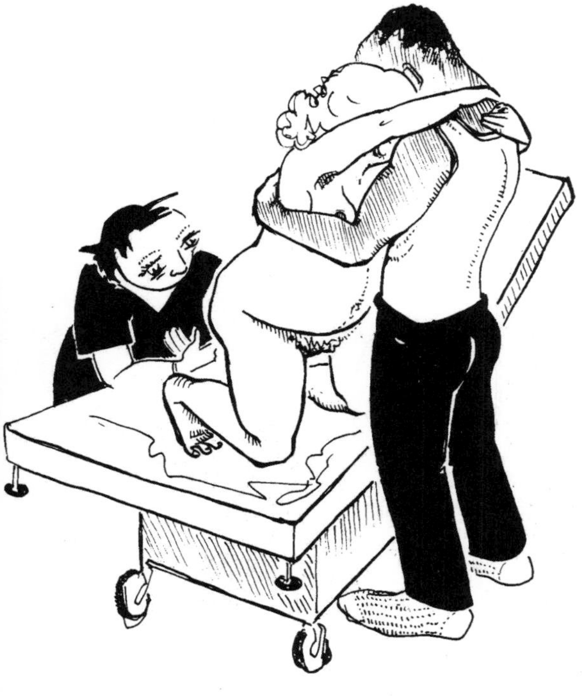

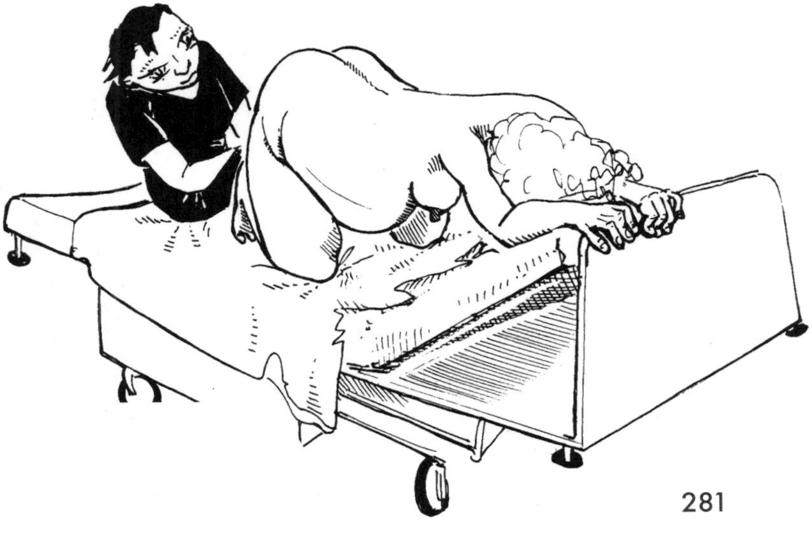

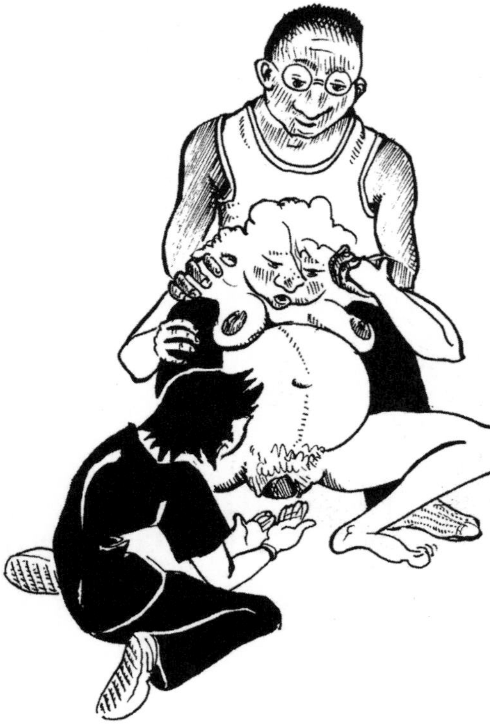

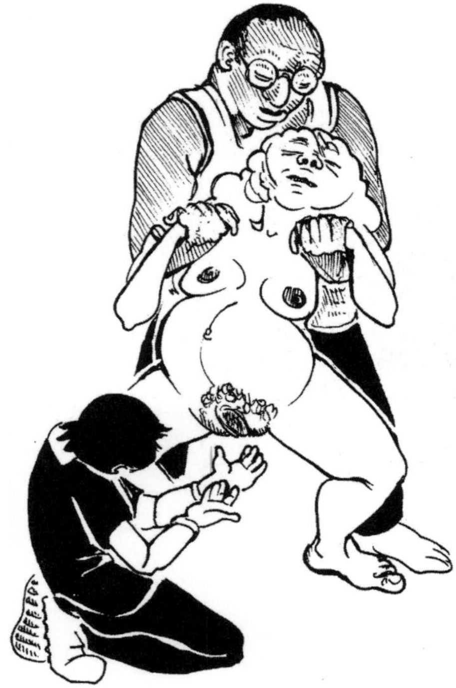

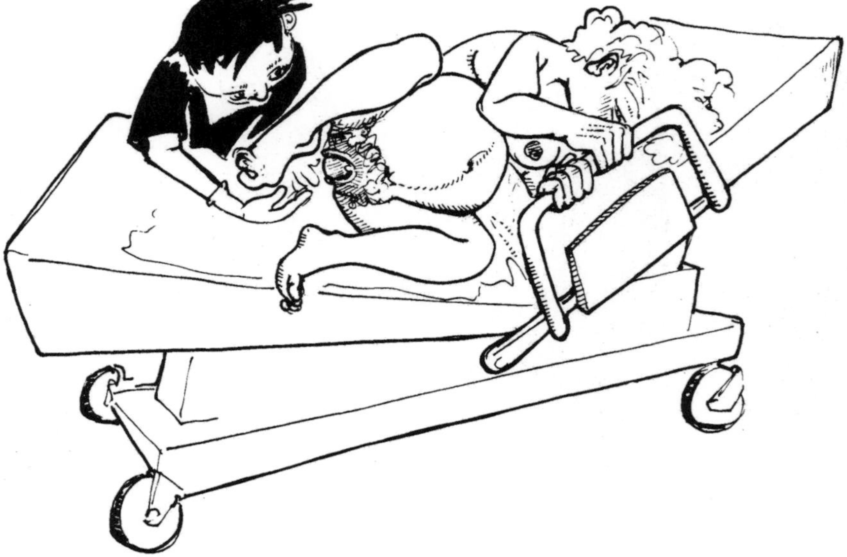

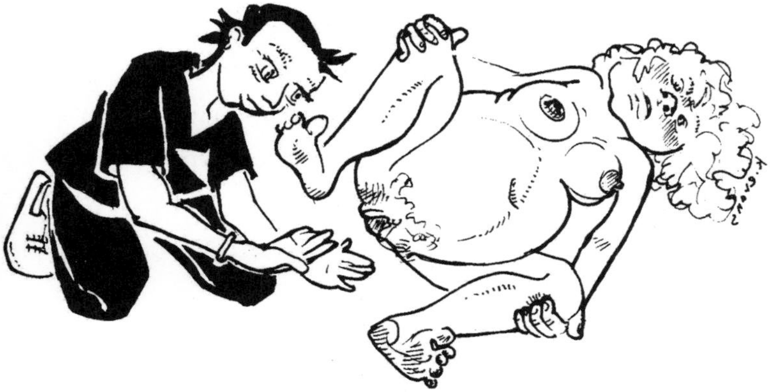

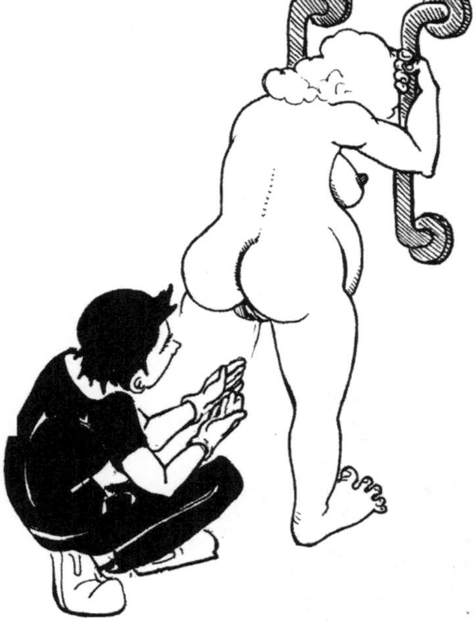

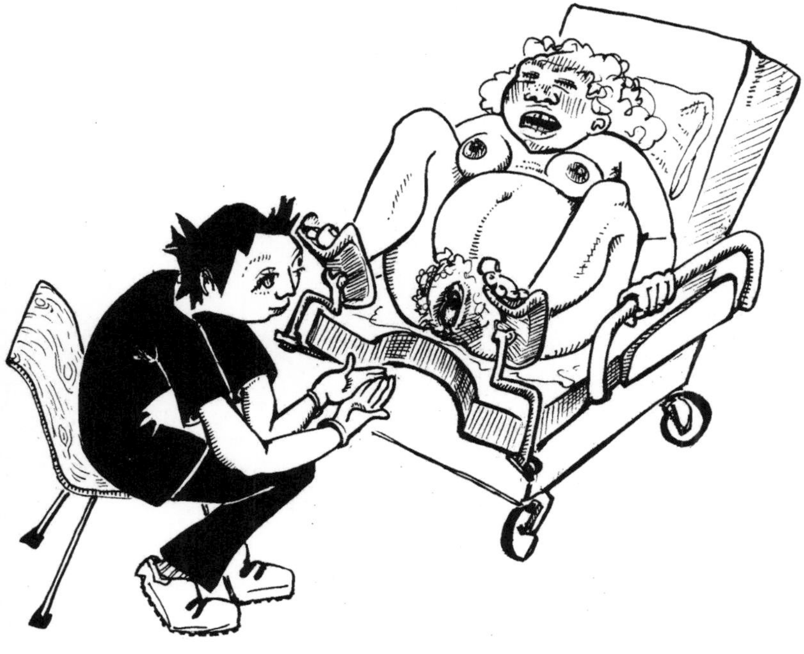

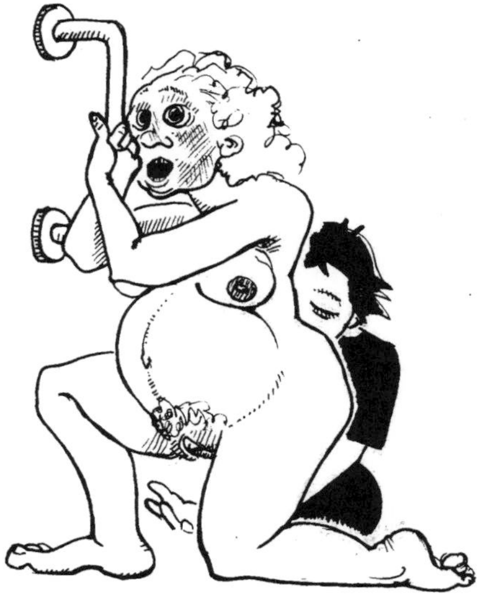

The Caesarean section

2   1

Caesarean rates keep climbing. Here in the UK they have doubled since 1990, with no improvement in outcomes for mothers or babies.[1] One baby in four is now born by Caesarean, in the US it's one baby in three, and in China one in two.[2] Contrast these rates with the 7% achieved by the maternity hospital at Pithiviers, France, and you can see the scale of the problem.[3] The Caesarean has become the default mode of operation in a world that has lost faith in women's ability to birth.

The media like to blame mothers for this rise. They run snide stories about the demand for elective sections. 'Too posh to push!' run the headlines. Push off! If a woman makes an informed choice to undergo major surgery for the birth of her child, it's her body, and her right.

But really, what choices are women given? From a doctor's perspective, Caesarean is convenient, predictable, quick, and well paid, and high-risk women are steered towards it. Can such women choose to be supported and respected by their doctors if they don't choose Caesarean?

Can any of us choose to be part of a culture that values birth as part of women's sexuality, that acknowledges the power of women's genitals as men's playthings?

Are women guaranteed their choice of birth attendant if they opt for vaginal birth? A pre-planned Caesarean is the only way most NHS patients can get continuity of care around birth, and that stinks.

It is doubly insulting to frame the Caesarean debate around women's choices when, for the vast majority of women being raced to the operating theatre, this is precisely what they didn't want. It represents the moment when choice was wrested from them – all their options dissected cleanly by the surgeon's knife. We know that unnecessareans are performed daily, yet at this moment the necessity for surgery is undeniable. There is no alternative.

Being sliced apart is not the easy option. It requires courage, and it involves pain. It takes women a long time to heal from a Caesarean section. So many are scarred by that uncertainty. What if…? If only…

Let's look again at Pithiviers' natural birth statistics. Thanks to Michel Odent's pioneering practice, 93% of babies there can be born by the traditional route. But that proves something profound. Some babies can't. Some need to be born by Caesarean. Yours might be one of them.

This is your baby, it's your birth, and you still have choices and can still have control…

The operating theatre. Scene of the primordial drama. Birth.

Forget 'ripped untimely from the mother's womb' – Shakespeare wasn't *au fait* with recent innovations in Caesarean surgery. It doesn't have to be clinical. It can be reverent and magical. Here's how…

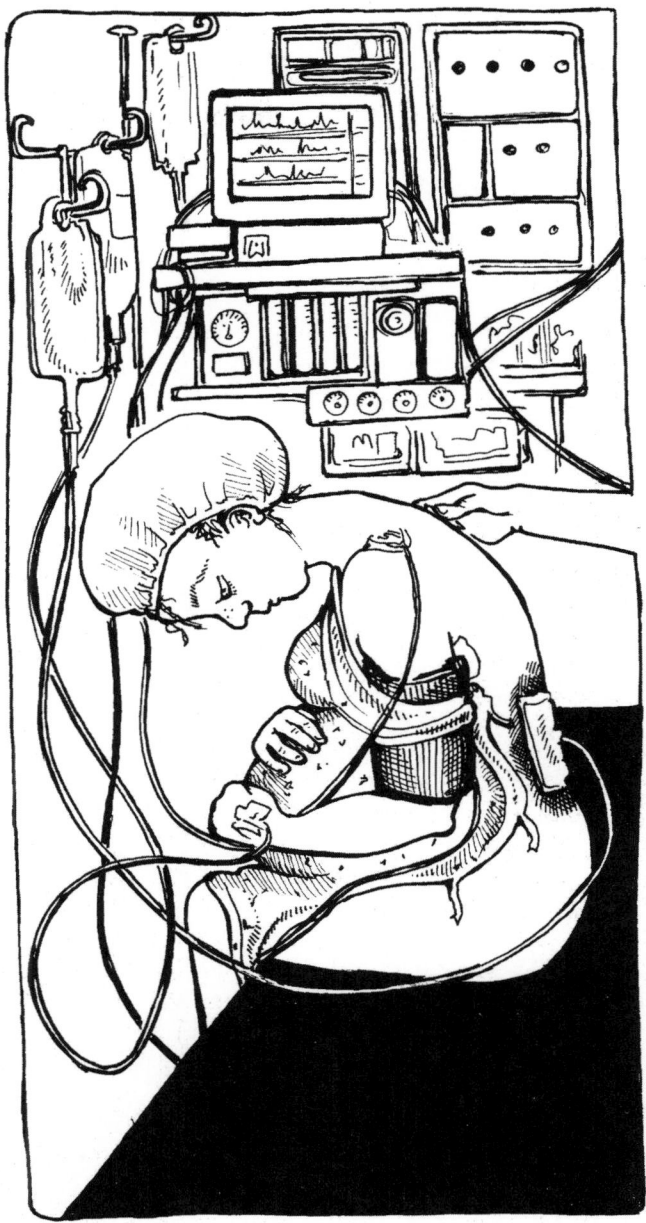

A little forward planning. As the mother is prepped for surgery, the heart monitor stickers are placed upon her sides and her shoulders, leaving her chest free from wires. With a drip in her left hand, and the oxygen saturation monitor attached to her toe, her right arm is freed from her gown.

The mother lies down.

The epidural trickles like cold water inside her spine.

The screens go up, and the lights are dimmed. This baby doesn't need the glare of the spotlight.

The surgeon rummages around in her belly, finds the baby's head, cups it in his hand and brings it out.

A wonderful moment of operating theatre. The curtain falls and the head of the bed is raised.

'Here's your baby!'

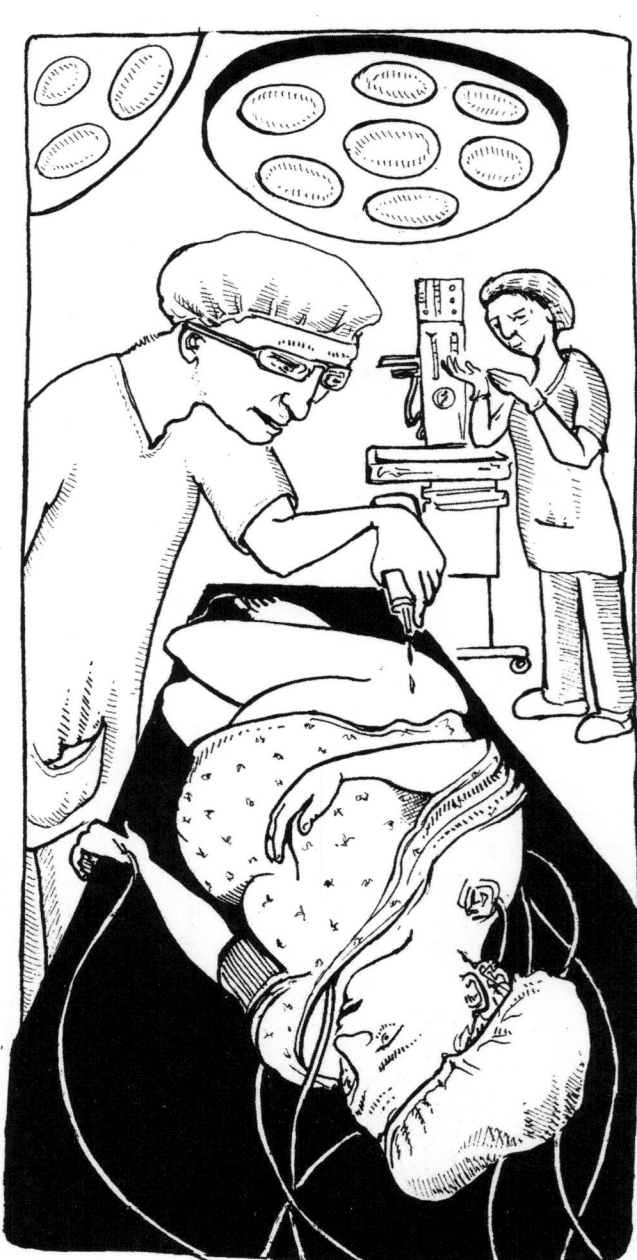

286

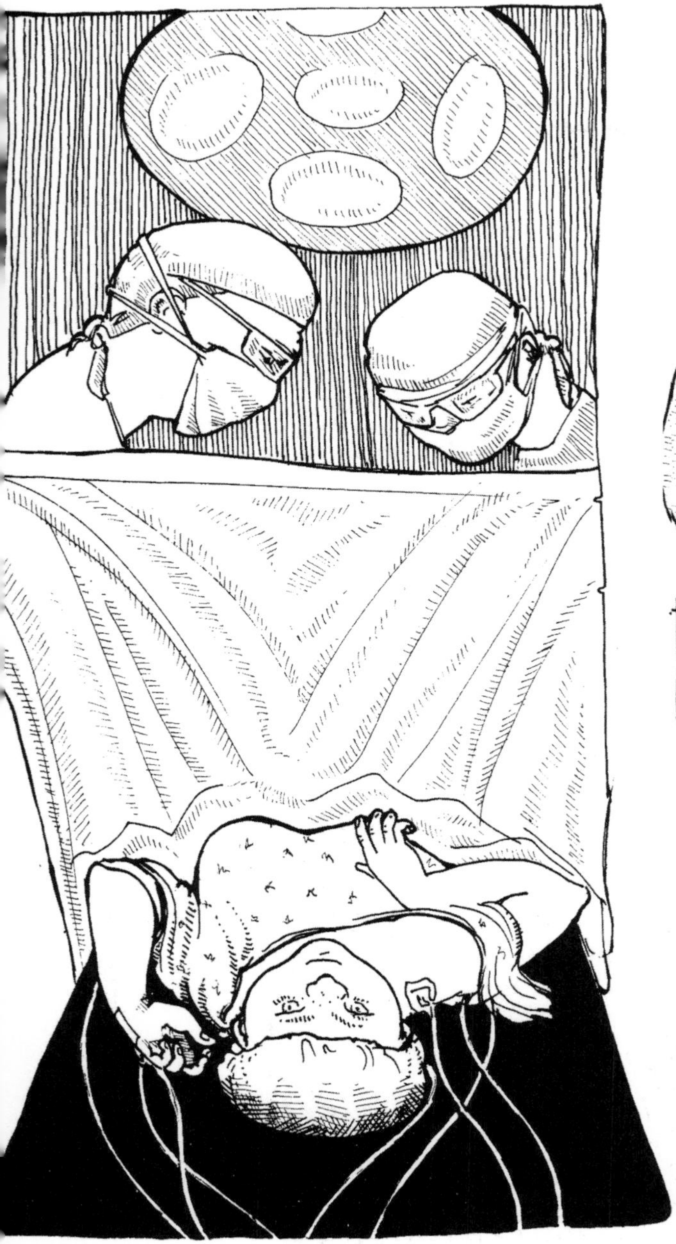

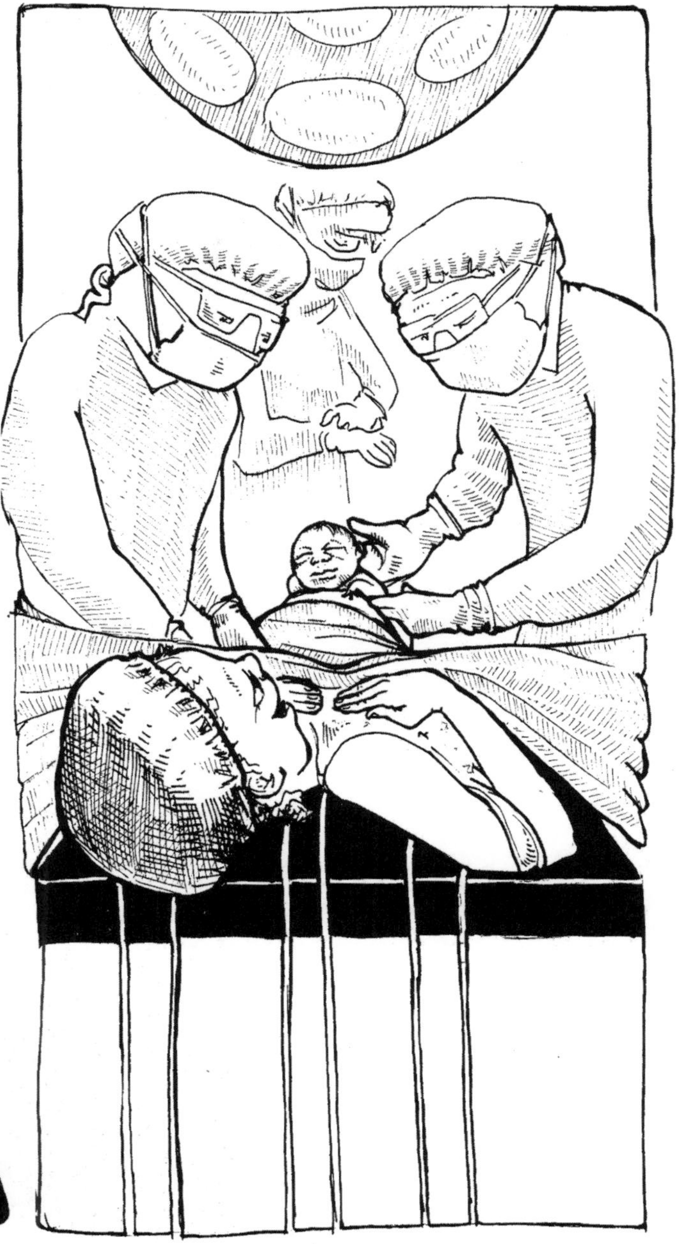

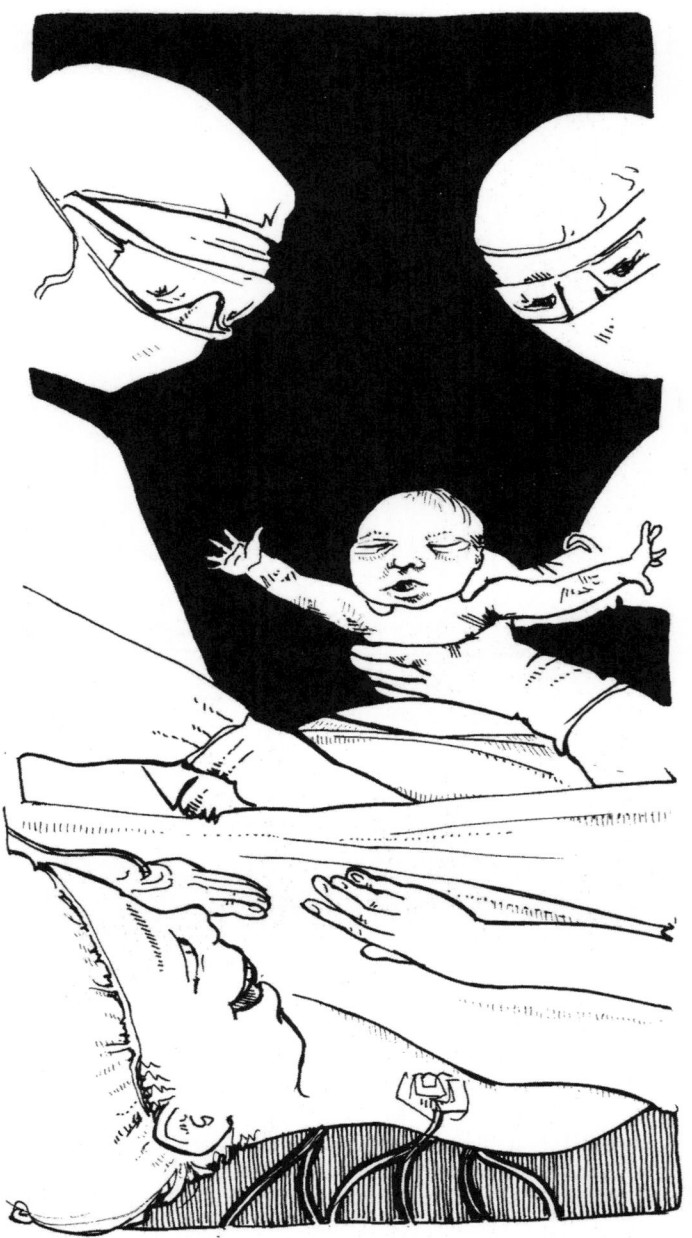

At the threshold of birth, the fluid drains from the baby's lungs. First one shoulder, then the other wriggles free.

The surgeon lifts the baby clear, so the mother can see the baby's sex.
She's a girl!
     The cord still pulses. Stem cells flood the baby's system.

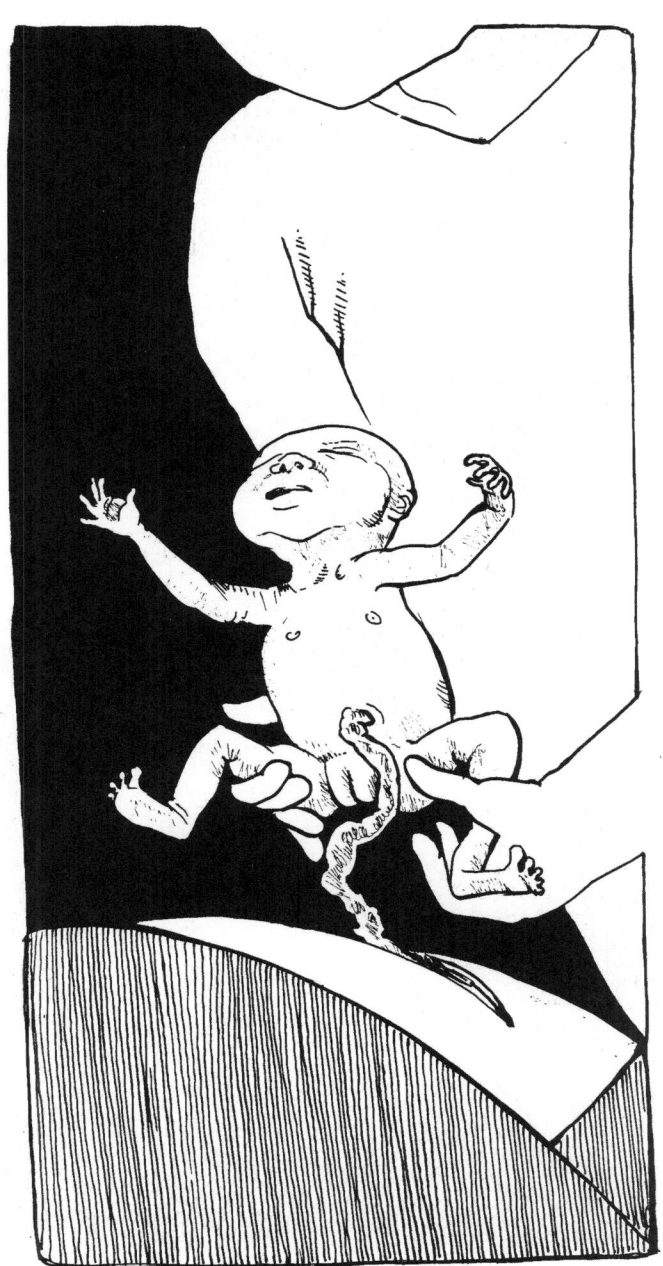

The midwife then brings the baby straight to the mother's bosom, where she can snuggle and nuzzle and suckle. Warm blankets are piled upon them both.

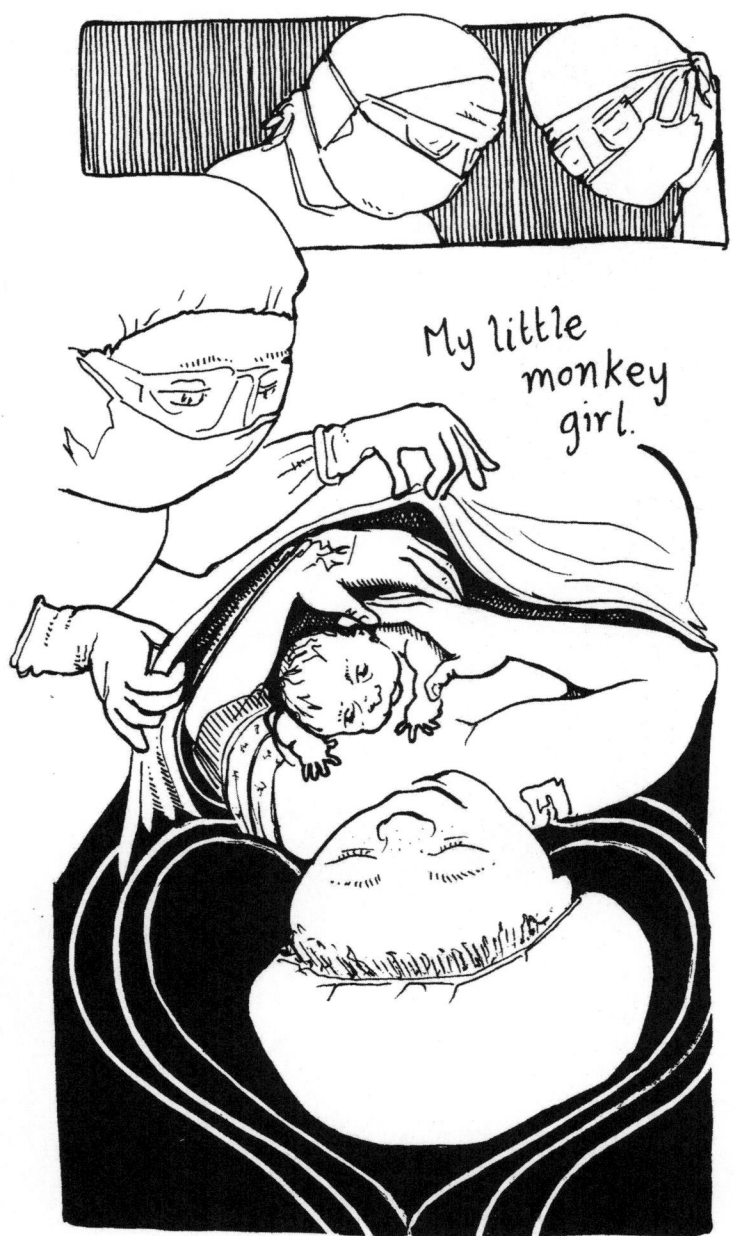

My little monkey girl.

The operation described here is a 'woman-centred Caesarean'[4] or 'gentle Caesarean'. It was developed for pre-planned surgery, but it can be used for emergency delivery too.[5]

- Banish inane chatter. Everyone present should respect the indelible significance of this occasion: the birth of your baby.
- A delayed 'incision to delivery time' gives the baby time to adjust. Unless there are very serious concerns for the baby's condition, it should be standard best practice for Caesarean surgery.
- As long as the placenta is still functioning, there is no need to cut the cord immediately – the benefits of 'delayed cord clamping' apply to all babies.[6]
- Keeping the mother and baby together during surgery and recovery is known as 'couplet care'. It has lasting benefits.[7]
- If the mother is very unwell or unconscious, the best place for the baby is on the father/other-mother. Skin-to-skin contact helps stabilise the baby's temperature, blood sugar and respiratory function.[8] (By the way, if you have an emergency general anaesthetic, you'll probably be sick when you wake up. Just so you know.)
- There is conflicting evidence on the best method for suturing the womb. Single layer closure is quicker and bleeds less, but double layer closure may be stronger in the long term. A modified mattress suture shows promising results.[9]

Write a birth plan with protocols for Caesarean, and be prepared to fight for it.
    Aim for the Caesarean birth you want.

22 *After birth*

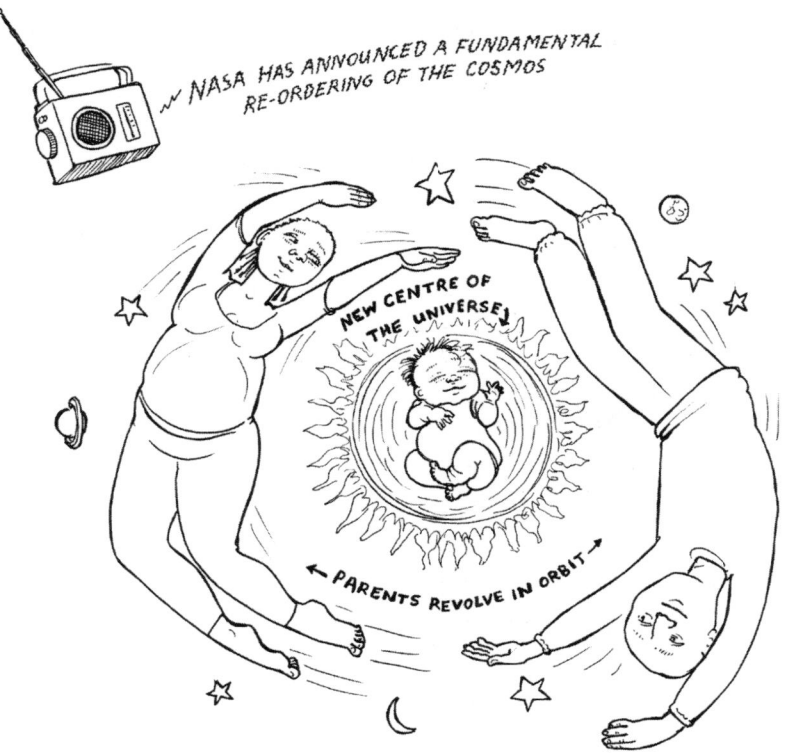

NASA HAS ANNOUNCED A FUNDAMENTAL RE-ORDERING OF THE COSMOS

NEW CENTRE OF THE UNIVERSE

← PARENTS REVOLVE IN ORBIT →

That was the easy bit. That was just making, growing and birthing a baby. Now you have to raise a child! Actually, newborn baby care is quite straightforward. It's an endurance test, but the basic principles are simple.

- Cuddle the baby lots.*
- Feed the baby lots.*
- Ignore the housework.
- Sleep when you can.

You might fall in love at first sight with your baby, or your feelings might take time to grow. Spend lots of time skin-to-skin, massage them and sniff their lovely baby smell.

* i.e., practically all the time.

No matter how long you have waited for your baby, sometimes it's hard to believe they're really here.

I hope your adventure in birth went well, but in the fairytale of life there can be dragons and demons as well as angels and rainbows.

Just as you can't predict how your birth will unfold, you also can't anticipate how it will make you feel. I had a nine-hour orgasm with a hospital birth on a CTG monitor and a saline drip, but was stunned and shocked by the next labour, in a beautiful birth-centre pool.

However you feel about your birth, it is valid to feel it. If you're traumatised, don't feel you have to rationalise this, and don't let your feelings be dismissed with the platitude, 'Well, at least you have a baby.' Instead, seek out someone who can help you process what has happened. Some midwives and doulas offer a specialist post-birth counselling service. Eye Movement and Desensitisation Reprocessing therapy gets good results.

Make time to write your birth story. It's a very special thing to make a record of.

And whether the birth was wonderful or terrible, or any combination of the two, give some feedback to the people involved in your care. They go out every day of their working lives and help people give birth. So much of their time is taken up with form-filling and box-ticking, and they are continually subject to pressure to conform to the latest protocol or learn the newest procedure. They need to hear how their actions affect birthing women, so if they did something that embarrassed or upset you, no matter how minor, then let them know what that was.

But when they do their job well, they support women in producing miracles, every day. Tell them if they helped make your happy-ever-after.

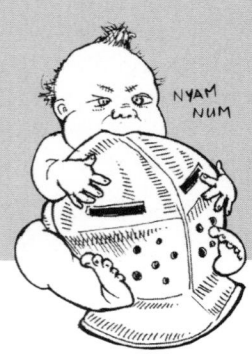

NYAM NUM

References
and
Index

References

This book doesn't have all the answers, but it might inspire you to further research.

If you are interested in natural childbirth, the writings of Sheila Kitzinger, Ina-May Gaskin, Michel Odent, Soo Downe and Denis Walsh are all excellent. Special mention should go to the blogs *Midwife Thinking* and *Evidence-based birth*.

A word about evidence. I have referenced Cochrane reviews wherever possible in the text. You can find them yourself at www.cochrane.org. The Cochrane Collaboration seeks out randomised controlled trials ('we gave one half this new thing and the other half the old thing and compared the results'), rates them according to how impartial they are, and plots all the results on a chart. This kind of meta-analysis is more conclusive than a single scientific study.

However, a Cochrane analysis is only as good as the studies that are fed into it, and, in birth, trials are only as good as the hospitals they are performed in. Randomised controlled trials aren't the only form of evidence. Descriptive and qualitative studies can be better for analysing how something feels, or how it works, which is part of what it does.

The science indicates what the average outcome is, but it won't tell you what will happen in your particular case. It's useful if you want to challenge outdated or illogical hospital protocols – a Cochrane review is a very powerful tool to wave at a doctor in this case.

But you don't have to be bound by what the average or recommended outcome is. There are many paths.

You can be as adventurous as you want to be.

1 The story of the egg and the fish

page 18 (1)–(14) These references can be found on page 18 itself.

page 25 (15) 'Herbal treatments for alleviating premenstrual symptoms: a systematic review', Dante, G and Facchinetti, F, *Journal Of Psychosomatic Obstetrics and Gynecology*, Vol 32, Issue 1, pp.42–51, March 2011.

page 27 (16) 'Capacitation as a regulatory event that primes spermatozoa for the acrosome reaction and fertilization', Eve de Lamirande, Pierre Leclerc and Claude Gagnon, *Molecular Human Reproduction*, Vol 3, Issue 3, pp.175–94, 1997. Also: *The Great Sperm Race*, Jennifer Beamish, Channel 4 and Wellcome Trust; and 'Watching sperm's striptease act', *New Scientist*, Issue 2127, 28 March 1998.

page 30 (17) and (18) 'Wild, energetic sex is key to conception', *Observer*, 22 March 2009.

page 31 (19) 'Semen acts as an anti-depressant', *New Scientist*, 26 June 2002.

(20) 'The secret life of semen', *New Scientist*, 5 August 2006.

page 32 (21) 'Sperm transport in the female reproductive tract', Suarez, SS and Pacey, AA, *Human Reproduction Update*, Vol.12, No.1, pp.23–37, 4 November 2005.

(22) 'Surfing sperm ride the womb's waves', *New Scientist*, 24 December 1994.

page 33 (23) *The Great Sperm Race*, Jennifer Beamish, Channel 4 and Wellcome Trust.

page 34 (24) *Mayes Midwifery*, ed. Betty R Sweet, Bailliere Tindall 1997.

3 You and your cycle

page 39 (1) *Taking Charge of Your Fertility*, Toni Weschler, Harper Collins 1995.

page 50 (2) *Taking Charge of Your Fertility*, ibid.

4 Trying for a baby

page 57 (1) 'Endless human eggs on demand', *New Scientist*, 3 March 2012.

page 58 (2) 'The secret life of semen', *New Scientist*, 5 August 2006.

(3) 'Daily sex "best for good sperm"', BBC News reporting an announcement by Dr David Greening to the European Society for Human Reproduction and Embryology, 30 June 2009.

(4) 'Wild, energetic sex is key to conception', *Observer*, 22 March 2009.

(5) 'The relationship between cervical secretions and the daily probabilities of pregnancy: effectiveness of the Two Day Algorithm', Dunson, DB, Sinai, I and Colombo, B, *Human Reproduction*, Vol 16, pp.2278–82, 2001.

page 61 (6) 'Shift work and subfecundity: a causal link or an artefact?', Zhu, JL *et al.*, *Occupational and Environmental Medicine*, Vol 60, Issue 9, September 2003.

(7) 'Optimizing natural fertility', Practice Committee of the American Society for Reproductive Medicine in collaboration with the Society for Reproductive Endocrinology and Infertility, *Fertility and Sterility*, Vol 90, S1–6, 2008.

page 62 (8) and (9) 'Optimizing natural fertility', *ibid*.

(10) 'Body mass index in relation to semen quality and reproductive hormones among 1,558 Danish men', *Fertility and Sterility*, Vol 82, pp.863–870, October 2004.

(11) 'Obesity and the polycystic ovary syndrome', Gambineri, A *et al.*, *International Journal of Obesity-Related Metabolic Disorders*, Vol 26, Issue 7, pp.883–96, July 2002.

(12) 'Effects of lifetime exercise on the outcome of in vitro fertilization', Morris, SN, Misssmer, SA, Cramer, DW *et al.*, *Obstetrics and Gynecology*, Vol 108, pp.938–45.

(13) 'Effects of age, cigarette smoking, and other factors on fertility: findings in a large prospective study', Howe, G *et al.*, *British Medical Journal*, Vol 290, p.1697, June 1985.

(14) 'Electronic cigarettes as a harm reduction strategy for tobacco control: A step forward or a repeat of past mistakes?', Zachary Cahn and Michael Siegel, *Journal of Public Health Policy*, Vol 32, pp.16–31, 2011.

(15) Cigarette Smoking Associated With Delayed Conception, Baird, DD and Wilcox, AJ, *Journal of the American Medical Association*, Vol 253, pp.2979–2983, May 1985.

(16) 'Sidestream smoking is equally as damaging as mainstream smoking on IVF outcomes', Michael S Neal *et al.*, *Human Reproduction*, May 2005.

page 63 (17) and (18) 'Optimizing natural fertility' *ibid*.

(19) 'Opiates and Sex', Ernest L Abel, *Journal of Psychoactive Drugs*, August 2012.

(20) 'Environmental Health Perspectives Supplements 101', Alex Vermeulen, *Environment, Human Reproduction, Menopause, and Andropause*, Supplement 2, pp.91–100, 1993.

(21) 'Effects of MDMA (Ecstasy) on Oocyte Quality and Fertilization Rate in Mice', Fatemeh Haji-Maghsoudi *et al.*, *Reproduction and Infertility*, Vol 11, Issue 2, No.43, July–September 2010.

(22) 'The Effects of LSD on Chromosomes, Genetic Mutation, Fetal Development and Malignancy', Stanislav Grof, Appendix II of *LSD Psychotherapy*, Stanislav Grof, Hunter House Publishers 1994.

page 65 (23) National average from www.fertilitysuccess.com.

(24) 'Recent thoughts on management and prevention of recurrent early pregnancy loss', Ai-Wei Tanga and Siobhan Quenby, *Current Opinion in Obstetrics and Gynecology*, Vol 22, pp.446–451, 2010.

(25) 'Reduction of blood flow impedance in the uterine arteries of infertile women with electro-acupuncture', Stener-Victorin, E *et al.*, *Human Reproduction*, Vol 11, pp.1314–17, 1996.

(26) 'A Pilot Study Evaluating the Combination of Acupuncture with Sildenafil on Endometrial Thickness', Yu, W *et al.*, presented at the Pacific Coast Reproductive Society Annual Conference 2007.

(27) 'A randomized, controlled, double blind, cross-over study evaluating acupuncture as an adjunct to IVF', Quintero, R *et al.*, *Fertility and Sterility*, Vol 81 (Supplement 3), S11–12,2004.

(28) 'Acupuncture and IVF Poor Responders: A Cure?', Magarelli, P and Cridennda, D, *Fertility and Sterility*, Vol 81 (Supplement 3), S20, 2004.

(29) 'Changes in serum cortisol and prolactin associated with acupuncture during controlled ovarian hyperstimulation in women undergoing in vitro fertilization–embryo transfer treatment', Magarelli, PC, Cridennda, D and Cohen, M, *Fertility and Sterility*, Vol 92, Issue 6, pp.1870–79, December 2009.

page 67 (30) 'Effect of Lepidium meyenii (MACA) on sexual desire and its absent relationship with serum testosterone levels in adult healthy men', Gonzales, GF *et al.*, *Andrologia*, Vol 34, Issue 6, pp.367–72, December 2002.

(31) 'Lepidium meyenii (maca) improved semen parameters in adult men', Gonzales, GF *et al.*, *Asian Journal of Andrology*, Vol 3, Issue 4, pp.301–3.

(32) 'Effect of maca supplementation on bovine sperm quantity and quality followed over two spermatogenic cycles', Clement, C *et al.*, *Theriogenology*, Vol 74, Issue 2, pp.173–83, 15 July 2010.

(33) 'Fertility and estrogenic activity of Turraeanthus africanus in combination with Lepidium meyenii (Black maca) in female mice', Lembe, DM *et al.*, *European Journal of Integrative Medicine*, Vol 4, Issue 3, E345–E351, September 2012.

(34) 'A prolactinoma masked by a herbal remedy', Joseph Gallagher, Frank Waldron Lynch and John Barragry, *European Journal of Obstetrics and Gynecology and Reproductive Biology*, Volume 137, Issue 2, pp.257–8, April 2008.

(35) 'Vitex agnus castus might enrich the pharmacological armamentarium for medical treatment of prolactinoma', Gianluca Tamagno, Maria C Burlacu, Adrian F Daly and Albert Beckers, *European Journal of Obstetrics and Gynecology and Reproductive Biology*, Vol 35, Issue 1, pp.139–40, November 2007.

(36) See note for page 25 (15).

(37) 'Fluoxetine versus Vitex agnus castus extract in the treatment of premenstrual dysphoric disorder', Atmaca, M, Kumru, S and Tezcan, E, *Human Psychopharmacology-Clinical and Experimental*, Vol 18, Issue 3, pp.191–5, April 2003.

(38) 'Vitex agnus-castus (Chaste-Tree/Berry) in the Treatment of Menopause-Related Complaints', van Die, MD *et al.*, *Journal Of Alternative and Complementary Medicine*, Vol 15, Issue 8, pp.853–62, August 2009.

(39) 'In vitro assays for bioactivity-guided isolation of endocrine active compounds in Vitex agnus-castus', Jarry, H *et al.*, *Maturitas*, Vol 55, Supplement 1, S26–S36, 1 November 2006.

(40) 'Casticin, a flavonoid isolated from Vitex rotundifolia, inhibits prolactin release in vivo and in vitro', Ye, Q *et al.*, *Acta Pharmacologica Sinica*, Vol 31, Issue 12, pp.1564–8, December 2010.

(41) 'Gynecological efficacy and chemical investigation of Vitex agnus-castus L. fruits growing in Egypt', Ibrahim, NA *et al.*, *Natural Product Research*, Vol 22, Issue 6, pp.537–46, 2009.

page 68 (42) 'In-vitro prolactin but not LH and FSH release is inhibited by compounds in extracts of agnus-castus – direct evidence for a dopaminergic principle by the dopamine-receptor assay', Jarry, H *et al.*, *Experimental and Clinical Endocrinology*, Vol 102, Issue 6, pp.448–54, 1994. See also 'Vitex agnus castus L. – Traditional drug and actual indications', Odenthal, KP, *Phytotherapy Research*, Vol 12, Supplement 1, S160–S161, 1998.

(43) 'Effectiveness of Vitex agnus-castus preparations', original title '*Zur Wirksamkeit von Vitex agnus castus-Praparaten*', Gorkow, C, Wuttke, W and Marz, RW, *Wiener medizinische Wochenschrift*, Vol 152, Issue 15–16, pp.364–72, 2002.

(44) http://medicinalplants.us/botanical-treatment-for-miscarriage.

(45) 'Effects of various heating methods on glucosinolate, carotenoid and tocopherol concentrations in broccoli', Eun-Sun Hwang and Gun-Hee Kim, *International Journal of Food Sciences and Nutrition*, Vol 64, Issue 1, pp.103–11, February 2013.

5 Up the duff

page 97 (1) 'Maternal pre-pregnancy underweight and fetal growth in relation to institute of medicine recommendations for gestational weight gain', Jeric, M *et al.*, *Early Human Development*, Vol 89, Issue 5, pp.277–8, 2015.

(2) 'Obesity in Pregnancy: A Big Problem and Getting Bigger', Mission, JF *et al.*, *Obstetrical and Gynecological Survey*, Vol 68, Issue 5, pp.389–99, 2013.

(3) 'Pregnancy after bariatric surgery – a review of benefits and risks', Kjaer, MM *et al.*, *Acta Obstetricia et Gynecologica Scandinavica*, Vol 92, Issue 3, pp.264–71, 2013.

page 98 (4) Information sourced from www.nhs.uk.

page 100 (5) www.examiner.com/article/smoking-during-pregnancy.

(6) 'Stereologic examination of placentas from mothers who smoke during pregnancy', Larsen, LG *et al.*, *American Journal of Obstetric Gynecology*, Vol 186, Issue 3, pp.531–7, 2002.

page 101 (7) 'Smoking During Pregnancy', *March of Dimes*, April 2008; and 'Teen Obesity Linked to Pre-birth Tobacco Exposure: Study', *The Gazette*, Canwest News Service, 27 April 2010.

(8) 'Fetal alcohol syndrome', http://www.ncbi.nlm.nih.gov/pubmedhealth/PMH0001909.

(9) 'Fetal Alcohol Exposure and IQ at Age 8: Evidence from a Population-Based Birth-Cohort Study', Luisa Zuccolo *et al.*, *Plus One*, November 2012.

page 104 (10) Fetal Abnormal Growth Associated With Substance Abuse, Soto, E, Bahado-Singh, R *et al.*, *Clinical Obstetrics and Gynecology*, Vol 56, Issue 1, pp142–53, March 2013. Also 'Duration of Methadone Maintenance Treatment During Pregnancy and Pregnancy Outcome Parameters in Women With Opiate Addiction', Peles, E *et al.*, *Journal of Addiction Medicine*, Vol 6, Issue 1, pp.18–23, March 2010. Also 'Neurobehavioral outcomes of infants exposed to MDMA (Ecstasy) and other recreational drugs during pregnancy', Singer, LT *et al.*, *Neurotoxicology and Teratology*, Vol 34, Issue 3, pp.303–10, March 2012. Also 'Infant With In Utero Ketamine Exposure: Quantitative Measurement of Residual Dosage in Hair', Pen-Hua Sul *et al.*, *Pediatric Neonatology*, Vol 51, Issue 5, pp.279–84, 2010.

(11) ' "Crack baby" study ends with unexpected but clear result', *Philadelphia Inquirer*, 22 July 2013.

(12) 'Transition to parenthood and substance use disorders: Findings from a 30-year longitudinal study', Fergusson, DM *et al.*, *Drug and Alcohol Dependence*, Vol 125, Issue 3, pp.295–300, October 2012.

(13) 'Birth outcomes associated with cannabis use before and during pregnancy', Hayatbakhsh, MR *et al.*, *Pediatric Research*, Vol 71, Issue 2, pp.215–19, February 2012.

(14) 'Marijuana use during pregnancy may reduce placental protective functions', Valeria Feinshtein *et al.*, *American Journal of Obstetrics and Gynecology*, Vol 204, Issue 1, Supplement, S59, January 2011.

(15) 'Intrauterine cannabis exposure leads to more aggressive behavior and attention problems in 18-month-old girls', El Marroun, H *et al.*, *Drug and Alcohol Dependence*, Vol 118, Issue 2–3, pp.470–74, November 2011.

(16) 'School achievement in 14-year-old youths prenatally exposed to marijuana', Goldschmidt, L *et al.*, *Neurotoxicology and Teratology*, Vol 34, Issue 1, pp.161–7 January 2012.

(17) 'Five-year follow-up of rural Jamaican children whose mothers used marijuana during pregnancy', Hayes, JS *et al*, *West Indian Medical Journal*, Vol 40, Issue 3, pp.120–23, September 1991.

(18) 'Cannabinoid hyperemesis syndrome: an under-reported entity causing nausea and vomiting of pregnancy', Schmid, SM *et al.*, *Archives of Gynecology and Obstetrics*, Vol 284, Issue 5, pp.1095–97, November 2011.

(19) 'Fetal Nicotine or Cocaine exposure, which one is worse?', Theodore A Slotkin, *Journal of Pharmacology and Experimental Therapeutics*, Vol 285, Issue 3, pp.931–45, June 1998.

page 114 (20) 'Change in Brain Size during and after Pregnancy: Study in Healthy Women and Women with Preeclampsia', Angela Oatridge *et al.*, *American Journal of Neuroradiology*, Vol 23, pp.19–26, 2002.

(21) 'Giving birth to a new brain: Hormone exposures of pregnancy influence human memory', Laura M Glynn, *Psychoneuroendocrinology*, Vol 35, Issue 8, pp.1148–55, September 2010.

(22) 'Emotional sensitivity for motherhood: Late pregnancy is associated with enhanced accuracy to encode emotional faces', Pearson, RM *et al.*, *Hormones and Behavior*, Vol 56, Issue 5, pp.557–63, November 2009.

(23) 'Attenuation of maternal psychophysiological stress responses and the maternal cortisol awakening response over the course of human pregnancy', Sonja Entringer *et al.*, *Stress*, Vol 13, No.3, pp.258–68, May 2010.

page 117 (24) 'Having a son or daughter with Down syndrome: Perspectives from mothers and fathers', Skotko BG *et al.*, *American Journal of Medical Genetics*, Vol 155, Issue 10, pp.2335–47, 2011.

6 Lost

page 126 (1) and (2) 'The condom broke!' Why do women in the UK have unintended pregnancies? Bury, L and Ngo, TD, Marie Stopes International, 2009.

(3) Surgical methods for first trimester termination of pregnancy' Kulier, R *et al*, Cochrane Fertility Regulation Group, July 2009.

(4) The risk of death as a result of childbirth is 14 times that of abortion. 'The comparative safety of legal induced abortion and childbirth in the United States', Raymond EG and Grimes DA, *Obstetrics and Gynecology*, Issue 119, Vol 2, Part 1, pp.215–19, February 2012.

(5) Induced abortion does not increase the risk of breast cancer, World Health Organisation, Fact Sheet No.240, June 2000.

(6) 'The effects of induced abortion on subsequent reproduction', Hogue, CJ *et al.*, *Epidemiologic Reviews*, Vol 4, pp.66–94, 1987.

page 128 (7) 'Abortion and long-term mental health outcomes: a systematic review of the evidence' Vignetta E Charles *et al.*, *Contraception*, Vol 78, pp.436–50, 2008.

7 Blooming marvellous!

page 147 (1) *Bumpology*, Linda Geddes, p.27.

8 Better shape up

page 148 (1) 'Association Between Preterm Delivery and Pre-pregnancy Body Mass (BMI), Exercise and Sleep During Pregnancy Among Working Women in Southern California', Guendelman, S *et al.*, *Maternal and Child Health Journal*, Vol 17, Issue 4, pp.723–31, 2013.

(2) 'Health Benefits of Physical Activity during Pregnancy: An International Perspective', Lanay M Mudd *et al.*, *Medicine and Science in Sports and Exercise*, accepted for publication July 2012.

(3) 'Scuba diving and pregnancy: can we determine safe limits?', St Leger Dowse, M *et al.*, *Journal of Obstetric Gynaecology*, Vol 26, Issue 6, pp.509–13, 2006.

page 150 (4) 'Postpartum sexual function of women and the effects of early pelvic-floor-muscle exercises', *Acta Obsterica et Gynecologica*, Vol 89, pp.817–22, 2010.

page 153 (5) and (6) 'The effects of yoga in prevention of pregnancy complications in high-risk pregnancies: A randomized controlled trial', Rakhshani, A *et al.*, *Preventive medicine*, Vol 55, Issue 4, pp.333–40, 2012. Also: 'Effect of the integrated approach of yoga therapy on platelet count and uric acid in pregnancy: A multicenter stratified randomized single-blind study', Jayashree, R *et al.*, *International Journal of Yoga*, Vol 6, Issue 1, pp.39–46, 2013.

(7) and (8) 'Mindfulness yoga during pregnancy for psychiatrically at-risk women: preliminary results from a pilot feasibility study', Muzik, M *et al.*, *Complementary therapies in clinical practice*, Vol 18, Issue 4, pp.235–40, 2012.

(9) 'Systematic Review of Yoga for Pregnant Women: Current Status and Future Directions', Curtis, K *et al.*, *Evidence-Based Complementary and Alternative Medicine*, 2012.

12 Baby, get down!

page 191 (1) 'Hands and knees posture in late pregnancy or labour for fetal malposition (lateral or posterior)', Hunter S *et al.*, *Cochrane Database of Systematic Reviews* Issue 1, 2009. The study only analyses the effect of getting on hands and knees for ten minutes twice a day, which may not be enough to make a difference.

page 194 (2) 'Cephalic version by moxibustion for breech presentation (Review)', Coyle, ME *et al.*, *Cochrane Database of Systematic Reviews*, Issue 5, 2012.

14 The waiting game

page 200 (1) 'Sexual intercourse for cervical ripening and induction of labour (Review)', Kavanagh, J *et al.*, *Cochrane Database of Systematic Reviews*, Issue 4, 2008. The study found that 86% of women and 93% of men wanted to know whether having sex works to bring on labour. I love the fact that the men were more keen to find out!

(2) 'Breast stimulation for cervical ripening and induction of labour (Review)', Kavanagh, J *et al.*, *Cochrane Database of Systematic Reviews*, Issue 1, 2010.

16 How Monkey Mama does it

The midwife in this chapter is a portrait of Mary Cronk.

page 228 (1) I am indebted to the work of Dr Sarah Buckley and her ebook *Ecstatic Birth: Nature's Hormonal Blueprint for Labor* for this synopsis of the hormonal interactions of birth. I have simplified things slightly.

High levels of beta-endorphin, produced in response to stress or severe pain, also have the ability to quell contractions. I couldn't fit that bit in.

page 229 (2) The word 'monkey' is used here to encourage women to connect with our evolutionary history: the fact that we have been giving birth since before we were human. The uniquely human part of the brain, the outer neo-cortex that controls our calculating, thinking and reasoning, actually impedes birth. The inner 'emotional' brain, the one that is structurally similar in all mammals, controls the hormones of birth, and surrendering to its dictates – feeling, rather than thinking – is the best way to let birth progress. Midwife Ina May Gaskin uses the same phrase when she exhorts birthing women to 'let your monkey do it'.

I can't think of a better word than 'monkey', but it is problematic. It has been used as a racist term of abuse, and within the discourse of Western colonialism indigenous mothers and midwives have been, and continue to be, labelled as 'animals', as 'less than human'. I have been careful to address this in my text. The representation of Monkey Mama is of a white woman, and the setting is in our pre-colonial past. The following chapter further deconstructs the racist stereotype of the white Western medical model as 'human' and indigenous birthing wisdom as 'animal' by portraying birth technicians in the hospital setting as silverback gorillas.

We truly are *all* monkeys (OK, apes, if you want to be pedantic) and I think we would do well to remember it. I want women to be able to reclaim the word. I accept that as a white woman I'm not the best person to lead the call. But neither do I want to self-censor words which may help women birth.

(3) *Mayes Midwifery*, Twelfth Edition ed. Betty Sweet, p.351, 1997.

page 230 (4) See the work of Robbie Davis-Floyd, who has reclaimed the phrase 'the oldest profession' for midwifery. (No, prostitution is not the oldest profession: it's the oldest capitalist exploitation. Humanity predates capitalism, and will hopefully outlive it too.)

(5) *Mayes Midwifery, ibid.* p.351

page 231 (6) 'Maternal hormone protects baby's brain during birth', *New Scientist*, 15 December 2006, reporting the work of animal experiments conducted by Yehezkel Ben-Ari, a neuroscientist at the Mediterranean Institute of Neurobiology in Marseille, France.

page 233 (7) 'Lunar cycles and birth rates: from a full Moon to a first quarter Moon effect', Arthur Charpentier, PhD France, CREM-Université, Rennes.

page 234 (8) *'I learned what is simple with my very first experience of childbirth as a medical student in 1953. At that time, a midwife had nothing to do. She was spending her life knitting. So, she was knitting when she was waiting for the baby, knitting when waiting for the placenta, knitting when there was no woman in labor. She had nothing else to do. In that respect, I realized the value of this traditional attitude.*

'Some scientists at Cambridge University in the UK explored the philological responses to a repetitive task. As an example of a repetitive task, they studied the task of knitting. When you are doing a repetitive task like knitting, you reduce your level of adrenaline. And that is the key to an easy birth – when the level of adrenaline of the midwife is low, because she is contagious. That helps the woman in labor to also be in a state of relaxation… and finally the birth is easier.' Michel Odent, in interview 'Rediscovering the Best Environment for an Easy Birth'.

page 235 (9) 'The purple line as a measure of labour progress: a longitudinal study', Ashley Shepherd *et al.*, *BMC Pregnancy and Childbirth*, Vol 10, p.54, 2010.

(10) The 'rest and be thankful' stage is described by Denis Walsh in the chapter 'Rhythms in the second stage of labour' in *Evidence and Skills for Normal Labour and Birth*, Routledge 2007, 2nd ed.2011.

page 236 (11) This phrase, and the description of the baby's descent, are inspired by Gloria LeMay's article 'Pushing for First-Time Moms', *Midwifery Today*, Issue 55, autumn 2000. This pattern of pushing could be typical of primagravida mothers – women who haven't had a baby before. A subsequent birth is likely to be more rapid.

page 237 (12) 'Perineal techniques during the second stage of labour for reducing perineal trauma', Aasheim, V *et al.*, *Cochrane Database of Systematic Reviews*, Issue 12, 2011.

(13) This is a description of the foetus ejection reflex, as identified by Michel Odent. I've had two. They exist.

page 238 (14) This baby has a nuchal cord (the umbilical cord wrapped around the neck). I was struck by the similiarity between the 'somersault manoeuvre' to free a nuchal cord and the movements that a mother would make to grasp her own baby at birth.

(15) 'Effect of timing of umbilical cord clamping of term infants on maternal and neonatal outcomes', McDonald, S and Middleton, P, *Cochrane Database of Systematic Reviews*, Issue 2, 2008.

page 239 (16) *Ecstatic Birth: Nature's Hormonal Blueprint for Labor*, ibid.

page 240 (17) 'Breast Crawl: a scientific overview', www.breastcrawl.org, January 2013.

17 Totally bananas

page 242 (1) *The Manner Born: Birth Rites in Cross-Cultural Perspective*, ed. Lauren Dundes, p.58, AltaMira Press 2003.

(2) 'Supine position compared to other positions during the second stage of labour: a meta-analytic review', De Jonge, A *et al.*, *Journal of Psychosomatic Obstetrics and Gynecology*, Vol 25, pp.35–45, 2004.

page 243 (3) (4) and (6) See previous reference. Also: 'Position for women in the second stage of labour', Gupta, JK *et al.*, *Cochrane Database of Systematic Reviews*, Issue 4, 2006.

(5) 'Factors Related To Perineal Trauma In Childbirth', Leah L Albers *et al.*, *Journal of Nurse-Midwifery*, Vol 41, Issue 4, pp.269–76, August 1996. Also: 'Maternal position and other variables: effects on perineal outcomes in 557 births', Meyvis, I *et al.*, *Birth*, Vol 39, Issue 2, pp.115–20, June 2012.

(7) On the subject of assisted birth in upright positions, Denis Walsh writes 'obstetricians… have to think through the direction of traction which is reversed from the conventional lithotomy pose. It does not make the procedure more technical or complex but does require them to move out of the comfort zone of convention.' *Evidence and Skills for Normal Labour and Birth*, Routledge 2007, 2nd ed. 2011, p.79.

page 244 (8) *Rediscovering Birth*, Sheila Kitzinger, Pinter and Martin 2011, p.234.

page 245 (9) 'Informed consent for epidural analgesia in labour: a survey of UK practice, Middle, J and Wee, Y, *Anaesthesia*, Vol 64, pp.161–4.

(10) *Ecstatic Birth*, Dr Sarah Buckley, p.8. Also: 'Plasma oxytocin levels in women during labor with or without epidural analgesia: a prospective study', Rahm, V *et al.*, *Acta Obstetrica et Gynecologica Scandivica*, Vol 81, pp.1033–9.

(11) 'Effects of epidural anaesthesia on plasma catecholamines and cortisol in parturition', Neumark, J *et al.*, *Acta Anaesthesia Scandinavia*, Vol 29, Issue 6, pp.555–9.

(12) 'Effects of epidural analgesia during labor on pelvic floor function after vaginal delivery', Sartore, A *et al.*, *Acta Obstetrica et Gynecologica Scandinavica*, Vol 82, pp.143–6.

(13) 'Epidural versus non-epidural or no analgesia in labour', Anim-Soumah, M *et al.*, *Cochrane Database of Systematic Reviews*, Issue 2, 2011.

(14) 'The effects of maternal epidural anesthesia on neonatal behavior during the first month', Sepkoski, CM *et al.*, *Developmental Medicine and Child Neurology*, Vol 34, Issue 12, pp.1072–80, 1992.

(15) 'Effects of epidural anesthesia on newborns and their mothers', Murray, AD *et al.*, *Child Development*, Vol 52, Issue 1, pp.71–82, 1981.

(16) 'Effect of labor epidural analgesia with and without fentanyl on infant breast-feeding: a prospective, randomized, double-blind study', Beilin, Y *et al.*, *Anesthesiology*, Vol 103, Issue 6, pp.1211–17, 2005.

(17) 'Diamorphine for pain relief in labour: a randomised controlled trial comparing intramuscular injection and patient-controlled analgesia', McInnes, R *et al.*, *British*

References

Journal of Obstetrics and Gyneacology, Vol 1119, Issue 10, pp.1081–9, 2004.

(18) *Pain in Childbearing and Its Control*, Mander, R, Wiley-Blackwell 2011.

(19) 'Parenteral opioids for maternal pain relief in labour', Ullman, R *et al., Cochrane Database of Systematic Reviews*, Issue 9, 2010.

(20) 'Maternal analgesia during labour disturbs newborn behaviour: effects on breastfeeding, temperature and crying', Ransjo-Arvidson, A *et al., Birth*, Vol 23, Issue 3, pp.136–4, 2001.

(21) *Evidence and Skills for Normal Labour and Birth*, Walsh, D, Routledge 2007, 2nd ed. 2011, p.97.

page 246 (22) 'Opiate addiction in adult offspring through possible imprinting after obstetric treatment', Jacobson, B *et al., British Medical Journal*, Vol 301, pp.1067–70, 1990. Also: 'Perinatal medication as a potential risk factor for adult drug abuse in a North American cohort', Nyberg, K *et al., Epidemiology*, Vol 11, Issue 6, pp.715–16, 2000.

(23) 'Nitrous oxide for relief of labour pain: a systematic review', Rosen, M, *American Journal of Obstetrics and Gynecology*, Vol 186, Issue 5, S110–S126, May 2002.

(24) Denis Walsh makes an important additional point that, since severe pain can be a sign of pathology, midwives should be familiar with undrugged normal birth in order to distinguish the abnormal. *Evidence and Skills for Normal Labour and Birth*, Walsh, D, Routledge 2007, 2nd ed. 2011, p.97.

page 247 (25) Stillbirth rates of 1 in 926 at 40 weeks, 1 in 645 at 37 weeks and 1 in 633 at 43 weeks. Figures from the Association for the Improvement in Maternity Services.

(26) 'Aging of the placenta', Fox, H, *Archives of Disease in Childhood*, Vol 77, F165–F170, 1997.

page 248 (27) *Evidence and Skills for Normal Labour and Birth*, Walsh, D, Routledge 2007, 2nd ed. 2011, p.42.

(28) 'Midwives' perspectives in 11 UK maternity units', Mead, M. In S. Downe (ed.), *Normal Childbirth: Evidence and Debate*, Churchill Livingstone 2008.

(29) Denis Walsh writes of syntocinon augmentation: *'To cope with this chemically enhanced pain, epidural anaesthesia is probably appropriate.' Evidence and Skills for Normal Labour and Birth*, Routledge 2007, 2nd ed. 2011, p88.

(30) and **[page 249]** (31) *Ecstatic Birth: Nature's Hormonal Blueprint for Labor*, Buckley, S, p.8.

(32) 'Outcome in obstetric care related to oxytocin use: a population-based study', Oscarsson, M *et al., Acta Obstetrica et Gynecologica*, Vol 85, Issue 9, pp.1094–8.

(33) 'Continuous cardiotocography (CTG) as a form of electronic fetal monitoring (EFM) for fetal assessment during labour', Alfirevic, Z *et al., Cochrane Database of Systematic Reviews*, Issue 3, 2006. *'The review is dominated by one large, well-conducted trial of almost 13,000 women who received one-to-one care throughout labour. In this trial, the membranes were ruptured artificially (amniotomy) as early as possible and oxytocin stimulation of contractions was used in about a quarter of the women.'* This analysis of the (in)effectiveness of continuous versus intermittent monitoring is particularly relevant to women who have been given syntocinon, and the serious risk of increased interventions balanced against questionable benefit to the baby applies.

(34) 'Oxytocin versus no treatment or delayed treatment for slow progress in the first stage of spontaneous labour (Review)', Bugg, GJ *et al., Cochrane Database of Systematic Reviews*, Issue 6, 2013.

(35) 'Re-evaluation of Friedmann's labour curve: a pilot study', Cesario, S, *Journal of Obstetric, Gynecologic and Neonatal Nursing*, Vol 33, pp.713–22, 2004.

(36) 'The natural history of the first stage of labour', Zhang, J *et al., Obstetrics and Gynecology*, Vol 115, Issue 4, pp.705–10, 2010.

(37) 'Understanding birth and Sphincter Law', Gaskin, IM, *British Journal of Midwifery*, Vol 12, Issue 9, 2004.

page 250 (38) This is the subject of a forthcoming review of available evidence by the Cochrane Collaboration, which should provide an answer to this question.

(39) *'Knowing the precise amount of cervical dilation does not appear to be a good predictor of how labour progress may proceed'* – a quote from 'Routine vaginal examinations for assessing progress of labour to improve outcomes for women and babies at term (Protocol)', Downe, S *et al.*, *Cochrane Database of Systematic Reviews*, Issue 9, 2012.

(40) 'How reliable is the determination of cervical dilation? Comparison of vaginal examination with spatial position-tracking ruler', Nizard, J *et al.*, *American Journal of Obstetrics and Gynecology*, Vol 200, Issue 4, No.402, 2009.

(41) 'Effect of partogram use on outcomes for women in spontaneous labour at term (Review)', Lavender, T *et al.*, *Cochrane Database of Systematic Reviews*, Issue 7, 2013.

(42) 'Amniotomy for shortening spontaneous labour (Review)', Smyth, RMD *et al.*, *Cochrane Database of Systematic Reviews*, Issue 6, 2013.

page 251 (43) The National Institute for Clinical Care and Excellence *'Do not do recommendations: Induction of labour'* – Guidance ID CG70, Recommendation ID 282.

(44) 'Restricting oral fluid and food intake during labour (Review)', Singata, M *et al.*, *Cochrane Database of Systematic Reviews*, Issue 11, 2012.

(45) *Rediscovering Birth*, Sheila Kitzinger, Pinter and Martin 2011, p.224.

(46) and (47) 'Continuous cardiotocography (CTG) as a form of electronic fetal monitoring (EFM) for fetal assessment during labour', Alfirevic, Z *et al.*, *Cochrane Database of Systematic Reviews*, Issue 3, 2006.

(48) *'After adjustment for potential confounders, the risk of postpartum death was 3.6 times higher after cesarean than after vaginal delivery,'* 'Postpartum Maternal Mortality and Cesarean Delivery', Deneux-Tharaux, C *et al*, *Obstetrics and Gynecology*, Vol 108, Issue 3, pp.541–48, 2006.

(49) *'Women having an emergency caesarean section had more than six times the risk of developing postpartum depression at three months postpartum.'* 'Increased risk of postnatal depression after emergency caesarean section', Boyce, MP and Todd, AL, *The Medical Journal of Australia*, Vol 157, pp.172–4, 1992.

(50) 'Previous caesarean increases women's risk of miscarriage: Mode of delivery and future fertility', Hall, MH *et al.*, *BJOG: An International Journal of Obstetrics and Gynaecology*, Vol 96, Issue 11, pp.1297–1303, 1989.

(51) 'Comparison of a trial of labor with an elective second caesarean section', McMahon, MJ *et al.*, *New England Journal of Medicine*, Vol 335, Issue 10, pp.689–95, 1996. Also: 'Previous caesarean increases women's risk of miscarriage: Mode of delivery and future fertility', Hall, MH *et al.*, *BJOG: An International Journal of Obstetrics and Gynaecology*, Vol 96, Issue 11, pp.1297–1303, 1989.

(52) 'Uncertain value of electronic fetal monitoring in predicting cerebral palsy', Nelson, K *et al.*, *New England Journal of Medicine*, Vol 334, pp.659–60, 1996.

page 252 (53) *'professionals... recognised that the CTG offered a false sense of security'*, 'Continuous cardiotocography (CTG) as a form of electronic fetal monitoring (EFM) for fetal assessment during labour', Alfirevic, Z *et al.*, *Cochrane Database of Systematic Reviews*, Issue 3, 2006.

page 253 (54) *The impact of CTG monitoring on caesarean section in low-risk and high-risk populations appears to be virtually identical, which is contrary to recommendations from many professional bodies providing guidance on intrapartum fetal monitoring.'* Quoted from 'Continuous cardiotocography (CTG) as a form of electronic fetal monitoring (EFM) for fetal assessment during labour', Alfirevic, Z *et al.*, *Cochrane Database of Systematic Reviews*, Issue 3, 2006.

(55) 'Intrapartum electronic fetal monitoring vs. intermittent auscultation in post caesarean pregnancies', Madaan, M and Trivedi, S, *International Journal of Gynecology and Obstetrics*, Vol 94, pp.123–5, 2006.

(56) 'Bioengineering principles of hydrotherapy', Edlich, RF *et al.*, *Journal of Burn Care and Rehabilitation*, Vol 8, Issue 6, pp.580–4, 1987.

(57) 'Observing position and movement in hydrotherapy: a pilot study', Stark, M and Miller, M, *Journal of Obstetric, Gynecologic and Neonatal Nursing*, Vol 37, pp.116–22, 2008.

References

(58) 'Warm tub bathing during labor: maternal and neonatal effects', Ohlsson, G *et al.*, *Acta Obstetricia et Gynecologica Scandinavica*, Vol 80, pp.311–14, 2001.

(59) 'The effects of maternal hyperthermia on maternal and fetal cardiovascular and respiratory function', Cefalo RC *et al.*, *American Journal of Obstetrics and Gynecology*, Vol 131, Issue 6, pp.687–94, 1978.

(60) *Evidence and Skills for Normal Labour and Birth*, Walsh, D, Routledge 2007, 2nd ed. 2011, p.144 and p.147.

(61) 'Immersion in water in labour and birth (Review)', Cluett, ER and Burns, E, *Cochrane Database of Systematic Reviews*, Issue 2, 2012.

page 254 (62) 'Staying in control: women's experiences of labour in water', Hall, SM and Holloway, IM, *Midwifery*, Vol 14, Issue 1, pp.30–36, 1998.

(63) 'Immersion in water in labour and birth (Review)', Cluett, ER and Burns, E, *Cochrane Database of Systematic Reviews*, Issue 2, 2012.

(64) 'Birth under water: to breathe or not to breathe', Johnson, P, *BJOG: An International Journal of Obstetrics and Gynaecology*, Vol 103, Issue 3, pp.202–208, 1996.

(65) *Evidence and Skills for Normal Labour and Birth*, Walsh, D, Routledge 2007, 2nd ed. 2011, p.144.

(66) 'Underwater Birth: Missing the Evidence or Missing the Point?', Bowden *et al.*, *Pediatrics*, Vol 112, Issue 4, pp.972–3, 2003.

(67) 'Warm tub bathing during labor: maternal and neonatal effects', Ohlsson, G *et al. Acta Obstetricia et Gynecologica Scandinavica*, Vol 80, pp.311–14, 2001.

(68) '*When you put a birth pool on a hospital unit, [staff] have not been oriented to the natural phenomenon of women labouring in ecstasy.*' Barbara Harper, founder of Waterbirth International, interviewed for oneworldbirth. net. YouTube: 'Waterbirths and Hospitals'.

(69) The one trial to investigate this issue found that getting in the birthing pool in early labour can speed labour up, not slow it down: 'Randomised controlled trial of labouring in water compared with standard of augmentation for the management of dystocia in first stage of labour', Cluett *et al.*, *British Medical Journal*, Vol 328, pp.314–20, 2004.

(70) 'Underwater Birth: Missing the Evidence or Missing the Point?' Bowden *et al.*, *Pediatrics*, Vol 112, Issue 4, pp.972–3, 2003.

(71) 'Underwater Births' Committee on Fetus and Newborn', 2004–2005, Daniel G Batton *et al.*, *Pediatrics*, Vol 115, Issue 5, pp.1413–14, 2005.

(72) This tradition can be traced back to François Mariceau, an early populariser of the lithotomy position, who included the practice in his textbook *Traité des Maladies des Femmes Grosses et Accouchées* of 1668.

page 255 (73) The descent of the presenting part of the baby past the ischial spines is posited as a more useful point from which to measure the beginning of the second stage of labour than full cervical dilation. This allows for a pause between the first and second stages, as illustrated on page 235.

(74) There are four randomised controlled trials that compare the speed of the second stage with directed versus spontaneous pushing. Two found that the second stage was shorter with spontaneous pushing, and two found it was shorter with directed pushing. That's a draw. The trials are: 'Pushing techniques in the second stage of labour', Thomson, A, *Journal of Advanced Nursing*, Vol 18, pp.171–7, 1993; 'Pushing method in the expulsive stage of labour: a randomised trial', Parnell, C *et al.*, *Acta Obstetrica et Gynecologica Scandivica*, Vol 72, Issue 1, pp.31–5, 1993; 'A randomized trial of coached versus uncoached maternal pushing during the second stage of labor', Bloom *et al. American Journal of Obstetrics and Gynecology*, Vol 194, pp.10–13, 2006; 'Effects of pushing techniques on mother and fetus: a randomized study', Yildirim, G and Beji, N, *Birth*, Vol 35, Issue 1, pp.25–30, 2008.

(75) 'Contemporary patterns of spontaneous labor with normal neonatal outcomes', Zhang, J *et al.*, *Obstetrics and Gynecology*, Vol 116, Issue 6, pp.1281–7, 2010. This is a non-randomised study.

(76) 'The effects of maternal pushing on fetal cerebral oxygenation and blood volume during the second stage of labour', Aldrich, C *et al.*, *British Journal of Obstetrics and Gynaecology*, Vol 102, Issue 6, pp.448–53, 1995.

(77) 'The "push" for evidence: management of the second stage', Roberts, J, *Journal of Midwifery and Women's Health*, Vol 47, Issue 1, pp.2–15, 2002. Also: 'Effects of pushing techniques in birthing chair on length of second stage of labour', Knauth, D and Haloburdo, E, *Nursing Research*, Vol 35, pp.49–51, 1986.

(78) 'Active pushing versus passive fetal descent in the second stage of labour: a randomised controlled trial', Hansen, S *et al.*, *Obstetrics and Gynecology*, Vol 199, pp.29–34, 2002.

(79) 'Spontaneous pushing during birth: relationship to perineal outcomes', Sampselle, C and Hines, S, *Journal of Midwifery and Women's Heath*, Vol 44, Issue 1, pp.36–9, 1999.

(80) 'A randomized trial of the effect of coached vs uncoached maternal pushing during the second stage of labor on postpartum pelvic floor structure and function', Schaffer, J *et al.*, *American Journal of Obstetrics and Gynecology*, Vol 194, pp.1692–6, 2005.

(81) '*Increased maternal satisfaction*' is one of the outcomes of spontaneous pushing cited in 'Effects of pushing techniques on mother and fetus: a randomized study', Yildirim, G and Beji, N, *Birth*, Vol 35, Issue 1, pp.25–30, 2008.

page 256 (82) Denis Walsh writes: '*I don't think there is one other area of normal birth where the research evidence is so unequivocal. There is no justification for the continued practice of coached pushing and it is probably putting women and babies at unnecessary risk.*' *Evidence and Skills for Normal Labour and Birth*, Routledge 2007, 2nd ed. 2011, p.106.

(83) 'Early pushing urge in labour and midwifery practice: A prospective observational study at an Italian maternity hospital', Borrelli, SE *et al.*, *Midwifery*, Vol 29, Issue 8, August 2013, pp.871–5, August 2013.

(84) 'The Prophylactic Forceps Operation', DeLee, JB, 1920, reprinted in *American Journal of Obstetrics and Gynecology*, Vol 187, Issue 1, pp.254–5, 2002.

(85) *Rediscovering Birth*, Sheila Kitzinger, Pinter and Martin 2011, p.112.

(86) A 96% episiotomy rate is quoted in 'Episotomy and the perineum: a random controlled trial', House, MJ *et al.*, *Journal of Obstetrics and Gynaecology*, Vol 7, pp.107–10, 1986.

(87) *Birthing Your Baby: the Second Stage*, Nadine Pilley Edwards and Beverley Beech, AIMS 2001, p.73.

(88) See 'Newborn Birth Injuries: the Untold Story' on YouTube for a succinct explanation of the iatrogenic brachial plexus injuries that result.

(89) Routine episiotomy also increases the likelihood of a severe tear, and leads to decreased pelvic floor strength, increased pain, and higher incidence of sexual dysfunction after the birth. Denis Walsh, *Evidence and Skills for Normal Labour and Birth*, Routledge 2007, 2nd ed. 2011, p.119.

(90) and **page 257** (91) 'Effect of timing of umbilical cord clamping of term infants on maternal and neonatal outcomes', McDonald, S and Middleton, P, *Cochrane Database of Systematic Reviews*, Issue 2, 2008.

(92) 'Neonatal Transitional Physiology: A New Paradigm', Mercer, JS and Skovgaard, R, *Journal of Perinatal and Neonatal Nursing* Vol 15, Issue 4, pp.56–75, 2002.

(93) In response to the question, can delayed cord clamping (DCC) lead to dangerously high levels of neonatal jaundice? Dr Mark Sloan writes: '*Since bilirubin, the source of neonatal jaundice, originates in red blood cells, it seems logical that the increased blood volume associated with delayed clamping could lead to severe hyperbilirubinemia. Yet while some studies have demonstrated mildly increased bilirubin levels in DCC babies in the first few days postpartum, most have found no significant difference between DCC and ICC [immediate cord clamping]. This seeming paradox – relatively stable bilirubin levels in the face of substantially increased blood*

volume – may have to do with increased blood flow to the neonatal liver that comes with the higher total blood volume associated with DCC. Yes, more blood means more bilirubin, which in turn could mean more jaundice, but better blood flow allows the liver to process bilirubin more efficiently.' 'Common Objections to Delayed Cord Clamping – What's The Evidence Say?', scienceandsensibility.org, 13 November 2012.

(94) 'Effect of delayed versus early umbilical cord clamping on neonatal outcomes and iron status at 4 months: a randomised controlled trial', Andersson, O et al., British Medical Journal, Vol 343, 2011.

(95) 'Timing of umbilical cord clamping: effect on iron endowment of the newborn and later iron status', Chaparro, CM, Nutrition Reviews, Vol 69, Issue Supplement S1, pages S30–S36, November 2011.

(96) 'Evidence for Neonatal Transition and the First Hour of Life', Judith Mercer and Debra Erikson-Owens, from Intrapartum Care (Essential Midwifery Practice), ed. Soo Downe and Denis Walsh, Blackwell 2010.

(97) RCOG statement on the benefits of delayed cord clamping: 'Delayed cord clamping (more than 30 seconds) may benefit the neonate in reducing anaemia, and particularly the preterm neonate by allowing time for transfusion of placental blood to the newborn infant. For the mother, delayed clamping does not increase the risk of postpartum haemorrhage. However, early clamping may be required if there is postpartum haemorrhage, placenta praevia or vasa praevia, if there is a tight nuchal cord **or if the baby is asphyxiated and requires immediate resuscitation**.' [my emphasis].

page 258 (98) There are instances of babies pronounced dead at birth being revived by maternal touch: 'Jamie Ogg, Baby Pronounced Dead Then Revived By Mother's Touch, Celebrates Second Birthday This Month', Huffington Post, 3 September 2012.

(99) 'Outcome of infants born with nuchal cords', Miser, WF, Journal of Family Practice, Vol 34, Issue 4, pp.441–5, 1992.

(100) 'Cutting the umbilical cord before birth is an intervention that has been associated with hypovolemia, anemia,

shock, hypoxic-ischemic encephalopathy, and cerebral palsy. This article proposes use of the somersault maneuver followed by delayed cord clamping for management of nuchal cord at birth.' 'Nuchal cord management and nurse-midwifery practice', Mercer, JS et al., Journal of Midwifery and Women's Health, Vol 50, Issue 5, pp.373–9, 2005.

(101) 'Delayed Cord Clamping in Very Preterm Infants Reduces the Incidence of Intraventricular Hemorrhage and Late-Onset Sepsis: A Randomized, Controlled Trial', Mercer, J et al., Pediatrics, Vol. 117, Issue 4, pp.1235–42, 2006.

(102) I saw a brilliant TV programme about this years ago. If any readers have more precise sources of ethnopediatric research, please get in touch.

(103) 'The Breast Crawl', summarised at www.breastcrawl.org/science.

page 259 (104) Feeding formula milk was associated with a fourfold increased risk of death. This isn't because poorly babies are less likely to breastfeed at birth – the finding holds true when examining babies who had nothing wrong with them. 'Delayed Breastfeeding Initiation Increases Risk of Neonatal Mortality', Edmond, K et al., Pediatrics, Vol. 117, Issue 3, e380–e386, 2006.

(105) 'Active versus expectant management for women in the third stage of labour (Review)', Begley, CM et al., Cochrane Database of Systematic Reviews, Issue 11, 2011.

(106) Birthing Your Placenta: the Third Stage, Pilley Edwards, N and Wickham, S, Association for Improvements in the Maternity Services, AIMS 2011, p.57.

page 260 (107) and (108) 'Risk of Severe Postpartum Hemorrhage in Low-Risk Childbearing Women in New Zealand: Exploring the Effect of Place of Birth and Comparing Third Stage Management of Labor', Davis, D et al., Birth, Vol 39, Issue 2, pp.98–105, June 2012. Also: 'Holistic physiological care compared with active management of the third stage of labour for women at low risk of postpartum haemorrhage: A cohort study', Fahy, K et al., Women and Birth, Vol 23, pp.145–52, 2010. The protocol is from this study by Fahy et al.

(109) Royal College of Obstetricians and Gynaecologists Green Top Guideline 52: 'Prevention and Management of Postpartum Haemorrhage', April 2009.

18 Risky business

page 262 (1), (2) and (3) *'for low-risk pregnancies both home and hospital births are sufficiently safe for safety no longer to be of overriding importance.'* 'Planned hospital birth versus planned home birth (Review)', Olsen, O and Clausen, JA, *Cochrane Database of Systematic Reviews*, Issue 2, 2013.

(4) Actually, it's more complicated than that, because planned home births that end up as emergency transfers to hospital really should be included in the home birth statistics. But then, if a woman changes her mind in early labour and decides to go to hospital for no particular medical reason, that's a hospital birth, not a home birth. Confusing.

(5) 'Maternal and newborn outcomes in planned home birth vs planned hospital births: a meta analysis', Wax, JR *et al.*, *American Journal of Obstetrics and Gynecology*, Vol 203, Issue 3, 2010. This research is flawed. Please see: 'Safety of planned home births. Findings of meta-analysis cannot be relied on', Gyte, G *et al.*, *British Medical Journal*, Vol 341, c4033, 2010.

(6) 'Perinatal mortality and morbidity in a nationwide cohort of 529,688 low-risk planned home and hospital births', DeJonge, A *et al.*, *BJOG: An International Journal of Obstetrics and Gynaecology*, Vol 116, Issue 9, pp.1177–84, 2009. Also: 'Outcomes of planned home birth with registered midwife versus hospital birth with midwife or physician', Janssen, P *et al.*, *Canadian Medical Association Journal*, Vol 181, Issue 6–7, pp.377–83, 2009.

page 263 (7) 'Alternative versus conventional institutional settings for birth (Review)', Hodnett, ED *et al.*, *Cochrane Database of Systematic Reviews*, Issue 8, 2012.

(8) 'Continuous support for women during childbirth', Hodnett, ED *et al.*, *Cochrane Database of Systematic Reviews*, Issue 2, 2011.

page 264 (9) 'Why does the Albany Midwifery Model work?', Edwards, N, *AIMS Journal*, 2010, Vol 22, No.1, 2010.

(10) 'Response to the Department of Health on the Vision for Nursing and Midwifery', p.5, Royal College of Midwives, November 2012.

(11) '£20bn NHS cuts are hitting patients', *Guardian*, 17 October 2011.

(12) A shortfall of 5,000 midwifery posts has persisted since the last election. A Conservative promise to increase the numbers of midwives by 3,000 has been translated into an actual increase of 145 posts. 'Nick Clegg denies government "deception" over midwife numbers', BBC News, 1 April 2013.

(13) 'Midwives attack hysteria over home births', Randeep Ramesh, *Guardian*, 16 August 2010.

(14) Disclaimer: I'm not actually serious here.

(15) 'Response to the Department of Health on the Vision for Nursing and Midwifery', p.5, Royal College of Midwives, November 2012.

page 265 (16) *'Ethnographic studies of large obstetric-led labour wards have revealed their hierarchical, institutional and medically led ethos that make the carving out of a "birth as normal" space in their midst problematic indeed.'* *Evidence and Skills for Normal Labour and Birth*, Walsh, D, Routledge 2007, 2nd ed. 2011.

(17) 'The lessons from the Savage inquiry', *British Medical Journal*, Vol 293, p.285, 1986.

(18) 'Why does the Albany Midwifery Model work?', Edwards, N, *AIMS Journal*, Vol 22, No.1, 2010.

(19) 'A happy birthday every day', Lucy Atkins, *Guardian*, 24 July 2007.

page 266 (20) 'Critique of the CMACE Report on the Albany Midwifery Practice', Edwards, N and Davies, S, *AIMS Journal*, Vol 22, No.3, 2010.

(21) 'Midwife Agnes Gereb taken to court for championing home births', Amelia Hill, *Guardian*, 22 October 2010.

(22) 'Extreme childbirth: Freebirthing', Anna Gosline, *New Scientist*, Issue 2585, 6 January 2007.

page 267 (23) 'Planned home versus planned hospital births: Adverse outcomes comparison by reviewing the international literature', Faucon, C and Brillac, T, *Gynecologie Obstetrique and Fertilite*, Vol 41, Issue 6, pp.388–93, June 2013. Also: 'Are First-Time Mothers Who Plan Home Birth More Likely to Receive Evidence-Based Care? A Comparative Study of Home and Hospital Care Provided by the Same Midwives', Miller, S and Skinner, J, *Birth-Issues In Perinatal Care*, Vol 39, Issue 2, pp.135–44, June 2012 (they do receive more evidence-based care.)

page 268 (24) 'Health and Social Care Bill 2011: a legal basis for charging and providing fewer health services to people in England', Pollock, AM *et al.*, *British Medical Journal*, Vol 344, e1729, 2012.

(25) Figures for 2008–2012 from data.worldbank.org

(26) Figure for national wealth from Wikipedia. *'This figure is an important indicator of a nation's ability to take on debt and sustain spending.'*

page 269 (27) See 'Tales of loss', pp.45–58, *Birth Stories for the Soul*, ed. Walsh, D and Byrom, S, Quay Books 2009.

(28) 'Home delivery: why independent midwives are key to the fight for birth freedom', Milli Hill, *Daily Telegraph*, 25 March 2013. Also: 'Independent midwives – and home births – are under threat', Notes and Theories, *Guardian*, 15 May 2013.

(29) 'Urgent meeting request with Independent Midwives UK (IMUK), Daniel Poulter and Jeremy Hunt – re PII for Independent Midwives', www.independentmidwives. org.uk.

(30) 'NHS patients to be treated by Virgin Care in £500m deal', *Daily Telegraph*, 30 March 2012.

(31) 'NHS reform leaves Tory backers with links to private healthcare firms set for bonanza', *Daily Mirror*, 19 January 2011.

19 Birth rights

page 270 (1) Ternovsky v Hungary (Application no. 67545/09), European Court of Human Rights, Strasbourg, 14 December 2010. The court found that, in denying Anna Ternovsky the choice of home birth, the Hungarian Goverment breached her right to private life under Article 8 of the Convention.

'24. ...*the mother is entitled to a legal and institutional environment that enables her choice...*'

'26. *Sections 15 and 20 of the Health Care Act 1997 recognise patients' right to self-determination in the context of medical treatment, including the right to reject certain interventions [...] In this welfare system practically everything is regulated; regulation is the default, and only what is regulated is considered safe and acceptable. Suddenly, in the absence of positive regulation, what was a matter of uncontested private choice becomes unusual and uncertain. In a very densely regulated world some disadvantages emerge for freedoms without regulatory endorsement [...] Private life includes a person's physical and psychological integrity, and the State is under a positive obligation to secure its citizens their right to effective respect for this integrity.*'

page 274 (2) 'Continuous support for women during childbirth', Hodnett, ED *et al.*, *Cochrane Database of Systematic Reviews*, Issue 2, 2011.

(3) It works out as $566.74 (Australian dollars) cheaper per woman. 'Caseload midwifery care versus standard maternity care for women of any risk: M@NGO, a randomised controlled trial', Tracy, SK *et al.*, *The Lancet Early Online Publication*, 17 September 2013.

(4) '*due to the exclusion of [some] women [...] caution should be exercised in applying the findings of this review to women with substantial medical or obstetric complications.*' This means that this model hasn't been tested on high-risk women, not that it isn't suitable. 'Midwife-led continuity models versus other models of care for childbearing women (Review)', Sandall, J *et al.*, *Cochrane Database of Systematic Reviews*, Issue 8, 2013.

(5) 'Practical applications and theoretical considerations in normal labour', Jenkins, MW and Pritchard, MH, *British Journal of Obstetrics and Gynaecology*, Vol 100, Issue 3, pp.221–6, 1993.

page 275 (6) 'Continuous support for women during childbirth', Hodnett, ED *et al.*, *Cochrane Database of Systematic Reviews*, Issue 2, 2011.

20 More than one good way to have a baby

page 276 (1) and (2) *'the post-test probability of detecting a macrosomic fetus in an uncomplicated pregnancy is variable, ranging from 15% to 79% with sonographic estimates of birth weight, and 40 to 52% with clinical estimate'*. So they're guessing. They don't know how much babies weigh before birth. *'Among uncomplicated pregnancies suspicion of macrosomia is not an indication for induction or for primary cesarean delivery.'* 'Suspicion and treatment of the macrosomic fetus: a review', Chauhan, SP *et al.*, *American Journal of Obstetrics and Gynecology*, Vol 193, Issue 2, pp.332–46, 2005. Also: 'Induction of labour for suspected fetal macrosomia', Irion, O and Boulvain, M, *Cochrane Database of Systematic Reviews*, Issue 2, 2000.

(3) 'Suspected macrosomia? Better not tell', Sadeh-Mestechkin, D *et al.*, *Archives of Gynecology and Obstetrics*, Vol 278, Issue 3, pp.225–30, 2008.

(4) 'Evaluation of predictors of neonatal infection in infants born to patients with premature rupture of membranes at term', Seaward, R, *American Journal of Obstetrics and Gynecology*, Vol 179, Issue 3, pp.635–639, 1998.

(5) 'Planned early birth versus expectant management (waiting) for prelabour rupture of membranes at term (37 weeks or more)', Dare, MR *et al.*, *Cochrane Database of Systematic Reviews*, Issue 1, 2009.

(6) 'Antibiotics for prelabour rupture of membranes at or near term (Review)', Flenady, V and King, JF, *Cochrane Database of Systematic Reviews*, Issue 3, 2012.

page 277 (7) 'Induction of labour for improving birth outcomes for women at or beyond term (Review)', Gülmezoglu, AM *et al.*, *Cochrane Database of Systematic Reviews*, Issue 6, 2012.

(8) 'Continuous cardiotocography (CTG) as a form of electronic fetal monitoring (EFM) for fetal assessment during labour', Alfirevic, Z *et al.*, *Cochrane Database of Systematic Reviews*, Issue 3, 2006.

page 279 (9) 'Randomised controlled trial of labouring in water compared with standard of augmentation for the management of dystocia in first stage of labour', Cluett *et al.*, *British Medical Journal*, Vol 328, pp.314–20, 2004.

page 280 (10) World Health Organization: Guidelines on basic newborn resuscitation.

21 The Caesarean section

page 284 (1) Statistic from NHS Institute for Innovation and Improvement.

(2) UK: 24%, US: 33%, China: 46%.

(3) Cited in *Easing Labor Pain*, Adrienne B Lieberman, p.290, Harvard Common Press.

page 290 (4) 'The natural caesarean: a woman centred technique', Fisk, N *et al.*, *BCOG*, Vol 115, Issue 8, pp.1037–42, July 2008.

(5) There is an example of a couple insisting on modification of standard operating practice at http://cord-clamping.com/2012/07/29/birth-story-woman-centred-emergency-c-section-with-delayed-clamping.

(6) See http://cord-clamping.com/2011/09/08/cesarean-delayed-clamping.

(7) 'Early contact versus separation: effects on mother-infant interaction one year later', Bystrova, K *et al.*, *Birth*, Vol 36, Issue 2, pp.97–109, 2009.

(8) 'Early skin-to-skin contact for mothers and their healthy newborn infants (Review)', Moore, ER *et al.*, *Cochrane Database of Systematic Reviews*, Issue 5, 2012. Also: http://evidencebasedbirth.com/the-evidence-for-skin-to-skin-care-after-a-cesarean and 'Kangaroo mother care: a practical guide', World Health Organization.

(9) 'Uterine Closure in Cesarean Delivery: A New Technique', Babu, KM and Magon, N, *North American Journal of Medical Sciences*, Vol 4, Issue 8, pp.358–61, 2012.

Index

Well done.

You have just undergone the most physically and emotionally exhausting process of your life.

You have successfully subdivided.

You have a baby.

You can take it home with you.

Unlike a library book, which you have to return after three weeks, this child is yours for years and years.

But what do you do with it?

What next?

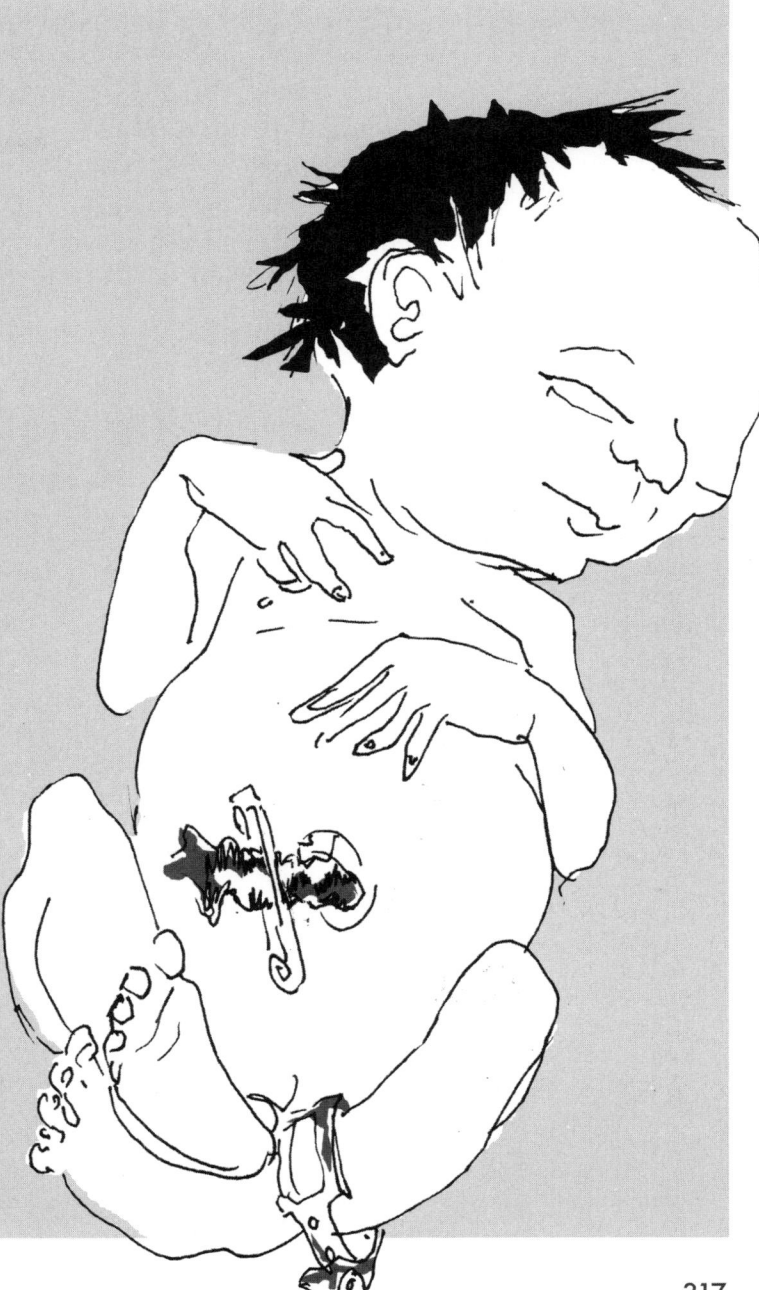

The Food of Love is a fresh and funny guide to parenthood. Kate Evans explains everything you'll need to know to breastfeed successfully, and a lot more.

New mothers say:
'It changed my life. It made me feel good about what I was doing.'
'I am getting more sleep, and so is my boy!'

Healthcare professionals say:
'As a GP and mother I highly recommend this book – all the facts are spot on!'
'Refreshing, beautiful, informative and, best of all, funny!'

ISBN: 978 0 954930 95 0

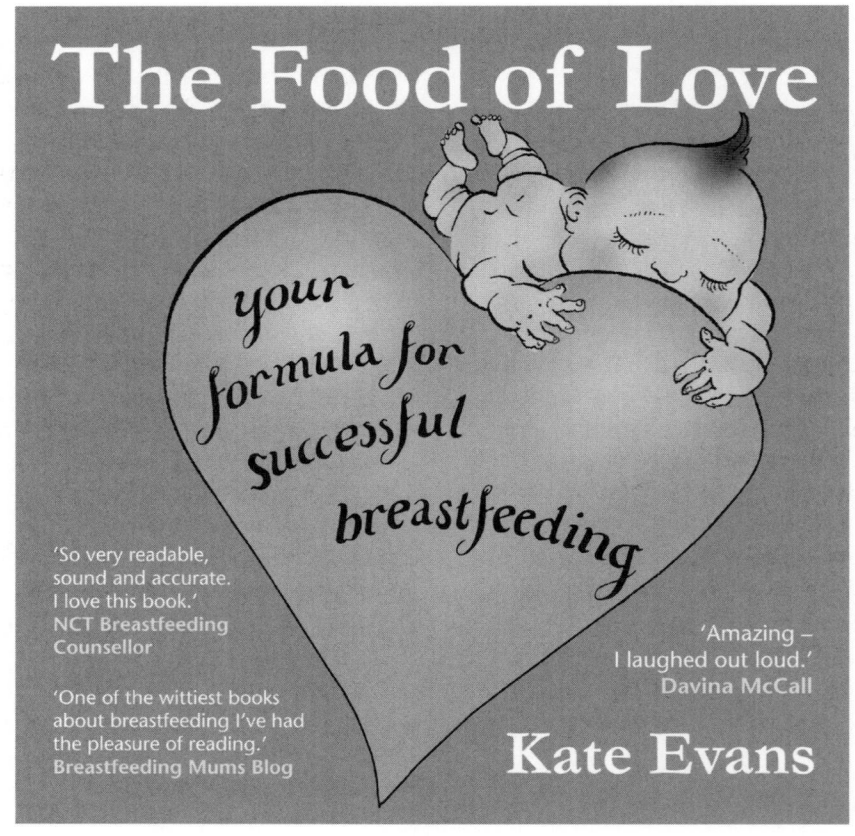

'Vibrant, exciting, funny – and based on up-to-date research.' **Sheila Kitzinger**

'One of the wittiest books about breastfeeding I've had the pleasure of reading... extremely well-written and bursting with thoroughly researched breastfeeding information. Covering everything from the first feeds to co-sleeping, it explains all you need to know about breastfeeding in a very comforting and inspirational fashion. A fabulous read... If you're looking for a great gift to give an expectant mother or a new mother who is breastfeeding, then this is the one.' **Breastfeeding Mums Blog**

'Honest advice and easy-to-follow diagrams, including a hilarious chapter on "Mama Sutra" explaining advanced breastfeeding positions... A laugh-out-loud approach to encourage mums to persevere with breastfeeding.' **Press Association**

'What a fantastic book! More like a chat over a coffee with a good friend than a text book, Evans' approach – although completely pro-breastfeeding – is totally non-threatening or "preachy" and is packed full of really useful advice and tips. The NHS should provide every pregnant woman with a copy.' *The Holistic Parent*

'I'd decided I wanted to breastfeed but I was a bit scared. Here were all the answers to questions I wanted to ask. It's transformed my approach. I just wanted to say thank you.' **Expectant mother of twins**

'I love this book. It is refreshing in so many ways: beautiful to look at (the cartoons are wonderful); informative and – best of all – funny. I genuinely haven't been as excited about a breastfeeding book since *Fresh Milk*.' **Association of Breastfeeding Mothers**

'Reading this book really does feel like chatting to a friend.' *Association of Breastfeeding Mothers Magazine*

'A funny, handy guide to help new mothers enjoy their baby and a valuable addition to the existing literature. Cartoon drawings successfully convey the message that breastfeeding is lovely and easy, yet Kate Evans also includes the latest facts and research surrounding breastfeeding as well as a useful section on further resources and references. Full of practical tips, it will meet the needs of many new mums and be of use to breastfeeding counsellors, antenatal teachers, midwives and health professionals.' *New Digest*, **NCT Magazine**

'Delightful... genuinely hard to put down, because it was so very readable. Kate's book is also sound and accurate – she uses research-based evidence as well as personal experience and shows how many mothers cope with a variety of initial difficulties and overcome them. As a breastfeeding counsellor and trainer of peer supporters I love this book – it is truly mother-and-baby-centred.' **NCT Breastfeeding Counsellor**

NEW WAYS OF SEEING FROM MYRIAD EDITIONS

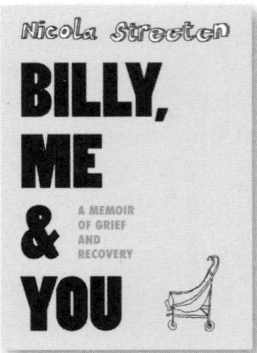

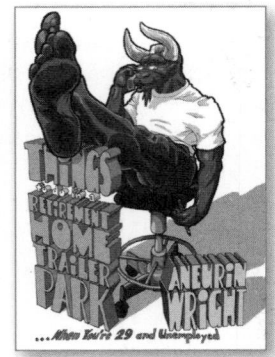

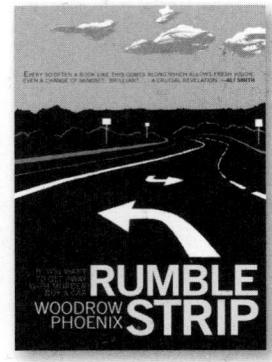

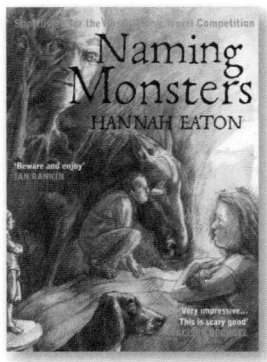

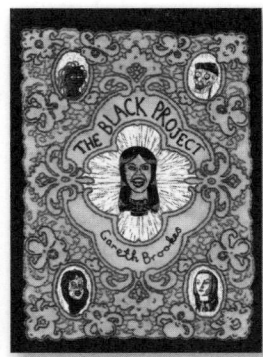

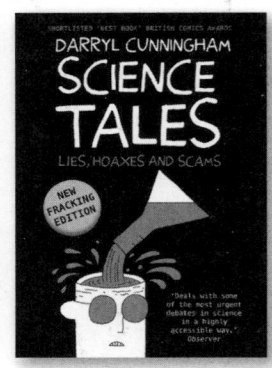

Also by Kate Evans

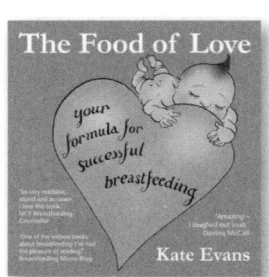

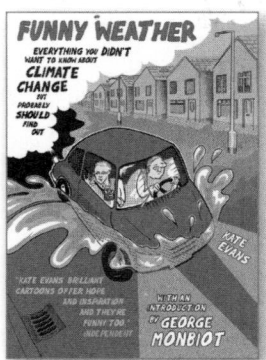

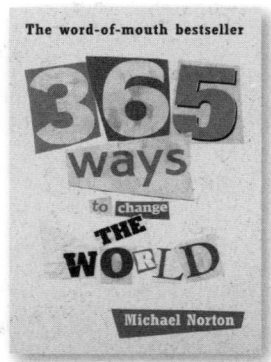